618.92
BYA

This book is due for return on or before the last date shown below.

Sudden Infant Death Syndrome

Problems, Progress and Possibilities

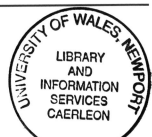

Edited by

ROGER W. BYARD MD

Specialist Forensic Pathologist, Forensic Science Centre; Clinical Associate Professor, Departments of Paediatrics and Pathology, University of Adelaide; Consultant Paediatric Forensic Pathologist, Child Protection Unit, Women's and Children's Hospital, Adelaide, South Australia, Australia.

and

HENRY F. KROUS MD

Director of Pathology, Childrens Hospital-San Diego, San Diego; Adjunct Professor, Departments of Pathology and Pediatrics, University of California, San Diego School of Medicine, La Jolla, California, USA

A member of the Hodder Headline Group

LONDON

First Published in Great Britain in 2001
by Arnold, a member of the Hodder Headline Group,
338 Euston Road, London NW1 3BH

http://www.arnoldpublishers.com

Co-published in the United States of America by
Oxford University Press Inc.,
198 Madison Avenue, New York, NY10016
Oxford is a registered trademark of Oxford University Press

British Library Cataloguing in Publication Data
A catalogue record for this book is available from the British Library

Library of Congress Cataloguing-in-Publication Data
A catalog record for this book is available from the Library of Congress

ISBN 0 340 75917 8 (hb)

2 3 4 5 6 7 8 9 10

Commissioning Editor: Georgina Bentliff
Development Editor: Tim Wale
Production Editor: Lauren McAllister
Production Controller: Martin Kerans

Typeset in 10pt Times by
J&L Composition Ltd, Filey, North Yorkshire
Printed and bound by MPG Books Ltd, Bodmin, Cornwall

What do you think of this book? Or any other Arnold title?
Please send your comments to feedback.arnold@hodder.co.uk

Dedication

To my parents, William and Mary Byard,
and to Renée (RWB).

To the memory of my twin brother Philip Krous,
my parents Elwyn and Elizabeth Krous,
and to my beloved Karen (HFK).

'To live in hearts we leave behind,
Is not to die'

Hallowed Ground
Thomas Campbell (1777–1844)

Contents

Colour plates appear between pages 178–9

Contributors — vii

Foreword *J. Bruce Beckwith* — ix

Preface — xiii

Acknowledgements — xiv

1. **Sudden infant death syndrome – a change in philosophy** *Roger W. Byard and Henry F. Krous* — 1

2. **Definition and pathologic features** *Torleiv O. Rognum* — 4

3. **Changing epidemiology** *Fern R. Hauck* — 31

4. **Death scene investigation** *Randy Hanzlick* — 58

5. **Respiratory mechanisms and hypoxia** *Thomas G. Keens and Sally L. Davidson Ward* — 66

6. **QT prolongation and SIDS – from theory to evidence** *Peter J. Schwartz* — 83

7. **Arousal and brain homeostatic control** *Ronald L. Ariagno and Majid Mirmiran* — 96

8. **Brain research in SIDS** *Hannah C. Kinney and James J. Filiano* — 118

9. **Rebreathing of exhaled air** *James S. Kemp and Bradley T. Thach* — 138

10. **Airway inflammation and peripheral chemoreceptors** *Ernest Cutz and Adele Jackson* — 156

11. **A microbiological perspective** *Caroline C. Blackwell, Donald M. Weir and Anthony Busuttil* — 182

12. **Differential diagnosis of sudden infant death** *Roger W. Byard and Henry F. Krous* — 209

13. **Specific pathologic problems and possible solutions** *Roger W. Byard and Henry F. Krous* — 228

14. **The rise and fall of several theories** *Susan M. Beal* — 236

15. **The role of monitoring** *Christian F. Poets* — 243

16. **Mother–infant cosleeping: toward a new scientific beginning** *James J. McKenna and Sarah Mosko* — 258

17. **Taking a Strategic approach to SIDS prevention in Maori communities – an indigenous perspective** *David Tipene-Leach, Caroline Everard and Riripeti Haretuku* — 275

18. **Recurrence of sudden unexpected infant death in a family** *Susan M. Beal* — 283

19. **SIDS and infanticide** *Richard Firstman and Jamie Talan* 291

20. **SIDS years later – how families survive** *Debbie Gemmill* 301

21. **The 'Reduce the Risks' Campaign, SIDS International, the Global Strategy Task Force and the European Society for the Study and Prevention of Infant Death** *Kaarene Fitzgerald* 310

Appendices:

I **International Standardized Autopsy Protocol** 319

II **Sudden Unexplained Infant Death Investigation Report Form (SUIDIRF)** 334

Contributors

Ronald L. Ariagno MD Division of Neonatal and Developmental Medicine, Department of Pediatrics, Stanford University School of Medicine, Palo Alto, CA, USA.

Susan M. Beal MBBS, MD Department of Ambulatory Paediatrics, Women's and Children's Hospital, Adelaide, Australia.

Caroline C. Blackwell PhD, DSc, FRCPath Department of Medical Microbiology, University of Edinburgh, Edinburgh, UK.

Anthony Busuttil MD, FRCPath, DMJ(Path), FRCP(Ed), FRCP(Glas) Forensic Medicine Unit, University of Edinburgh, Edinburgh, UK.

Roger W. Byard MD Forensic Science Centre and Departments of Paediatrics and Pathology, University of Adelaide, Adelaide, Australia.

Ernest Cutz MD, FRCPC Department of Pediatric Laboratory Medicine, Division of Pathology, The Hospital for Sick Children and University of Toronto, Toronto, Ont., Canada.

Sally L. Davidson Ward MD Department of Pediatrics, University of Southern California School of Medicine and Division of Pediatric Pulmonology, Childrens Hospital of Los Angeles, Los Angeles, CA, USA.

Caroline Everard Department of Maori and Pacific Health, School of Medicine and Health Sciences, University of Auckland, Auckland, New Zealand.

James J. Filiano MD Department of Pediatrics, Children's Hospital at Dartmouth, Dartmouth Hitchcock Medical Center, Lebanon, NH, USA.

Richard Firstman Author *The Death of Innocents*, Northport, NY, USA.

Kaarene Fitzgerald AC SIDS Victoria, Malvern, Australia.

Debbie Gemmill Author, Escondito, CA, USA.

Randy Hanzlick MD Chief Medical Examiner's Office, Fulton County Medical Examiner's Center and Emory University School of Medicine, Atlanta, GA, USA.

Riripeti Haretuku DipBus Department of Maori and Pacific Health, School of Medicine and Health Sciences, University of Auckland, Auckland, New Zealand.

Fern R. Hauck MD, MS Department of Family Medicine, University of Virginia School of Medicine, Charlottesville, VA, USA.

Adele Jackson PhD Department of Pediatric Laboratory Medicine, Division of Pathology, The Hospital for Sick Children and University of Toronto, Toronto, Ont., Canada.

Thomas G. Keens MD Department of Pediatrics, University of Southern California School of Medicine and Division of Pediatric Pulmonology, Children's Hospital of Los Angeles, Los Angeles, CA, USA.

James S. Kemp MD Department of Pediatrics and the Pediatric Research Institute, St Louis University School of Medicine, St Louis, MO, USA.

Hannah C. Kinney MD Departments of Pathology and Neurology, Children's Hospital and Harvard Medical School, Boston, MA, USA.

Henry F. Krous MD Pathology Department, Children's Hospital-San Diego, San Diego and Departments of Pathology and Pediatrics, University of California, San Diego School of Medicine, La Jolla, CA, USA.

Majid Mirmiran MD, PhD Division of Neonatal and Developmental Medicine, Department of Pediatrics, Stanford University School of Medicine, Palo Alto, CA, USA and Netherlands Institute for Brain Research, Amsterdam, The Netherlands.

James J. McKenna PhD Mother–Baby Behavioural Sleep Laboratory, University of Notre Dame, Notre Dame, IN, USA.

Sarah Mosko PhD Department of Neurology, University of California, Irvine, Orange, CA, USA.

Christian F. Poets MD Departments of Neonatology and Paediatric Pulmonology, Medical School, Hannover, Germany.

Torleiv O. Rognum MD, PhD Institute of Forensic Medicine, University of Oslo, Oslo, Norway.

Peter J. Schwartz MD Department of Cardiology, Policlinico S. Matteo IRCCS and University of Pavia, Pavia, Italy.

Jamie Talan Author *The Death of Innocents*, Northport, NY, USA.

Bradley T. Thach MD Department of Pediatrics, Washington University School of Medicine, St Louis, MO, USA.

David Tipene-Leach BHB, MBChB, D.ComH, MCCM(NZ) Department of Maori and Pacific Health, School of Medicine and Health Sciences, University of Auckland, Auckland, New Zealand.

Donald M. Weir MD, FRCP(Ed) Department of Medical Microbiology, University of Edinburgh, Edinburgh, UK.

FOREWORD by **J. Bruce Beckwith** MD, FRCPath (Hon).

Foreword

It is an interesting experience to peruse this volume from the perspective of more than four decades of involvement in sudden infant death syndrome (SIDS). This is a topic that engenders profound emotional reactions. Certainly no other activity in my professional life has engendered such intense feelings, both of achievement and of disappointment. As pointed out by several authors in this volume, the very term SIDS, which I introduced in 1969,[1] has been a mixed blessing. It served to focus the attention of the world upon a largely unrecognized problem, and helped to stimulate scientific research and the development of effective support systems for families victimized by this tragedy. On the downside, because SIDS was recognizable only as a syndrome and not a specific disease, its definition was necessarily imprecise. As a result, the term became a catchall that was applied too liberally to unexpected sudden deaths in early life. A spectacular variety of causes and mechanisms for certain cases of sudden infant death have been recognized in subsequent decades, many of which are touted as causes for 'SIDS', when it would have been more appropriate to have labeled them as causes for *sudden and unexpected infant death* (SUID). The reader will find proposed explanations for 'SIDS' in the present volume that might better have been labeled as explanations for SUID. This failure to clearly distinguish SUID from SIDS has led some workers to question the existence of SIDS, recalling that ancient admonition not to discard the baby while throwing out the bathwater.

At the 1969 conference, I argued for the inclusion of age range, sleep, and autopsy findings in the proposed definition, but most of the attendees felt it would be premature to define this condition too rigorously. It was also noted that a more inclusive definition would facilitate the development of management systems and scientific research into sudden infant death. Though the collective decision to adopt a looser, exclusion-based definition was probably a good one in 1969, I was confident it would soon be supplanted by more precise criteria, including a specified age range and association with presumed or apparent sleep (i.e. the infant is either found dead or *in extremis* after having been put down to sleep). It has been profoundly disappointing, more than 30 years later, to see how little progress has been made toward developing a more rigorous descriptive definition for SIDS. In my opinion this failure has resulted in many of the misleading clues to causation, and contributes significantly to present controversies concerning the nature, even the very existence, of SIDS.

The concern that a more rigorous definition might exclude many families from SIDS management and support systems is a legitimate one. One potential solution would be to adopt a two-tiered approach to the definition of SIDS that retains the advantages of a more permissive definition for *management* purposes, while at the same time raising the bar for the use of this term in *scientific* publications and presentations. Dr Rognum's excellent discussion of the definition problem (Chapter 2 of the present volume) includes a proposed definitional approach, based upon this concept, that I presented at the SIDS International meeting in Australia in 1992. Though this was not accepted by the large group present at that meeting, I still contend that the usage of this term in *scientific reports* must be more rigorously limited, even if death management systems continue to be based upon more liberal definitional criteria. Using this approach, a significant fraction of the contributions to the literature (including several chapters in this book) that are touted as explanations for SIDS would have been labeled as explanations for SUID, either because they do not fit the profile of 'typical' SIDS, or because they contain insufficient information about reported deaths to determine whether they fit that profile. It is one of the great regrets of my life that I was not more effective in advocating for a more restrictive definition of SIDS for use in scientific publications, since this failure contributed to so much of the confusion and controversy surrounding this topic.

Another regrettable aspect of the SIDS movement, in both the scientific and management arenas, has been the intensely personal and ego-driven manner in which some participants have advocated for their views. This is in part a manifestation of the intense emotions engendered by this topic. Scientists defending their concepts or attacking the concepts of others, and organizations defending their turf, have sometimes engaged in heated, unseemly, and destructive conflict. These conflicts consumed energies that could have been used more productively in other ways, creating more heat than light. They have also produced an atmosphere so distasteful that it drove dedicated individuals away from continuing involvement in SIDS. This problem became especially manifest during the period when infant apnea and home monitoring occupied center stage in the SIDS arena. Unhappily, it continues to be a significant deterrent to progress in a field that has in general been outstanding for its positive aspects.

On the positive side of the ledger, the SIDS movement has had beneficial effects in arenas far beyond its own boundaries. It has contributed to increased sensitivity and awareness of humanitarian issues on the part of forensic pathologists, law enforcement agencies, first responders, nurses, physicians, and the media. It has advanced the scientific study of post-neonatal infant biology, and brought scientists, lay groups, and administrative agencies together in remarkably effective collaborative efforts. The most gratifying result of all has been the significant reduction in the incidence of SIDS, especially the subgroup of 'typical' SIDS. Though the ultimate mechanism for this decline remains uncertain, it has been temporally associated with changes in the sleeping position and sleeping environment of infants during the early months of life. This changing incidence of SIDS is also shifting the pattern from predominantly 'typical' SIDS toward the more atypical cases, many of which represent SUID but perhaps not SIDS. It is a humbling demonstration of the limitations of modern science that we seem to have found a way to decrease the incidence of SIDS without understanding the reason for our success.

Many of the best results of the energy and commitment devoted to the SIDS problem are exemplified in the present volume. Between its covers will be found the wisdom of physicians and scientists with long experience with the tragedy of sudden infant death, the passion and insights of investigators who have devoted years to the investigation of specific aspects of the problem, and the perspective of individuals who have experienced this tragedy on the personal level. It also presents a variety of opinions upon the potential nature and causes of SIDS. The diversity of these opinions, and the fact that many of them are mutually contradictory, accurately reflects the general state of affairs at the present time. I applaud the editors upon their choice of contributors and topics, and for their personal contributions to this book, which are among its most valuable features. Nobody can agree with everything in this book, but every reader will find much of interest and value.

This volume demonstrates how far we have come in the past few decades, but it also shows how long and tortuous is the road ahead. May those of you who travel that road into the future find the hills less steep, the forks and byways less misleading, and the bandits along the route fewer in number, than we encountered on the first part of the journey. Those who choose to travel that road will find gratification in easing the suffering of souls along the way, and in helping to open the way for those who will follow. And if you are very fortunate, you may have that ultimate joy – of finding yourself at the end of that road, in a world where SIDS no longer exists, and many causes of SUID are also under control.

J. Bruce Beckwith, MD, FRCPath (Hon)
Professor Emeritus, Pathology and Human Anatomy
Loma Linda University School of Medicine

Reference

1. Beckwith JB. Terminology. In: Bergman AB, Beckwith JB, Ray CG: *Sudden Infant Death Syndrome*. Proceedings of the Second International Conference on Causes of Sudden Death in Infants. University of Washington Press, Seattle and London, 1970, pp. 14–15.

Preface

Given the tremendous changes that have occurred in our understanding and perception of sudden infant death syndrome (SIDS) in recent years, it seems appropriate to try to draw together in a single text some of the threads that form the tapestry of this enigmatic and confusing entity.

As the number of deaths from SIDS have fallen, new theories have arisen and older theories have been clarified or discarded. Vigorous debates have occurred regarding the definition, and even the validity, of the term 'SIDS'. In this text we have attempted to reflect the nature of the most important recent developments, with chapters on such diverse aspects as pathologic features, pathophysiology, epidemiology, parental concerns, medicolegal issues and indigenous perspectives. We have also allowed contributors considerable leeway in expressing individual, sometimes quite contentious and emotive, viewpoints as we consider that this most accurately reflects the current issues concerning SIDS in the international community. The reader may, therefore, find this an unusual text containing a wide variety of topics and viewpoints dealing with issues in very different, and sometimes contradictory, ways. The style of authors of different chapters varies from very traditional scientific approaches to very personal anecdotes and points of view. Once we had seen the range of chapters being submitted for the text we felt that any attempt to impose a uniform approach would have been to unduly simplify the tremendously complex ramifications that SIDS deaths have.

An important point to emphasize is that the SIDS arena is extraordinarily multidisciplinary. Not only do SIDS data reflect complex epidemiologic phenomena, and SIDS deaths cause puzzling pathologic problems, but each 'case' represents a grieving family that has lost a baby. This point should not be lost on researchers and for this reason the content of the text has been left deliberately eclectic, sometimes straying well outside the boundaries of usual scientific literature.

Ultimately, however, readers will have to decide for themselves how valid many of these arguments, opinions and hypotheses are. Although not all viewpoints are endorsed by the editors, they have been included to encourage the vigorous debate that has been so necessary for the development of our understanding of SIDS in the past, as we now enter the new century, with all of its potential promises and perceived problems. If this book provokes even a small amount of critical debate in this important area then the editors will have in part achieved their aim.

R.W. Byard and H.F. Krous
Adelaide and San Diego
July 2000

Acknowledgements

The authors gratefully acknowledge the editorial assistance, advice and support of Renée Amyot.

CHAPTER 1

Sudden infant death syndrome – a change in philosophy

ROGER W. BYARD AND HENRY F. KROUS

Introduction   1
Historical tradition   1
Recent research   2
References   3

Introduction

In recent years there has been a decline in the rates of sudden infant death syndrome (SIDS) reported from a number of centers around the world, associated with the identification of specific environmental risk factors. This has been shown to be due to a genuine decrease, rather than as a result of significant changes in diagnostic practices.[1] There has also been recognition of the complexity of the relationship among environmental, socioeconomic and biological factors that may influence the vulnerable infant.[2,3] This indicates the development of a more sophisticated conceptual approach to SIDS than has characterized previous years.

Historical tradition

The historical tradition in investigating the cause of SIDS was to seek out a potential single cause that could then be held responsible for all cases that occurred.[4] This led to an approach in which one factor would be zealously sought to explain all the possible epidemiologic and pathologic findings. For example, the earliest records attribute the cause of SIDS to suffocation of an infant by an adult who was sleeping in the same bed as the dead child. The first description of SIDS demonstrates this in the Judgement of Solomon where a bereaved mother is described as having lost her child due to 'overlaying' in bed.[5]

Later investigators found themselves being led reluctantly away from the possibility of accidental asphyxia, when cases of unexpected death occurred in infants who were known to be sleeping alone in their cots at the time of the lethal episode.[6] In spite of the divergence away from overlaying, the 'single cause' philosophy prevailed, and in the late nineteenth century death was attributed to *status thymolymphaticus*. In this condition sudden death was thought to have been caused by compression of the upper airway by abnormally large thymus glands. Subsequent studies have convincingly demonstrated, however, that the size of the thymus glands in infants who die of SIDS is no different from healthy age-matched controls, and that the error had occurred because ill infants in hospital with atrophic thymus glands had been selected as 'normal' controls.

Recent research

Although a great deal of more recent research has also focused on promoting a single elusive cause of SIDS, with toxic, infective, metabolic, nutritional, endocrine, cardiac, respiratory and neurologic disorders being blamed, it now appears to the authors that the 'syndrome' is most likely a heterogeneous entity, with not all the previous proposed causes playing significant roles.[7] Thus the term refers not to a specific disease process, but to a lethal situation in which an infant, who may be physiologically compromised in poorly understood ways, is subject to the additive effects of a number of risk factors at a particularly vulnerable time of life. This has been referred to as the 'triple risk model' of SIDS which holds that the unexpected death of an infant occurs only when a vulnerable infant is subjected to external stressors during a critical developmental stage.[8] It is also quite possible that different infants may not have the same inherent vulnerabilities and may not respond identically to the same environmental stresses. This further complicates assessment of causes of SIDS and the development of possible predictive tests.

The interactions between the infant's immature and possibly defective neurophysiological pathways and risk factors such as prone sleeping position and passive smoking[9] are, therefore, undoubtedly highly complex and variable from individual to individual. This, combined with the relative rarity of cases, makes antemortem and postmortem studies difficult, as it is possible that investigation of small subsets of SIDS infants may produce divergent or even contradictory results. This would explain certain apparent inconsistencies in the literature, as well as the not infrequent headline in the popular press of yet another 'cause' of SIDS being discovered.

If it is accepted that SIDS is an amalgam of subtle tendencies, risk factors and defects, it would now seem appropriate for researchers to concentrate on identifying the characteristics of particular subgroups of SIDS infants with the aim of modifying specific features in at-risk infants. This approach abandons the tradition of 'single cause' research, and instead concentrates on developing an overall understanding of the complexities of infant physiological and pathologic responses to a variety of intrinsic and extrinsic factors. Each additional factor that is identified may, therefore, hold clues to the further understanding of mechanisms of infant death, with the potential for prevention of death for more, but undoubtedly not all, vulnerable children. The following chapters deal in detail with these issues.

References

1. Byard RW, Beal SM. Has changing diagnostic preference been responsible for the recent fall in incidence of sudden infant death syndrome in South Australia? *J Paediatr Child Health* 1995;31:197–9.
2. Malloy MH, Hoffman HJ. Prematurity, sudden infant death syndrome, and age of death. *Pediatrics* 1995;96:464–71.
3. Byard RW. Sudden infant death syndrome – a 'diagnosis' looking for a disease. *J Clin Forens Med* 1995;2,121–8.
4. Byard RW. Sudden infant death syndrome – historical background, possible mechanisms and diagnostic problems. *J Law Med* 1994;2:18–26.
5. Byard RW, Cohle SD. *Sudden Death in Infancy, Childhood and Adolescence,* Cambridge University Press, Cambridge, 1994.
6. Fearn SW. Sudden and unexplained death of children. (Letter) *Lancet* 1834;2:246.
7. Byard RW. Possible mechanisms responsible for the sudden infant death syndrome. *J Paediatr Child Health* 1991;27:147–57.
8. Filiano JJ, Kinney HC. A perspective on neuropathologic findings in victims of the sudden infant death syndrome. *Biol Neonate* 1994;65:194–7.
9. Mitchell EA, Taylor BJ, Ford RPK *et al*. Four modifiable and other major risk factors for cot death: the New Zealand study. *J Paediatr Child Health* 1991;28 (Suppl. 1):S3–8.

CHAPTER 2

Definition and pathologic features

TORLEIV O. ROGNUM

Definitions   4
Definition by inclusion   5
Definition by exclusion   9
Attempts to standardize the diagnosis of SIDS   13
Is there a syndrome at all?   16
The grey zone   17
Borderline SIDS   17
Autopsy findings   19
Familial clustering of infant deaths   24
Future perspectives   25
References   27

Definitions

DEFINITION: BY PATHOLOGIC FEATURES OR EXCLUSION OF IDENTIFIABLE CAUSES?

Despite the fact that the phenomenon of sudden unexpected death in infancy has been known since Biblical times,[1] the mechanism of death is not yet understood. Although typical features are present at the autopsy in many cases, the specificity of these features has been intensely debated.

PREVIOUS MISINTERPRETATIONS OF FEATURES PRESENT AT AUTOPSY

Throughout the centuries, misinterpretations of normal anatomical structures have caused erroneous ideas concerning the mechanism of death. One example is the 'abnormally' large thymus gland which was supposed to have compressed the airway behind it, thus asphyxiating the child. The condition was named *status thymolymphaticus.*[2,3] However, the fact that all infants have large thymuses clearly demonstrates the classic problem in SIDS research: the lack of suitable controls. The misunderstanding that a 'pathologically enlarged thymus' might cause cot death, led to the mistake of reducing the size of the thymus in healthy infants by means of x-rays. Some of these unfortunate children later developed cancer of the thyroid as a result of the radiation.[4] Another reported pathologic feature claiming to explain sudden unexpected death in infancy was a lack of parathyroid glands[5]; however this was discarded in a control study.[6]

INTRATHORACIC PETECHIAE – A PREREQUISITE?

Some pathologists have regarded the presence of intrathoracic petechiae a prerequisite for the diagnosis of 'true' or 'classic' SIDS[7] (Fig. 2.1a–c). This contrasts with the consensus of the National Institute of Child Health and Human Development (NICHD) multicenter epidemiologic study which found that only 52% of SIDS had thymic petechiae.[8]

TYPICAL AGE DISTRIBUTION – A DISTINCTIVE FEATURE OF SIDS?

In all studies SIDS shows an age distribution with a peak between two and four months of age[9] (Fig. 2.2); an attempt to narrow the definition of SIDS based on age distribution has been proposed by Beckwith.[10] He defined typical (category 1) SIDS as occurring in infants aged between 3 weeks and 8 months – a selection including 95% of cases in most previously published series[10]. However, the age distribution has changed after the recent decrease in SIDS rate (Fig. 2.2); the typical age peak between 2 and 4 months has become less significant, whereas the proportions of unexplained deaths during the first weeks after birth, as well after 6 months of age, have increased (Fig. 2.2). From our own observations at the Institute of Forensic Medicine in Oslo, it can be seen that although sudden death due to definable disease dominates in the first week after birth (Fig. 2.3), the percentage of sudden unexplained deaths during the 3 weeks after birth increased from 1% of all SIDS cases in the period between 1984 and 1989, to 7% after 1990. Furthermore, Vege *et al.*[9] have demonstrated that the significant reduction in deaths between 2 and 4 months after 1989 has occurred because there are now fewer prone sleeping infants with signs of infection found dead in that particular age group. Since it seems that the shift in risk factor profile has caused changes in the age distribution of SIDS, it is obviously impossible to apply age *per se* as a consistent pathologic feature.

Definition by inclusion

During the Second SIDS International Conference in Sydney 1992[10] Beckwith proposed a three-tiered definition of SIDS which represented a detailed description of features common to most cases, i.e:

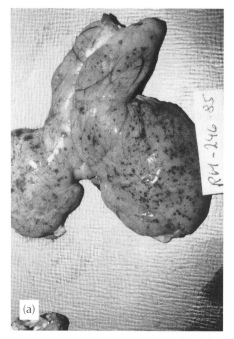

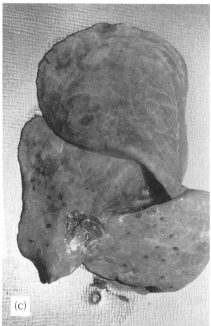

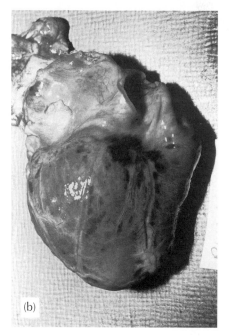

Fig. 2.1 Thymus (a), heart (b) and the right lung (c) from a case of SIDS. Petechiae are abundantly present on the thymus and to a lesser degree on the heart and lung. The lung has a variegated appearance due to partial atelectasis.

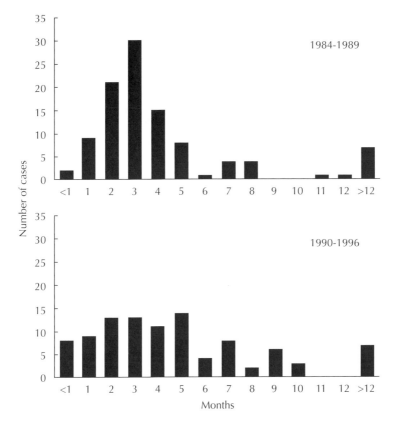

Fig. 2.2 Age distribution of SIDS victims in southeast Norway during the period with high SIDS rates (1984–1989) and the period with low SIDS rates (1990–1996). The typical age peak between 2 and 4 months of age is less significant in the latter period.

The sudden, unexpected death of an infant under 1 year of age, which remains unexpected after a thorough case investigation, including performance of a complete autopsy, examination of the death scene, and review of the clinical history. Minor inflammatory infiltrates or other abnormalities insufficient to explain the death are acceptable.

CATEGORY I SIDS

An infant death that, in addition to meeting the above criteria, meets the following standards:

- Age between 3 weeks and 8 months.
- Death, or onset of the lethal episode, apparently occurred during sleep (i.e., the infant was not observed to be awake at the time).

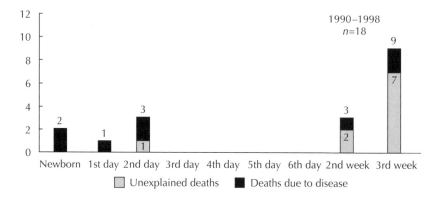

Fig. 2.3 Age distribution of sudden unexpected deaths during the first 3 weeks after birth investigated at the Institute of Forensic Medicine, Oslo, in the time period 1990–1998. Only one out of six deaths (17%) occurring during the first week after birth was unexplained, whereas during the second and third week as many as nine out of 12 deaths (75%) remained unexplained.

- No similar deaths in siblings or other first-degree relatives.
- No evidence of significant stress in the thymus, adrenal glands, or other organs.
- Intrathoracic petechial hemorrhages are a supportive, but not an obligatory finding.

CATEGORY II SIDS

Cases meeting the criteria for Category I SIDS, but differing in one or more of the following features:

- Age under 1 year, but outside the 3 week to 8 month range.
- Similar deaths have occurred in siblings or other close relatives.
- Inflammatory lesions or other abnormalities found during the autopsy or case investigation are thought to be more severe than for Category I, but are debatably sufficient to explain the death.
- Infants found in extremis who are temporarily and partially resuscitated, but die later, and who would otherwise fit the criteria for Category I or II SIDS; the designation 'temporarily interrupted SIDS' is appropriate for such cases.

CATEGORY III SIDS

These are cases that seem to meet clinical criteria for SIDS, where autopsy and/or other required studies are not performed.

The latter group (Category III) recognizes that there are sometimes economic, logistic, religious, or other barriers to the performance of a postmortem examination.

Incorporated into the proposed definition are specified features such as age less than 8 months, death occurring during sleep, no similar deaths in siblings, no evidence of stress in internal organs. Beckwith[10] uses the phrase inclusionary criteria which is based upon more than 20 years of descriptive clinical, epidemiologic and pathologic studies.

These additional features stress the requirements of a negative family history and furthermore contain references to current hypotheses and theories about the mechanism of death.[11] The approach proposed by Beckwith in 1992[10] would mean a departure from the philosophy of the 1969 definition[12] which was based on an exclusion of explainable causes of death. This was immortalized in verse by Sylvia Limerick in Toronto in 1973[13]:

> When theories compete in profusion,
> Then the experts conclude, in confusion,
> There'll be flaws in all laws
> Of this unexplained cause
> Till the problem is solved by exclusion.

Definition by exclusion

In spite of lack of unequivocal pathognomonic features present at autopsy, sudden infant death syndrome (SIDS) has been recognized as a diagnostic entity since Beckwith proposed the definition in 1969 as:

The sudden death of an infant or young child, which is unexpected by history, and in which a thorough postmortem examination fails to demonstrate an adequate cause of death.[12]

This definition has been the dominating one during the last 30 years and was endorsed during the Second Global Strategy Meeting in Stavanger in 1994.[14] In spite of its widespread acceptance, it is an intriguing fact that SIDS rates show a dramatic variability (Fig. 2.4). There may be several reasons for this scatter, however it is most probably due to differences in the reporting of sudden infant deaths. For example, it has been claimed that in some countries a doctor being called to a case of sudden infant death may fabricate a diagnosis for the death certificate to avoid autopsy, because of local cultural or religious practices. In addition, differing opinions among pathologists as to which pathologic findings may be considered lethal also constitutes a problem and a great challenge (Table 2.1).

The definition from 1969 contains two exclusion criteria:

1 The infant seems to have been healthy before death.
2 No cause of death can be found at autopsy.

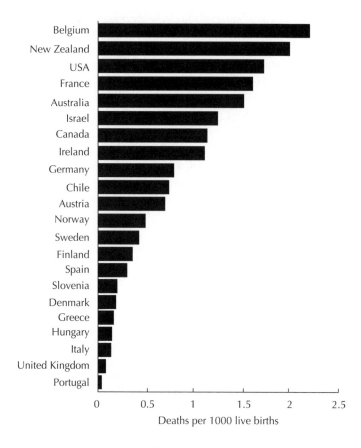

Fig. 2.4 SIDS rates in countries of the world. WHO, 1996. *World Health Statistics Annual,* Geneva, 1998.

Table 2.1 Percentage of sudden deaths in infancy that are diagnosed by various authors as pure SIDS

Helweg-Larsen *et al.* (1992)[16]	70%
Arneil *et al.* (1985)[17]	45%
Rajs (1993)[18]	26%
Knowelden *et al.* (1984)[19]	17%
Imbert *et al.* (1992)[20]	17%
Taylor *et al.* (1990)[21]	17%
Cheron *et al.* (1993)[22]	4.5%
Hatton *et al.* (1995)[23]	2.5%

However, from a forensic point of view, the circumstances under which death takes place is of paramount importance. This is probably why The National Institute of Child Health and Human Development (NICHD) in the 1989 definition required that an examination of the death scene should be performed before a diagnosis of SIDS could be made[24]: SIDS was defined as:

The sudden death of an infant under one year of age which remains unexplained after a thorough case investigation, including performance of a complete autopsy, examination of the death scene, and review of the clinical history.

Guntheroth *et al.*[25] have criticized the NICHD definition, claiming that wide implementation would result in a marked reduction in the number of cases diagnosed (i.e reducing the sensitivity of diagnosis) with only a small improvement in specificity. The compulsory death scene investigation may also cause problems in some countries. In Norway the Director General of Public Prosecutions in 1991 instructed the police to await the result of the forensic autopsy before undertaking any further investigations, such as death scene investigation and questioning of the family. If no suspicious conditions were found, the forensic pathologist was instructed to forward the results of the autopsy directly to the health personnel involved, and the police to close the case without further investigation.[11,26] However, after the decline in SIDS rates, other causes of sudden infant death have become more prominent. The percentage of deaths due to neglect, abuse and murder in southeast Norway has thus increased from approximately 2.3% of all sudden unexpected deaths in the period 1984–1989, to 6% in the period 1990–1998 (Fig. 2.5).[27]

The significance of death scene investigation for detecting both accidents and neglect/abuse is well documented.[28,29] Therefore, when a death scene investigation is performed only in cases that seem suspicious from the beginning it is very likely that a number of cases of accidents and homicides will be missed. Out of 289 cases of sudden unexpected deaths in infants and small children (0–3 years) investigated at The Institute of Forensic Medicine in Oslo from 1984 to 1998, investigation of the scene combined with a reconstruction of the event revealed three accidental deaths, three cases of neglect and one case of murder. In comparison, the autopsy itself revealed four cases of abuse, one case of neglect, one accident and one case of poisoning (TO Rognum, unpublished observations). Given that autopsies were performed in all cases, and death scene investigation took place in less than 10% of the cases, the importance of the latter should not be underestimated. Recently, a thorough investigation of one scene revealed a plastic bag with the lip marks of the deceased baby and biological material with the DNA-profile of the baby, as well as the fingerprints of the mother.

An initiative to reintroduce compulsory death scene investigation has now been undertaken, and the initiative is strongly supported by the Norwegian SIDS Society and by the ombudsman for children.

To avoid problems with different legislation and cultural traditions, a new definition was proposed as a compromise during the Third SIDS International Conference in Stavanger, Norway, 1994. The 'Stavanger-definition' stresses the importance of examination of circumstances of death, but avoids the term

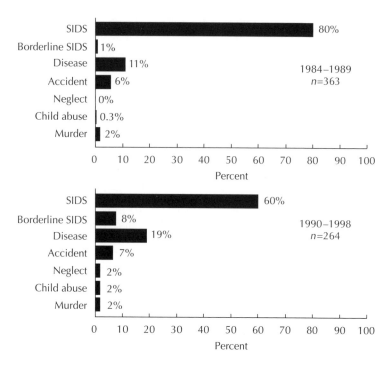

Fig. 2.5 Distribution of modes of sudden infant death in southeast Norway in the two time periods 1984–1989 and 1990–1998. SIDS was the dominant category of death in both periods, but in the latter period all other causes together amount to nearly 40%.

death scene investigation. The definition of SIDS which was proposed by a panel co-ordinated by Marie Valdes-Dapena and Marion Willinger was:

Sudden death in infancy unexplained after review of the clinical history, examination of the circumstances of death and postmortem examination.

During the subsequent SIDS Global Strategy Meeting in Stavanger, the new 'Stavanger-definition' failed to be adopted by a narrow margin. The original definition from 1969 received the most votes.[11] The resistance to restricting the diagnosis of SIDS to the first year after birth also contributed to the re-endorsement of the 1969 Seattle definition.[30]

WIDE VARIATION IN SIDS RATES

SIDS rates in different countries show great variations[15] (WHO Health Statistics 1996) (Fig. 2.4). Are these due to ethnic differences, different risk profiles or classification problems? Differences in ethnicity have been claimed to play a role

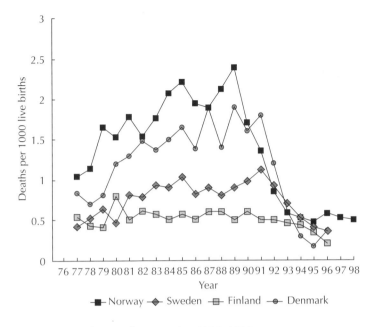

Fig. 2.6 SIDS rates in the Nordic countries 1976–1998.

in these divergent rates. For example, even when correcting for prone sleeping, Native Americans have 2.3 times the SIDS rate of the white population in North Dakota.[31] However, great variations in SIDS rates have also been observed between populations with similar ethnicity. During the years of the rapid increase in SIDS rates in the 1980s, Norway had more than twice the SIDS rate of Sweden and more than four times that of Finland.[32,33] Nevertheless, after the anti-prone sleeping campaign was launched in 1989[32] the SIDS rates in all Nordic countries dropped and are now approximately 0.5 deaths per 1000 live births[32,33] (Fig. 2.6). From this observation it may be concluded that risk factors are more important for the SIDS rate than ethnicity.

However, the most important reason for the variation in SIDS rates throughout the world (Fig. 2.4), is most likely problems with classification and the difficulties with reporting in some countries. For SIDS research it is thus of great importance to reach a consensus on standardizing the diagnosis and classification of the syndrome.[30,34]

Attempts to standardize the diagnosis of SIDS

Several attempts have been made to standardize the classification of SIDS. The results of a large multicenter study initiated by the NICHD in the 1980s have been compiled and published by the US Federal Government in association with the Armed Forces' Institute of Pathology[35] in 1993, as the *Histopathology Atlas of the Sudden Infant Death Syndrome*. This manual has already set the standard for the histologic diagnosis of SIDS. Applying these criteria, d'Espaignet and McFeeley[36] were able to demonstrate a high degree of reproducibility between pathologists in Australia and in the United States, examining the same Australian material from sudden infant death cases.

Another attempt to standardize SIDS classification was initiated in the Nordic countries in 1990. The NORD SIDS study was an initiative by the Nordic Council of Ministers and consisted of three working parties: NORD PAT, NORD EPI and NORD FYS.[32] The pathology working party reached a consensus on diagnostic exclusion criteria for the lung, heart and brain,[37] and from 1992 onwards the criteria were implemented in routine diagnostic work in Denmark, Sweden, Finland and Norway. To examine whether different diagnostic criteria could explain the differences in SIDS rates between the Nordic countries, 127 randomly selected sudden unexpected infants deaths from all Nordic countries from 1970 to 1995 were re-evaluated blindly by 10 forensic pathologists from Denmark, Sweden, Finland and Norway. The study showed that neither the increase in the SIDS rates in the 1970s and 1980s, nor the decline of SIDS rates since 1989, seemed to be due to changed diagnostic practices. However, for Denmark, Finland and Norway, the revised diagnoses of cases from the period 1970–1991, showed a higher proportion of SIDS cases than the original diagnoses ($P<0.01$) (Fig. 2.7). After 1992 no significant differences between the original and revised diagnoses were found[33] (Fig. 2.7). In Sweden there was little discrepancy between the original and revised diagnoses throughout the period 1970–1995[33] (Fig. 2.7). One explanation for the latter observation may be that SIDS as a concept may have been accepted earlier in Sweden than in the other countries.

Berry has suggested[38] that different groups of pathologists are likely to adopt their own pragmatic criteria for the diagnosis of SIDS. Hospital pathologists may apply criteria with reference to similar cases that they have seen in routine hospital practice.[38] Forensic pathologists are likely to use the quite variable histopathologic findings present in victims of accidents and homicides as a 'normal reference'.[34] In the Nordic countries, autopsies in cases of sudden unexpected infant death are almost always performed by forensic pathologists, which may explain why it has been possible to reach such a high degree of consensus. The great variation in histologic findings that may be incidental to the cause of death is illustrated by the case of an 11-month-old girl. Although she was apparently well when she was put to bed, 25 minutes later she was found lifeless by her 5 year old sister with an electric cable around her neck. Classic signs of asphyxiation were present with petechial hemorrhages in the conjunctivae and in the skin of the face (Fig. 2.8a). The autopsy also revealed bronchopneumonia, small septic foci within the liver and significant myocarditis (Fig. 2.8b). The cause of death would certainly have been septicemia with myocarditis, if one had not considered the fatal circumstances. Cable marks around the neck and petechiae in the conjunctiva proved that the death was caused by suffocation. Furthermore, in spite of the severe histopathologic findings, the infant had been apparently healthy prior to death. This case clearly demonstrates the problem of

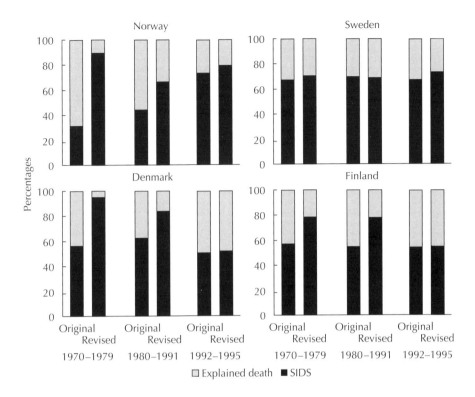

Fig. 2.7 Distribution of original and blindly revised diagnoses of SIDS and explained death from the Nordic countries in the periods 1970–1979, 1980–1991, and 1992–1995. SIDS was under-diagnosed in the first two periods in all countries except Sweden, whereas after 1992, when the Nordic criteria were in general use, there were almost no differences between original and revised diagnoses. (From Vege and Rognum, *Acta Paediatr* 1997;86:391–6.)

normal variation, and the importance of the synthesis of clinical history, circumstances of death, and autopsy findings. It is simply not possible to make the diagnosis of SIDS based on microscopic slides alone.

The cultural 'differences' in classifying SIDS are demonstrated by Hatton *et al.*, 1995.[23] Out of 1503 sudden deaths in infancy in France in 1987, the authors have derived 281 cases in which autopsies, including histologic examination, had been performed. The authors were able to find explainable death in 47.7% of the cases; 49.8% were grouped as unexplained SIDS with associate findings, whereas only 2.5% were regarded as unexplained SIDS without anomaly. Hatton *et al.*[23] also presented the distribution of diagnoses in the series of sudden unexpected infant deaths published by other authors (Table 2.1). The percentage of pure SIDS varies from 70% to 2.5% out of the total population of sudden unexpected deaths.[16–22]

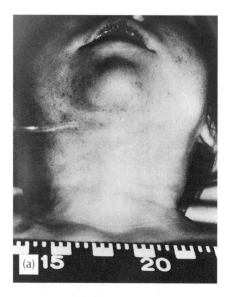

Fig. 2.8 (a) Eleven-month-old girl who was accidentally strangled by an electric cable: Note ligature mark and petechiae of the skin on the face. (b) Histologic section from the heart shows myocarditis.

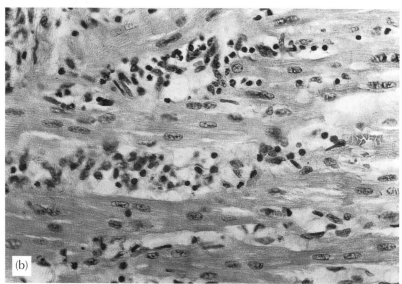

Is there a syndrome at all?

Most pathologists probably still agree that SIDS should be a diagnosis based on the exclusion of findings and circumstances that are generally recognized as causes of death. Nevertheless, Emery[39] raised the question of whether SIDS is really a diagnosis – or just a diagnostic dustbin? Huber (1993)[40] went one step further and claimed that SIDS as a concept 'does not and cannot exist'. He therefore wanted to leave out the 'S' in SIDS, using merely the descriptive term SID. His view has been adopted as the official one by the editorial board of *European Journal of Pediatrics*. During a panel discussion on the definition of SIDS at the Third SIDS International Conference in Stavanger 1994, Huber described sudden infant death (SID) as:

That part of infant mortality where the clinical presentation of death occurs more or less suddenly and unexpectedly. Postmortem examination which ideally should consist of a history of gestation, delivery and postnatal evaluation, a death scene, a family psycho-social history, a complete autopsy, and a confidential case conference:

● may reveal pathologic changes that alone *or* in combination – constitute a sufficient cause of death *or*
● may reveal changes that even when clearly present are not sufficient to explain death *or*
● fail to demonstrate any abnormalities.

The last line represents what the supporters of the 'syndrome' would name SIDS.

The grey zone

Like Huber, many pathologists realize that there is a group of 'in between' cases in which there are pathologic findings – either morphologic or microbiologic ones – or information from the history or the circumstances of death, that are significant, but most likely not sufficient to explain death. This borderline group is also recognized by pathologists who use the term SIDS. In spite of the obvious existence of such a grey zone, which may include neglect, abuse and even murder, the existence of an entity or a syndrome for these virtually unexplained cases may have been fruitful for research efforts in the field of sudden unexpected infant death. These research efforts have revealed knowledge about the risk factors which has saved thousands of lives. The great challenge now is to unveil the dangerous mechanisms behind risk factors like prone sleeping position, increased ambient temperature and smoking. To abolish SIDS as a registerable cause of death would mean putting the clock back to 1960.[39] It may force pathologists to apply obscure diagnoses such as pneumonitis or interstitial pneumonia to avoid the 'shame' of writing 'unexplained'. Such a development would in turn be extremely counter-productive for research, pulling down a smoke screen over this still important part of infant mortality.

Borderline SIDS

In the borderline cases there is information in the history, morphologic or microbiologic findings or circumstances that cannot be considered normal. In the Nordic SIDS study[37] sudden infant death is divided into the following three categories:

1 Pure SIDS cases in which the autopsy and clinical information do not reveal any cause of death.
2 Borderline SIDS cases in which pre-existing congenital disorders or clinical symptoms and/or postmortem findings are not severe enough to explain the cause of death.
3 Non-SIDS cases in which the cause of death is explained according to clinical information and/or the results of the postmortem examination.

The criteria for these three categories in the Nordic SIDS study are defined with regard to morphologic changes in lungs, heart and brain,[37] but an initiative has been undertaken to continue the NORD PAT study, expanding it to include better standardized information about the history and the circumstances of death.

It has become increasingly evident that obscure circumstances may also add to the borderline group.[41] In southeast Norway (2.5 million inhabitants) the bor-

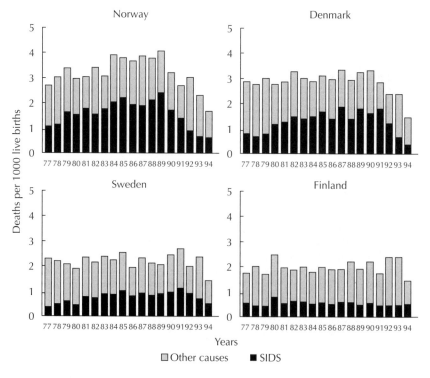

Fig. 2.9 Infant mortality after the fourth week of life in the Nordic countries 1977–1994. The total infant mortality is approximately 30% lower in Sweden and Finland than in Norway and Denmark. The difference appears to be almost entirely due to the different SIDS rates.

derline group increased from 1% of the total population of sudden unexpected death in infancy in the period from 1984 to 1989, to 8% in the time period 1990 to 1998 (Fig. 2.5). During the same time periods deaths due to neglect, abuse or murder increased from 2.3% to 6% (Fig. 2.5).

Furthermore, pure SIDS cases were reduced from 80% to 60% (Fig. 2.5). It is not yet clear whether the modest increase in deaths due to neglect or abuse reflects a real increase or merely a relative increase due to the 80% drop in the SIDS rate (Fig. 2.6). It cannot be totally excluded that increased awareness may have played a role in revealing more cases of abuse and neglect. Nevertheless, it is evident that the decrease in SIDS rates in the Nordic countries has been paralleled by a corresponding decrease in total infant mortality[33] (Fig. 2.9).

Autopsy findings

MACROSCOPIC

More than half of the infants who succumb suddenly and unexpectedly are found in the prone sleeping position.[42] Not infrequently, the baby has been dead for some hours before being found. In these cases lividity is observed in the face, on the chest and on the abdomen (Fig. 2.10). Pink foam may be seen in nose, throat and trachea. The same material may be found on the cot sheet, corresponding to where the face was placed.

Recently, Meadow [43] has suggested that the presence of frank blood from the nose and/or mouth may be suggestive of imposed suffocation. Twenty-seven out of 70 children who had been killed by their parents were reported to have been found with blood apparent in the mouth, nose and face. On examination by medical staff, stale blood was seen in 20 of those 27 children. Meadow stresses that care was taken to establish that the finding was of frank blood, rather than

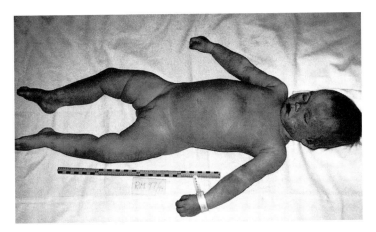

Fig. 2.10 A SIDS victim found dead in the prone position showing anterior lividity.

the common sero-sanguineous froth that can be present in moribund children, particularly when subjected to resuscitation. Interestingly, Southall *et al.*[44] observed bleeding from nose and/or mouth in 11 out of 39 cases of life-threatening child abuse revealed by covert video recordings, whereas petechiae in the face were only found in three cases.

In 187 SIDS cases investigated at The Institute of Forensic Medicine, University of Oslo, between January 1984 and July 1999, frank blood from the nose and/or the mouth was seen in 8% of the cases. White-red froth in the nose and/or mouth had been recorded in 7% of the SIDS cases. These percentages are low, probably due to the practice in Norway of admitting infants found unexpectedly dead to the nearest hospital, where the nursing staff wash and clean the babies thoroughly before they are forwarded to autopsy. In countries with other practices the percentage of SIDS victims with white-red foam from the nose and mouth is more than 30% (Kleeman W, personal communication).

It seems clear to the author that it is not possible to differentiate between imposed suffocation and SIDS in individual cases based on the presence or absence of frank blood in the nose and mouth.

An increasing proportion of sudden infant death takes place during cosleeping with an adult.[32,42] There are of course several ways to cosleep. To share a bed with a mother who smokes seems dangerous.[45] A hazardous variant may also be to place the baby between the back of a sofa and the back of an adult (Fig. 2.11).

In half of the cases of sudden infant death the body temperature is increased in the hours after death.[46] Not infrequently, these infants have had symptoms of

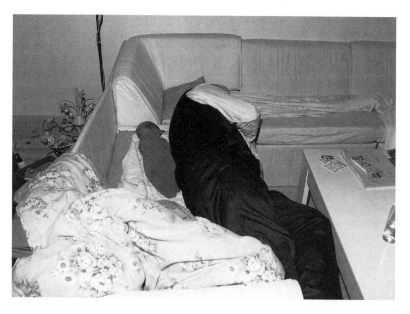

Fig. 2.11 Sofa sharing with an adult may be an unsafe sleeping practice for infants.

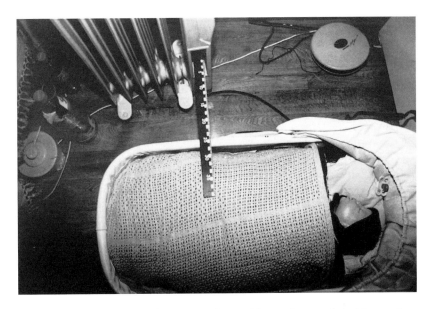

Fig. 2.12 Overheating. An infant put to sleep with two layers of clothing and a cap, into a sleep skin bag with a quilt on the top. The bag was placed 20 cm from an electric oven. Three hours after the baby was found dead the rectal temperature was 41.5°C.

a cold during the days before death. We have seen cases in which young inexperienced mothers have been instructed by their own mothers to keep the babies warm, especially when they have a cold (Fig. 2.12).

A total of 70% of the SIDS victims (TO Rognum, personal observation) have petechial haemorrhages on the thymus (Fig. 2.1a). Petechiae are also frequent on the surface of the lungs (Fig. 2.1c), especially between the lobes and on the surface of the heart (Fig. 2.1b). The cause of these petechiae is heavily debated. Some authors claim that they are due to suffocation because of obstruction of the upper airways,[47,48] whereas others think that petechiae may be due to a combination of airway obstruction and infection.[49]

In recent studies of intrathoracic petechiae related to the position of the face when found dead, Krous concludes that the presence of petechiae argues against external airway obstruction, but does not exclude internal airway or nasal obstruction, or rebreathing.[50] Macroscopically the lungs show dark and light areas in a variegated pattern due to partial atelectasis (Fig. 2.1c).

MICROSCOPIC

Alveolar edema and intraseptal lymphocytes

Histologic sections from the lungs often show edema fluid within alveoli, with congestion and aggregation of macrophages (Fig. 2.13). Not infrequently, small aggregates of lymphocytes are found around the bronchioli and occasionally within the alveolar septae (Fig. 2.13). Partial atelectasis, a frequent finding in SIDS, might further strengthen the impression of increased cellularity of the septae. Twenty-five years ago these observations often led to pathologists diagnosing interstitial pneumonia as a cause of death.[51] Later studies have shown that such collections of lymphocytes in lung tissue are common in infants and thus do not explain death. This experience demonstrates the importance of having access to a large reference collection to show the extent of normal variation, and of having generally accepted exclusionary diagnostic criteria.[51,37,33] From the standpoint of the researcher, however, it cannot be excluded that minor infections causing inflammatory changes in the respiratory tract or in the intestinal mucosa may induce the release of interleukin-6 (IL-6) in the cerebrospinal fluid, thereby contributing to factors that may play a role in the pathogenesis of SIDS.[52–55] In combination with a prone sleeping position, especially with the face down in the mattress, such minor infections may cause fever and thus overheating, bradycardia, irregular breathing, inefficient gasping and finally coma and death.[54–56] It is, however, extremely important to stress that such opinions about a possible mechanism of death, should not be implemented in routine diagnostic work. Conversely, the use of unconfirmed theories and individual viewpoints of the pathogenesis and etiology of SIDS in diagnostic work may impede further research.[11] For instance, diagnoses such as positional asphyxia are of little help when trying to classify sudden infant death.

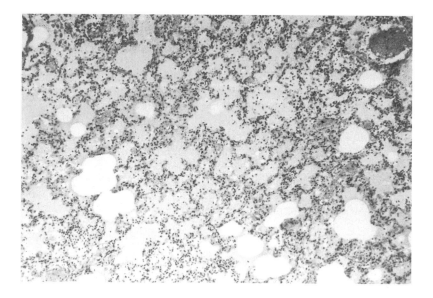

Fig. 2.13 Lung section from a SIDS case. Note edema and a slight thickening of the alveolar septae. (See also colour plate section)

Intra-alveolar hemorrhage

Recently Yukawa *et al.*, 1999[57] reported that intra-alveolar hemorrhage covering more than 5% of the total lung surface area was indicative of suffocation due to smothering (Fig. 2.14). Five out of 11 cases (45%) in which smothering was either admitted or was a possibility (45%) showed significant intra-alveolar hemorrhage.[57] In our own series from The Institute of Forensic Medicine, University of Oslo, six out of 11 cases (35%) in which suffocation was the cause of death, showed intra-alveolar hemorrhage (35%) (TO Rognum, unpublished observations). However, the same was true for 15% of the SIDS cases and for 23% of cases of sudden death due to natural disease (TO Rognum, unpublished observations). We therefore agree with Berry[58] that more than 5% of alveoli showing hemorrhage is neither a necessary, nor a specific, criterion for the diagnosis of deliberate suffocation. Moreover, Berry[58] points to the fact which can be seen from the work of Yukawa *et al.*[57] that intra-alveolar hemorrhage seems to be a feature of younger babies that die suddenly and unexpectedly, regardless of the cause of death.

Interstitial hemosiderin

In 1985 Stuart *et al.*[59] proposed that interstitial hemosiderin in the lungs of sudden infant death syndrome was a histologic hallmark of 'near miss' episodes. This assumption has been supported by Byard *et al.*, 1993[60] and Valdes-Dapena *et al.*, 1993.[61]

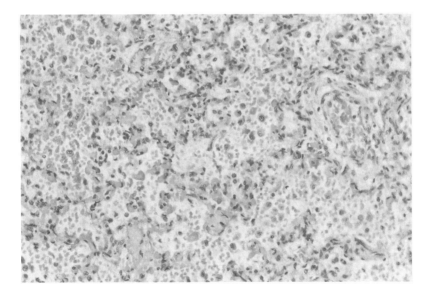

Fig. 2.14 Lung section from a SIDS case. Note intra-alveolar hemorrhage and macrophages. (See also colour plate section)

Becroft and Lockett[62] studied the lungs of two pairs of siblings, who had hospital admissions for life-threatening events (ALTEs) before dying suddenly at home. A mother and a babysitter were subsequently convicted of their murder and manslaughter respectively. Staining of lung sections for iron showed previously overlooked intra-alveolar siderophages widely distributed in the lungs of the two pairs of siblings.[62] No siderophages were found in the lungs in a fifth infant whose death was included in the murder charge, but who had not had ALTEs reported.[62] Moreover, bleeding from the mouth or nose was observed during six of 10 previous ALTEs suffered by these children, and in three unrelated infants in the same care.

Becroft and Lockett[62] concluded that intra-alveolar siderophages can be a marker of previous abuse. However, when studying lung sections from 158 infants diagnosed as SIDS, these authors also report that alveolar siderophages were found in the lungs of seven of them (4.5%). Nevertheless, they recommend that specific staining of lung sections for iron should be performed in all sudden deaths of infants who have a history of previous ALTE, particularly those leading to hospital admission, or associated with external bleeding. Such examinations should also be performed in infants who have had siblings dying in similar circumstances or when other causes give rise to suspicions that death was not natural.[62]

In a recent case of four sibling deaths in Norway, massive intra-alveolar hemorrhage was seen in all cases (TO Rognum, personal observation). However, none of the lung sections showed significant iron-positive macrophages. The mother had always been alone with the infants when they were found dead. Until the last death, no death scene investigation had been performed. However, after the last death, death scene investigation revealed a plastic bag in the garbage. The plastic bag had lip marks from the baby and biological material with an identical DNA profile to that of the baby, in addition to fingerprints from the mother. The mother was convicted of homicide of the last baby, but was acquitted in a higher court half a year later. In spite of the findings on the plastic bag, the jury found her not guilty due to a possible genetic predisposition for sudden death.[63] The mother and the two fathers, as well as all four dead babies had been investigated for mutations in five of the genes associated with long QT-syndrome, and in the case in which the plastic bag was found, the baby turned out to have a new, not previously described, mutation in the KCNH2 gene.[63]

Familial clustering of infant deaths – genetic predisposition or homicide?

A family who has lost one child to SIDS has a sixfold increased risk of losing the next child when compared with all other families.[64,65] Since Schwartz *et al.*[66] published that half of their SIDS deaths may be due to long QT-syndrome and DNA markers are now available to characterize long QT-syndrome, this theory has become a hot issue.[67] The possibility of a genetic predisposition has become re-acknowledged.

After the scandal of multiple infant deaths incorrectly attributed to SIDS in the United States,[13] it became unfashionable to mention a possible genetic factor in SIDS. The quotation from DiMaio: 'one case of sudden infant death in a family may be SIDS, two deaths in one family is suspicious, whereas three deaths in the same family is equal to homicide'[13] has been accepted by several pathologists. A recent infant death necropsy protocol from Ontario, Canada[68] carried on its first page, the message, printed in bold: 'THINK DIRTY!' The protocol advises all concerned to treat every 'so-called SIDS death' as a possible homicide until proved otherwise. In a recent editorial, Green[69] strongly supports this view. Furthermore, he recommends that in cases in which pathologists are uncomfortable with SIDS as a diagnosis, they should use the phrase 'not ascertained' and hope that social services will be made aware of the circumstances, through the coroner, and that any future child born into the family should then be closely supervised. However, the recent focus on the long QT-syndrome and sudden infant deaths has given the hypothesis of a genetic predisposition for SIDS a renaissance.

Future perspectives

The 'grey-zone' cases between SIDS and totally explained deaths seem to have become more frequent, a fact which is a challenge for forensic pathologists, and also implies the necessity of cooperation with other experts. The exclusion of explained causes of death demands expertise in forensic medicine as well as in pediatric pathology, neuropathology, radiology, pediatrics, microbiology, and toxicology.

What types of examination lead to exclusion from the SIDS group?

Out of the total population of 289 cases of sudden unexpected death in infancy investigated at The Institute of Forensic Medicine, University of Oslo, between 1984 and 1998, 66 cases were excluded as explained death. The different modes of death in this non-SIDS group were 37 cases of natural disease, 13 accidents, six cases of abuse or neglect, and 10 cases of homicide (Fig. 2.15).

Information about the circumstances of death and the death scene were the most important factors, when diagnosing explained death (non-SIDS) (Fig. 2.16)

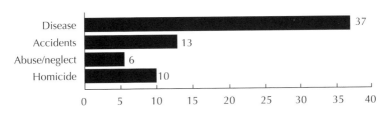

Fig. 2.15 Unexpected deaths in southeast Norway 1984–1998. Mode of death in 66 cases of explained deaths (non-SIDS).

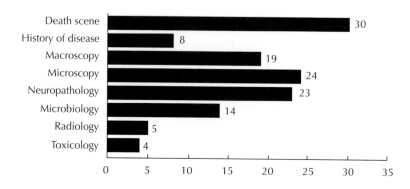

Fig. 2.16 Sudden unexpected infant death. What part of the investigation contributed to the diagnosis of explained death?

followed by microscopy, neuropathology and the gross pathology findings. Also microbiology, history of disease, radiology and toxicology contributed significantly to the diagnosis in a number of cases.

Death scene investigation and case conferences

There is an increasing understanding that death scene investigation and case conferences should be compulsory in cases of sudden infant death.[29] We think that the death scene investigation should preferably be performed by police officers with special training and by forensic pathologists. The aims of the death scene investigation are firstly to reveal criminal acts such as maltreatment. However, by ensuring a death scene investigation in every case of sudden unexpected death in infants and small children, gossip and suspicion towards bereaved families may be avoided. Secondly, the aim is to make the exclusion of all other known causes of death as qualified as possible and thus establish a sound basis for the study of the cause(s) of SIDS. Information about circumstances and risk factors may furthermore help generate new hypotheses as to possible mechanisms of death. Moreover new risk factors may be discovered by a thorough death scene investigation. The increasing number of SIDS victims who are found dead while bed-sharing in southeast Norway is an example: in the period 1996–1998, 42% died in bed with an adult whereas 25% of the case controls usually slept in bed with parents.[42] In addition, the prevention of accidents by revealing dangerous factors in infants' environments is an important issue.

In 1995 a mother who had lost five children – two of whom had been included in the famous publication by Steinschneider[70] that initiated the 'apnea monitor movement' – was convicted of murder. Bergman,[71] in a commentary, wrote that it would be sad if publicity about the infanticide cases should result in a return to the aura of suspicion that surrounded the families of the SIDS victims of the past. A more appropriate memorial to the slain infants, Bergman concluded,[41] would be an effort to both strengthen the death investigation system for all infants who die suddenly and unexpectedly, and to increase support for research aimed at reducing the number of such deaths.

References

1. The story of King Solomon. *The Bible*, 1.Kings 3:19.
2. Kopp JH. Denkwordichkeiten in der ärtzlichen Praksis, 1830. Cited by Lee CK. Art XII On the thymus gland, its morbid affections and the diseases that arise from its abnormal enlargement. *Am J Med Sciences* 1842;3:135–54.
3. Paltauf A. Plötzlichen Thymustod. *Wien Klin Wochenschr* 1889;II:877 and 1890: III: 172.
4. Valdes-Dapena M. A half century of progress: The evolution of SIDS research. In: Rognum TO (ed.) *Sudden Infant Death Syndrome. New Trends in the Nineties.* Scandinavian University Press, Oslo, 1995.
5. Geertinger P. Sudden unexpected death in infancy with special reference to the parathyroids. *Pediatrics* 1967;39:43–8.
6. Valdes-Dapena M, Weinstein D. The parathyroids in sudden unexpected death in infancy. *Acta Path Microbiol Scand* 1971;79:228–32.
7. Haas JE, Taylor JA, Bergman AB *et al*. Relationship between epidemiologic risk factors and clinicopathologic findings in SIDS. *Pediatrics* 1993;91:106–12.
8. Valdes-Dapena M. A pathologist's prospective on possible mechanisms in SIDS. *Ann NY Acad Sci* 1988;533:31–6.
9. Vege Å, Rognum TO, Opdal SH. SIDS – changes in the epidemiological pattern in Eastern Norway 1984–1996. *Forensic Sci Int* 1998;93:155–66.
10. Beckwith JB. A proposed new definition of sudden infant death syndrome. In: Walker AM, McMillen C (eds) *Second SIDS International Conference*. Perinatology Press, Ithaca, NY, 1993, pp. 421–4.
11. Rognum TO, Willinger M. The story of the 'Stavanger-definition'. In: Rognum TO (ed.) *Sudden Infant Death Syndrome. New Trends in the Nineties*. Scandinavian University Press, Oslo, 1995, pp. 17–20.
12. Beckwith JB. Discussion of terminology and definition of the sudden infant death syndrome. In: Bergman AB, Beckwith JB, Ray CG (eds) *Sudden Infant Death Syndrome. Proceedings of the Second International Conference on the Causes of Sudden Death in Infants*. University of Washington Press, Seattle, 1970, pp.14–22.
13. Firstman R, Talan J. *The death of Innocents*. Bantam Book, NY, 1997.
14. Hilton J, Berry JP. Pathology. In: Fitzgerald K (ed.) *Second SIDS Global Strategy Meeting*, Stavanger, Norway, August 5–6, 1994, p. 334. In: Rognum TO (ed.) *Sudden Infant Death Syndrome. New Trends in the Nineties*. Scandinavian University Press, Oslo, 1995.
15. World Health Organization (WHO). *World Health Statistics Annual*. Geneva, 1998.
16. Helweg-Larsen K, Knudsen LB, Gregersen M, Simonsen J. Sudden infant death syndrome (SIDS) in Denmark: Evaluation of the increasing incidence of registered SIDS in the period 1972 to 1983 and results of a prospective study in 1987 through 1988. *Pediatrics* 1992;89:855–9.
17. Arneil GC, Brooke H, Gibson AAM, *et al*. National post perinatal infant mortality and cot death study, Scotland 1981–82. *Lancet* 1985;1:740–3.

18. Rajs J. Differential diagnosis of SIDS from the medico-legal point of view. *Acta Paediatr Scan* 1993; (Suppl.) 389:80–1.
19. Knowelden J, Keeling J, Nicholl JP. *A Multicentre Study of Post Neo-natal Mortality.* Medical Care Research Unit, University of Sheffield, 1984.
20. Imbert MC, Briand E, Broyer M, *et al.* Intérêt de la comparison anatomo-clinique dans la mort subité du nourrisson. *Arch Fr Pediatr* 1992;49:311.
21. Taylor EM, Emery JL. Categories of preventable unexpected infant deaths. *Arch Dis Child* 1990;65:535–9.
22. Cheron G, Rambaud C, Rey C *et al.* Morts subités au berceau. *Arch Fr Pediatr* 1993; 50:293–9.
23. Hatton F, Bouvier-Colle MH, Barois A *et al.* Autopsies of sudden infant death syndrome – classification and epidemiology. *Acta Paediatr* 1995;84:1366–71.
24. Willinger M, James S, Catz C. Defining the SIDS: deliberations of an expert panel convened by the National Institute of Child Health and Human Development. *Pediatr Pathol* 1991;11:677–84.
25. Guntheroth WG, Spiers PS, Naeye RL. Redefinition of SIDS: the disadvantages. *Pediatr Pathol* 1994;14:127–32.
26. Rognum TO, Lier LA. Police investigation and SIDS: an improved system of co-operation between health personnel, forensic pathologists and the police? In: Rognum TO (ed.) *Sudden Infant Death Syndrome. New Trends in the Nineties.* Scandinavian University Press, Oslo, 1995; pp. 289–92.
27. Rognum TO, Vege Å. Plutselig uventet død i spedbarnsalder etter 'krybbedødepidemien'. *Scand J Forens Sci* 1999;5:20–23 (in Norwegian).
28. Byard RW, Carmichael E, Beal S. How useful is post mortem examination in sudden infant death syndrome? *Pediatr Pathol* 1994;14:817–22.
29. Byard RW, MacKenzie J, Beal SM. Formal retrospective case review and sudden infant death. *Acta Paediatr* 1997;86:1011–12.
30. Byard RW, Becker LE, Berry PJ *et al.* The pathological approach to sudden infant death – consensus or confusion. *Am J Forens Med Pathol* 1996;17:103–5.
31. Burd L. Prevalence of prone sleeping position and selected infant care practices of North Dakota infants: the comparison of whites and Native Americans. *Public Health Rep* 1994;109:446–9.
32. The Nordic Council: Irgens LM, Rognum TO, Lagercrantz H, Helweg-Larsen H, Norvenius G. Sudden infant death in the Nordic countries. *TemaNord* 1997: 600.
33. Vege Å, Rognum TO. Use of new Nordic criteria for classification of SIDS to re-evaluate diagnoses of sudden unexpected infant death in the Nordic countries. *Acta Pædiatr* 1997;86:391–6.
34. Rognum TO. SIDS or not SIDS? Classification problems of sudden infant death syndrome. *Acta Paediatr* 1996;85: 401–3.
35. Valdes-Dapena M, McFeeley PA, Hoffmann HJ *et al. SIDS: Histopathology Atlas of the Sudden Infant Death Syndrome.* Washington DC, Armed Forces Inst of Pathol, NICHD, 1993, pp. 339.
36. d'Espaignet ET, McFeeley P. Diagnosis of SIDS: reproducibility in Australia and comparability with diagnosis in the United States. In: Rognum TO (ed.) *Sudden Infant Death Syndrome. New Trends in the Nineties.* Scandinavian University Press, Oslo, 1995; pp. 59–66.
37. Gregersen M, Rajs J, Laursen H *et al.* Pathologic criteria for the Nordic Study of

Sudden Infant Death Syndrome. In: Rognum TO (ed.) *Sudden Infant Death Syndrome. New Trends in the Nineties*. Scandinavian University Press, Oslo, 1995, pp. 50–8.

38. Berry PJ. . . . and remains unexplained after a thorough postmortem examination. In: Rognum TO (ed.) *Sudden Infant Death Syndrome. New Trends in the Nineties*. Scandinavian University Press, Oslo, 1995, pp. 38–9.

39. Emery JL. Is sudden infant death syndrome a diagnosis? Or just a diagnostic dustbin? *Br Med J* 1989;299:1240.

40. Huber J. Sudden infant death syndrome: the new clothes of the emperor. *Eur J Pediatr* 1993;152:93–4.

41. Bergman AB. Wrong turns in sudden infant death research. *Pediatrics* 1997;99: 119–21.

42. Arnestad M, Andersen M, Vege Å, Rognum TO. Changes in the epidemiological pattern for sudden infant death syndrome (SIDS) in Southeast Norway 1984–1998. *Paper given at the Sixth SIDS International conference*. Auckland, New Zealand, February 8–11, 2000.

43. Meadow R. Unnatural sudden infant death. *Arch Dis Child* 1999; 80: 7–14.

44. Southall DP, Plunkett BM, Banks MW, Falkov AF, Samuels MP. Covert video recordings of life-threatening child abuse: Lessons for child protection. *Pediatrics* 1997;100:735–60.

45. Mitchell EA, Thompson JMD. Co-sleeping increases the risk of SIDS, but sleeping in parents' bedroom lowers it. In: Rognum TO (ed.) *Sudden Infant Death Syndrome. New Trends in the Nineties*. Scandinavian University Press, Oslo, 1995.

46. Stanton AN. Overheating and cot death. *Lancet* 1984;8413:1199–201.

47. Beckwith JB. Intrathoracic petechial hemorrhages: a clue to the mechanism of death in SIDS? *Ann NY Acad Sci* 1988;533:37–47.

48. Krous HF, Jordan J. A necropsy study of distribution of petechiae in non-SIDS. *Arch Pathol Lab Med* 1984B;108:75–6.

49. Guntherroth WG, Kawabori I, Breazeale DG, Galinghouse LE, van Hoosier GL. The role of respiratory infection in intrathoracic petechiae. *Am J Dis Child* 1980; 134:364–6.

50. Krous HK. Contribution of pathology to SIDS beginning the new millenium. *Plenary paper given at Sixth SIDS International Conference*. Auckland, New Zealand, February 8–11, 2000.

51. Løberg EM, Næss AB. Skyldes økningen i plutselig spedbarnsdød endrede diagnostiske kriterier? *Tidsskr Nor Lægeforen* 1991;111:2864–6.

52. Vege Å, Rognum TO, Scott H, Aasen A, Saugstad OD. SIDS cases have increased levels of Interleukin-6 in the cerebrospinal fluid. *Acta Paediatr* 1995;84:193–6.

53. Rognum TO, Saugstad OD. Biochemical and immunological studies in SIDS victims. Clues to the understanding of the mechanism of death. *Acta Paediatr (Suppl.)* 1993; 389:82–5.

54. Vege Å, Rognum TO, Ånestad G. IL-6 cerebrospinal fluid levels are related to laryngeal IgA and epithelial HLA-DR response in SIDS. *Pediatr Res* 1999;45:803–9.

55. Vege Å, Rognum TO. Inflammatory responses in sudden infant death syndrome – past and present views. *FEMS Immunol Medi Microbiol* 1999;25:67–78.

56. Poets CF, Meny RG, Chobanian R, Bonofiglo RE. Gasping and other cardiorespiratory patterns during sudden infant deaths. *Pediatr Res* 1999;45:350–4.

57. Yukawa N, Carter N, Rutty G, Green MA. Intra-alveolar haemorrhage in sudden infant death syndrome: a cause for concern? *J Clin Pathol* 1999;52:581–7.
58. Berry JP. Intra-alveolar heamorrhage in sudden infant death syndrome: a cause for concern? Editorial. *J Clin Pathol* 1999;52:553–4.
59. Stewart S, Fawcett J, Jacobsen W. Interstitial hemosiderin in the lungs of sudden infant death syndrome: a histological hallmark of 'nearmiss' episodes? *J Pathol* 1985; 145:53–8.
60. Byard RW, Telfer S, Moore L. Is interstitial hemosiderin deposition within the lungs in SIDS infants a useful marker of previous hypoxic episodes? (Abstract) *Lab Invest* 1993;68:2P.
61. Valdes-Dapena M, McFeeley PA, Hoffman HJ *et al. Histopathology Atlas for the Sudden Infant Death Syndrome.* Washington, DC: Armed Forces Institute of Pathology, 1993, Chapter 10, Summary of histologic findings and implications for future SIDS research.
62. Becroft DMO, Lockett B. Intra-alveolar pulmonary siderophages in sudden infant death: a marker for previous imposed suffocation. *Pathology* 1997;29:60–3.
63. Christiansen M *et al.* Long QT syndrome: Genotype–phenotype relationship and relation to sudden infant death syndrome (SIDS). Abstract. *Am J Hum Genet* 1999;65 (Suppl.), A289.
64. Guntheroth WG, Lohman R, Spiers PS. Risk of sudden infant death syndrome and subsequent siblings. *J Pediatr* 1990;116:520–4.
65. Øyen N, Skjærven R, Irgens LM. Population-based recurrence risk of sudden infant death syndrome compared with other infant and fetal deaths. *Eur J Epidemiol* 1996; 144:300–5.
66. Schwartz PJ, Stramba-Badiale M, Segantini A *et al.* Prolongation of the QT interval and the sudden infant death syndrome. *New Engl J Med* 1998;338:1709–14.
67. Towbin JA, Friedman RA (editorial). Prolongation of the QT interval and the sudden infant death syndrome. *New Engl J Med* 1998;338:1760–1.
68. Protocol for the investigation of sudden and unexpected deaths in children under 2 years of age. (*Memorandum No 631.*) Ontario: Ministry of the Solicitor General and Correctional Services, 1995.
69. Green MA. A practical approach to suspicious death in infancy – a personal view. *J Clin Pathol* 1998;5;561–3.
70. Steinschneider A. Prolonged apnea and the sudden infant death syndrome: clinical and laboratory observations. *Pediatrics* 1972;50:646–54.
71. Bergman AB (commentary). Wrong turns in sudden infant death syndrome research. *Pediatrics* 1997;99:119–21.

CHAPTER 3

Changing epidemiology

FERN R. HAUCK

Introduction   31
Rates of SIDS before and after risk reduction campaigns   31
Risk factors   33
Sociodemographic factors   33
Pregnancy related factors   37
Miscellaneous conditions of infant prior to death   39
Sleep environment   41
Changes in SIDS epidemiology following reductions in SIDS rates   48
Acknowledgements   50
References   50

Introduction

The dramatic decline in rates of SIDS following national and local education campaigns is a major achievement for epidemiology.[1] While researchers continue to search for the physiologic or anatomic abnormalities responsible for SIDS deaths, these campaigns, whose main messages were based on observational epidemiologic data, have been effective in reducing the risk for and rates of SIDS. This chapter provides a historical overview of the leading risk factors for SIDS, with particular attention to sleep position, other sleep environment factors, and smoking, and will identify emerging factors and the changing risk profile following reductions of SIDS rates resulting from the campaigns.

Rates of SIDS before and after risk reduction campaigns

Rates of SIDS for representative countries are shown in Table 3.1. All have reached record lows. Widespread risk reduction campaigns were initiated in Great Britain,[2] New Zealand,[3] and Australia[4,5] in 1991; in the Netherlands in

Table 3.1 SIDS rates in representative countries, 1987–1997

Year	Australia–1	Austria–2*	England/Wales–3	Netherlands–4	New Zealand–5	Norway–6	Scotland–7	Switzerland–8	USA–9
1987	2.49	1.63	2.40	0.91†	4.30	1.89	2.00	0.86	1.37
1988	2.32	1.66	2.50	0.58	4.40	2.12	2.00	0.92	1.40
1989	2.16	1.48	2.10	0.70	4.10‡	2.39†	2.20	1.23	1.39
1990	2.19	1.56	1.80	0.56	2.90†	1.70	2.00	1.18	1.30
1991	1.80†	1.13	1.60†	0.44	2.50	1.36	1.30†	1.02	1.30
1992	1.42	1.12	0.80	0.41	2.30	0.85	0.90	0.97†	1.20‡
1993	1.37	1.17	0.70	0.35	2.10	0.59	0.90	0.98†	1.17
1994	1.01	0.79	0.70	0.30	2.10	0.53	0.70	0.72	1.03†
1995	0.88	0.64	0.60	0.25	2.10	0.48	0.70	0.66	0.87
1996	0.90	0.60	0.70	0.26	1.90	n/a	0.80	0.44	0.78
1997	1.12**	0.58	0.60	0.17	1.50	n/a	0.90	n/a†	0.77

Ages	Source
1. All ages, including >1 yr	Australian SIDS Organizations.
2. Birth to 1 yr	1987–96: Austrian Demographic Reports, 1996. 1997: personal communication, Austrian Central Bureau for Demographic Statistics.
3. Birth to 1 yr	Office of Population and Census Surveys.
4. 1 wk to 1 yr	Dutch Bureau of Statistics, 1997.
5. All ages, including >1 yr	New Zealand Health Information Service, Fetal and Infant Deaths.
6. 1 mo to 1 yr	Vege A, Rognum TO. Use of new Nordic criteria for classification of SIDS to re-evaluate diagnoses of sudden unexpected infant death in the Nordic countries. *Acta Paediatr* 1997; 86, 391–6.
7. 1 wk to 1 yr	Scottish Cot Death Trust, 1999.
8. Birth to 1 yr	Federal Bureau of Statistics, Bern, March 1999.
9. Birth to 1 yr	National Center for Health Statistics, Centers for Disease Control and Prevention.

Key:

* Intervention strategies implemented at variable times in different regions, some in 1980s, others more recently.

** Provisional data.

† Year risk reduction campaign started.

‡ Other risk reduction activity (e.g. limited media, statements from professional organisations).

n/a Not available.

1987[6]; in the Scandinavian countries 1990–1992 (Norway 1990, Denmark 1991, and Sweden 1992)[7]; and in the United States in 1994.[8,9] The declines in SIDS rates of 50% or more shown for each of these countries can be attributed largely to reductions in placing babies prone (on their stomach) for sleep.[7,10–14] No significant changes were observed in other behaviors targeted by some of the campaigns, such as reducing smoking during pregnancy and increasing breastfeeding.[12,15]

Risk factors

A number of modifiable and non-modifiable factors have been found to be associated with increased (and decreased) SIDS risk (Table 3.2). Non-modifiable factors will be described briefly, since changes in these factors are either impossible or would require significant social change beyond the scope of the public health community.

Sociodemographic factors

FAMILIAL CHARACTERISTICS

While SIDS strikes infants from all socioeconomic backgrounds, research has consistently shown that lower socioeconomic status, variously measured by household income, unemployment, lower maternal education, single maternal marital status, or young maternal age, is associated with higher risk for SIDS.[16–21] Some differences have been found for indigenous populations where SIDS has not consistently been associated with single marital status or young maternal age, but this may relate to the poor discriminatory power of these variables under general conditions of extreme poverty.[22–24]

INFANT CHARACTERISTICS

Race-ethnicity

In the United States, one of the most ethnically and culturally diverse countries in the world, Native American and African–American infants have higher rates of SIDS than other racial–ethnic groups. In 1996, SIDS rates were as follows (number per 1000 live births): Native American 2.03; African–American 1.54; white 0.64; Hispanic 0.49; and Asian/Pacific Islander 0.44.[36] Among Hispanics, rates differ according to country of origin, with infants of Puerto Rican ancestry having about a twofold increased risk compared with those of Mexican and Central or South American ancestry (0.82, 0.47, and 0.31, respectively).

One explanation for the higher rate of SIDS among African Americans is the higher concentration of socioeconomic risk factors commonly associated with SIDS, such as young maternal age, single marital status, lower education and

Table 3.2.   Summary of risk factors for sudden infant death syndrome

Factor	Association	Comment
Sociodemographic		
Lower socioeconomic status	↑	
African–American	↑	
Indigenous populations	↑	
Asian/Pacific Islander	↓	In some reports
Age at death	↑	Peaks at 2–4 months
Male	↑	30-50% more likely to be affected than females
Cold season	↑	Attenuation with SIDS rate declines in some locations
Pregnancy		
Higher parity	↑	
Low birth weight, short gestation	↑	
Inadequate prenatal care	↑	
Maternal smoking	↑	
Smoking by father or other household member	↑	Difficult to separate effects from maternal smoking; probably no to small increased risk over maternal smoking
Maternal recreational drug use		
Opiates	↑	Difficult to evaluate drugs separately; probably stronger increased risk from opiates compared with cocaine
Cocaine	↑	
Maternal alcohol use (during and after pregnancy)	–	
Conditions post-birth		
Infections	–	Recent illness potentiates effects of prone position or overbundling
Passive smoke exposure	↑	Difficult to assess due to high correlation of smoking during and after pregnancy; probably small independent risk of passive exposure
Breastfeeding	–	Adjustment for other factors in most studies eliminates protective effect; may be slightly protective
Prone sleep position	↑	Well established risk factor
Unaccustomed prone, secondary prone	↑	Recent evidence of increased risk for these conditions in a few studies
Side sleep position	↑	Becoming more important as prone rates decline
Bed-sharing	↑	Risk greater with smoking mothers, on couches, with other children and in younger infants
Room-sharing	–	Few studies address
Soft sleep surfaces	↑	Pillows, comforters, sheepskins, polystyrene cushions and older or softer mattresses are associated with increased risk
Head/face covered by bedding	↑	Few studies address
Comforter (duvet) use	↑	Few studies address
Overheating	↑	May be more important factor for prone-sleeping infants
Pacifiers	↓	Consistent finding in all studies reporting use

Key:

↑ Increased risk

↓ Decreased risk

– Inconclusive or no apparent association.

poverty. The effect of race was eliminated in one study after controlling for family income and maternal education.[18] In another study, where only infants of college educated couples were included, there were no differences in the rates of SIDS, despite the twice higher incidence of low birth weight in African–American infants.[25] The higher rate of SIDS can also be explained, in part, by higher usage of the prone sleeping position by black mothers (43%) compared with white mothers (22%).[14] Other practices such as bed-sharing, which is more common among African Americans, may also contribute to the higher rate. [26,27]

Regarding indigenous peoples, Maori infants in New Zealand have been shown to be more likely to die from SIDS compared with infants of European ancestry (unadjusted odds ratio [UOR] 4.76, 95% confidence interval 3.12–7.27)* in a 1991–1993 case–control study.[19] In an earlier study including all live births in New Zealand 1987–1990, Maori infants had a four times higher risk of SIDS (UOR 3.81, 3.06–4.76).[28] The risk factors for Maori and non-Maori infants were similar, but the prevalence of many of the known risk factors were higher among the Maori, including mothers who were socio-economically disadvantaged, younger, and more likely to smoke, and infants who were of lower birth weight and more likely to bed-share.[28] Controlling for potential confounders found that being Maori did not significantly increase the risk for SIDS (adjusted odds ratio [AOR] 1.37, 0.95–2.01). More recent data (1996) confirm the persistent disparity, with rates of SIDS (per 1000 live births) as follows: Maori 4.6; Pacific Islander 1.9; and other (predominantly European) 0.7.[29]

In Australia, Aboriginal infants have the highest rates of SIDS of all racial–ethnic groups. For the period 1993–1996, the rate for Aboriginal infants was 4.6 per 1000 live births and for infants of European ancestry, the rate was 0.65 per 1000, resulting in a ratio of 7.1 to 1. (Personal communication, Dr. Susan Beal, May 1998). In a case–control study conducted in Western Australia, Aboriginal infants were found to have an almost fourfold increased risk of SIDS, but after adjusting for the increased frequency of most of the available risk factors, this reduced to 1.43 times higher risk (1.04–1.95).[30]

As previously described, of all racial–ethnic groups in the US, rates of SIDS among Native American infants are over three times higher than among white infants. In a study comparing Native American and white infants in Washington State, where the Native American infants were 3.25 times more likely to die from SIDS, adjustment for differences in age, marital status, parity, and smoking status during pregnancy reduced the relative risk to 1.82 (1.28–2.58).[31] Native Americans experience a higher level of poverty, adverse environmental home conditions, and alcoholism than other groups and these factors may contribute

---

* Throughout this chapter, the following conventions will apply when reporting odds ratios: the odds ratio will be provided first, followed by 95% confidence interval. It will be indicated if the odds ratio is unadjusted (unadjusted odds ratio [UOR]) or adjusted (AOR), if available from the reference cited.

to the higher rate of postneonatal mortality.[32] Further study is needed to determine their influence on the risk of SIDS.

Regarding Asian and Pacific Islanders, rates of SIDS in Hong Kong (0.3 per 1000 live births in 1987) and Japan (0.41 per 1000 in 1996), where prone sleeping is uncommon, are among the lowest reported throughout the world.[33,34] Data for the other Asian countries and Pacific islands have not been reported. In England, SIDS rates were lower among infants of Asian ancestry (predominantly from India, Pakistan and Bangladesh) than among white infants. In a study of infant care practices comparing the two groups prior to the country's risk reduction campaigns, Asian infants were more often placed supine (on their back) and less often placed prone for sleep. Almost all the Asian infants slept in their parents' room at night compared with 61% of whites, and 36% of the former group slept in their parents' bed compared with 11% of the latter. However, in a Swedish study, immigrant women from Southeast Asia and the Pacific Islands experienced significantly higher rates of SIDS than Swedish women, after controlling for a number of factors including smoking habits, parity and maternal age (AOR 1.61, 1.10–2.36).[35] In Australia, the rates for Asians are the lowest of all racial–ethnic groups (0.4 per 1000 live births for the period 1988–1997) (Personal communication, Dr Susan Beal, May 1998). This is true, also, for Asians and Pacific Islanders in the United States.[36]

Since risk reduction interventions have been instituted, in both Australia and New Zealand the gap in rates between indigenous and non-indigenous infants has increased.[37] In the United States, the gap in rates between African–American and white infants increased following the national Back to Sleep campaign (ratio of 2.5 to 1 in 1995), but recent data indicate that this trend may be reversing.[14,36] Further research is needed to evaluate the reasons for the continuing and, in some cases, worsening disparities in SIDS rates between different racial–ethnic groups within and across countries.

Age at death

The age at death distribution is one of the most characteristic features of SIDS; it is uncommon in the first month of life and peaks at 2–4 months of age.[38,39] Approximately 80% of SIDS deaths occur by 6 months.[39,40]

Sex

Generally, SIDS affects between 30% and 50% more males than females.[16–19,21,38,41] However, this male predominance has not been found among indigenous populations in Australia, New Zealand and the US.[42]

Season at death

SIDS occurs two to three times more commonly in the winter or cold season compared with the warmer months, for both the northern and southern hemispheres.[38,43,44] This seasonal variation has declined or disappeared in some countries following recent reductions in SIDS rates.[39,44] A seasonal attenuation was not found among African Americans in California, whose rates of SIDS declined only 20% between 1990 and 1995, but was suggested for other racial groups, whose rates declined 41%, implying that a threshold in reduced SIDS levels must be met in order to see the seasonal pattern changes.[45]

Pregnancy related factors

PARITY

SIDS infants are more likely to be of higher birth order, independent of their mother's age.[16,18,19,21,38,40] Likewise, a short interpregnancy interval confers a higher risk.[38]

BIRTH WEIGHT AND GESTATION

The incidence of SIDS is higher in infants with low birth weight, preterm birth/short gestation, or intrauterine growth retardation.[18,19,38,40] In the Nordic countries, unadjusted odds ratios for these factors, respectively, were 9.3 (5.1–17), 5.7 (3.5–9.4), and 3.1 (2.0–4.9), while in New Zealand the unadjusted odds ratio for low birth weight was 4.07 (1.95–8.44) and for gestation under 38 weeks 2.35 (1.38–3.98).[19,40]

PRENATAL CARE

SIDS mothers generally receive less prenatal care and initiate care later in pregnancy, with two to three times higher risk associated with late or no prenatal care.[16,18,19,21]

SMOKING

Maternal smoking during pregnancy has consistently been associated with increased risk for SIDS. Mitchell and Milerad reviewed over 50 studies reporting the relationship between maternal smoking in pregnancy and sudden infant death syndrome and conducted meta-analyses for two groups, namely, those done before intervention campaigns and those done after interventions where the prevalence of prone sleeping became low.[46] For the first analysis, the pooled relative risk associated with maternal smoking was 2.89 (2.81–3.00). For the latter, the pooled relative risk for eight studies was 4.67 (4.04–5.35), indicating the increased importance of smoking as a risk factor following declines in prone sleeping.

The effects of paternal smoking and smoking by other household members are more difficult to interpret, as they are highly correlated with maternal smoking. In order to evaluate the independent effect of paternal smoking, Mitchell and Milerad performed a meta-analysis with six studies in which paternal smoking was present and maternal smoking was absent in cases and controls, and the resulting pooled relative risk was 1.39 (1.11–1.74).[46] Since there was no adjustment for socioeconomic status, a known confounder, it is likely that this small effect would disappear after adjustment. They also reviewed four studies that examined smoking by other household members, where either adjustment for maternal smoking was done or only maternal non-smokers were included. Of these, two showed a small significantly increased risk and two showed no additional effect. Therefore, maternal smoking in pregnancy has been found to be the most influential smoking behavior in increasing risk for SIDS among offspring.

RECREATIONAL (ILLEGAL) DRUG USE

Maternal drug use (unspecified) during pregnancy was associated with a twofold increased risk of SIDS in the NICHD Cooperative Epidemiological Study (1978–1979) for cases compared with controls matched on birth weight, race and age.[21] In the UK case–control study, maternal use of illegal drugs (any combined) became non-significant in the multivariate model for use before, during or after pregnancy.[47] Paternal use of drugs after the baby's birth remained significant in the model (AOR 4.68, 1.56–14.05).

Increased rates of SIDS among offspring have been reported among mothers who used methadone, cocaine, heroin or other recreational drugs during pregnancy. A sevenfold increased risk was found among infants of substance-abusing mothers compared with drug-free mothers in Los Angeles.[48] Relative risks varied from 3.07 (0.43–21.74) for phencyclidine, 6.87 (4.04–11.68) for cocaine, to 15.10 (6.30–36.20) for opiates. A fivefold increased risk was found in a Detroit study among drug-using compared with non-using mothers of similar socioeconomic status. In this study, the principal drugs used were heroin and methadone, although other drugs and alcohol were often used as well.[49] Potentially confounding variables, aside from socioeconomic status in the latter, were not examined in these studies. The association between opiates and SIDS is much more consistent than for cocaine. In a New York study spanning 10 years of births and using vital record data, the SIDS rate was 5.83 per 1000 live births in the drug-exposed infants compared with 1.39 in the unexposed group.[50] After adjusting for race, teen mother, parity, maternal cigarette smoking, and birth weight, the following risk ratios were obtained: methadone only 3.7 (2.6–5.3); heroin only 2.3 (1.3–4.1); methadone and heroin 3.1 (1.2–8.4); cocaine only 1.3 (1.0–1.8); and cocaine and heroin or methadone 1.0 (0.5–2.5). In a meta-analysis of five studies comparing cocaine-exposed infants with drug-free infants, the pooled odds ratio for SIDS was 4.10 (3.17–5.30).[51] In another analysis of three studies comparing cocaine exposed to other drug-exposed infants, there was no increased risk of SIDS for cocaine use over other drug use (OR 2.67, 0.88–8.15).[51] With the exception of the New York study previously cited, none of the studies controlled for potentially confounding variables.

ALCOHOL USE (DURING AND AFTER PREGNANCY)

The majority of published studies to date have reported no association between maternal alcohol use during or after pregnancy and SIDS. Alcohol consumption has been found to be highly correlated with smoking and adjusting for this factor eliminates the independent effect of alcohol.[47] In a study by L'Hoir *et al.* in the Netherlands with 73 SIDS cases and 146 controls, maternal alcohol consumption in the 24 hours before the infant died carried a twofold (AOR 2.25, 1.01–6.34) to eightfold elevated risk (AOR 8.09, 2.25–29.11), depending on the model.[52] There was no risk associated with maternal alcohol use since the birth of the child, and no effect from paternal alcohol use for either period.

Miscellaneous conditions of infant prior to death

INFECTIONS

The possible role of upper respiratory infections (URI) in the etiology of SIDS has been considered for many years. Most of the earlier studies focused on the morphology of the lower respiratory tract. Kleemann and coauthors investigated the presence of URI in 56 SIDS cases and 26 controls who died from other causes.[53] No differences were found and at least two-thirds of each group had signs of URI. The authors suggested that infections of the nose in conjunction with other factors, such as prone sleeping, may play a role in the pathogenesis of SIDS. Likewise, in the US NICHD SIDS Cooperative Epidemiological Study, colds and related symptoms in the past 2 weeks were reported with equal frequency among cases and controls.[21] SIDS infants, however, had a higher prevalence of diarrhea and vomiting (29.3%) than each control group (17% and 19%, $P<0.001$). In Scotland, a range of symptoms in the previous week were not found to be associated with increased risk for SIDS in multivariate analysis (AOR 1.58, 0.83–3.01).[17]

No clear association has been identified between SIDS and specific viral or bacterial pathogens.[54] In a UK study, limited sampling from the upper respiratory tract and gastrointestinal tract (throat swabs and stool specimens) showed no excess in viral infection in the sudden unexpected death group compared with living controls (UOR 1.98, 0.9–4.5).[55]

Recent illness appears to interact with other factors to increase the risk of SIDS. In an Australian study, mild illness was not associated with an increased risk if the infant did not usually sleep prone (UOR 0.83, 0.27–2.6), but was associated with a sixfold increase among infants who usually slept prone (UOR 5.7, 1.8–19).[56] In a New Zealand study, the risk associated with prone sleeping increased by the level of illness.[39] In a British case–control study, among infants over 70 days of age, the combined effects of viral infection and wrapping in excess of 10 togs produced a UOR of 51.5 (5.64–471.5).[55] In the absence of heavy wrapping, the presence of a viral infection was not found to be a major risk factor for SIDS. Therefore, recent infectious illness does not appear to increase the risk for SIDS significantly, but may interact with other factors to potentiate the risk.

EXPOSURE OF THE INFANT TO PASSIVE SMOKE

It is extremely difficult to assess the independent effect of the infant's passive exposure to smoking, since parental smoking behaviors during and after pregnancy are highly correlated. Eleven studies were examined by Mitchell and Milerad and they found a correlation of 0.95 ($P<0.0001$) in maternal smoking between the two periods.[46] In only one study was the effect of maternal smoking after the infant was born examined in the absence of maternal smoking during pregnancy.[25] In this US study, only infants of normal birth weight were included. Among African–American infants the odds ratio for passive exposure was 2.33 (1.48–3.67) and for white infants 1.75 (1.04–2.95), adjusting for marital status, maternal education, and maternal age. One weakness of the study was that since pregnancy only consisted of the period in which the mother knew she was pregnant, it is possible that some of the mothers in the 'not smoking during pregnancy' group had in fact been exposed to tobacco early in pregnancy.

In another US study in which extensive data were collected on smoking during and after pregnancy by mother, father and other household members, the authors attempted to look at the independent effect of passive exposure by adjusting for maternal smoking during pregnancy.[57] This resulted in an odds ratio of 3.50 (1.81–6.75) after adjusting for that factor plus birth weight, breastfeeding, sleep position, prenatal care, and medical conditions at birth. However, since paternal smoking during pregnancy (41% among cases) and other household members (18%) were not controlled, it is still difficult to draw conclusions about the effect of passive smoking on the risk for SIDS independent of prenatal exposure. Nonetheless, the study demonstrates a strong dose response with the number of household smokers, the number of people smoking in the same room as the infant, and the number of cigarettes smoked, although confidence intervals were wide for the highest levels of each variable, indicative of the small numbers in those categories. In the UK study, a dose response was similarly found for passive postnatal smoke exposure for the number of smokers in the household, number of cigarettes smoked, and the number of hours the infant was exposed daily.[47] While this issue needs further study, it is prudent to recommend both cessation of smoking by the mother and other family members (or at least not smoking in the same room as the mother) during pregnancy and to avoid smoking near the infant, particularly in the same room.

BREASTFEEDING

The effect of breastfeeding on SIDS risk has been inconclusive. Early studies suggested a protective effect, but a larger number of studies have found that once other factors are taken into consideration, this effect becomes non-significant.[17–19,54,58] This, along with lack of a 'dose response' suggests that breastfeeding is a marker for lifestyle and/or socioeconomic status as opposed to a biologic effect.[58] In an earlier New Zealand study, SIDS cases were less likely to have been exclusively breastfed at discharge from hospital and in the last 2 days before death than control infants (AOR 0.52, 0.35–0.77 and 0.65,

0.43–0.91, respectively).[59] Following a national prevention campaign, breast-feeding was no longer found to be protective, but this may have been related to inadequate power to detect a difference, as breastfeeding rates are high in New Zealand.[19] In the United States, 'ever' breastfed infants in the NICHD study had about half the risk of SIDS compared with controls matched on age, low birth weight and race[21] and in a California study, the risk was lower only for infants who had non-smoking mothers (0.37, 0.19–0.72).[57] In Scandinavia, over the course of a 3-year case–control study during which SIDS rates declined in each country, bottle feeding became a risk factor for SIDS in the third year of the study (AOR 4.5, 1.4–14.7, adjusted for maternal smoking, usual infant sleep position, and infant age).[7] Finally, in the Netherlands, exclusive breastfeeding beyond 13 weeks was found to have a protective effect, after adjustment for a large number of variables (AOR 0.09, 0.01–0.88)[52] but in another publication by these authors, the same factor was found to be insignificant.[60] Although the effect of breastfeeding against SIDS is at best, mildly protective, breastfeeding is still the preferred method for infant feeding because of its many beneficial effects on infant health, and it should be encouraged for those reasons.[61]

Sleep environment

SLEEP POSITION

Prone

Prone sleeping has consistently been shown to increase the risk of SIDS and as described in the introduction to this chapter, its reduction has contributed in large part to the dramatic declines in SIDS rates globally. In 1991, Beal and Finch conducted a meta-analysis of six case–controls studies; for prone as the usual sleep position, the common odds ratio was 2.72 (2.27–3.26).[62] The American Academy of Pediatrics Task Force on Infant Positioning and SIDS published a review in 1992 on which they based their recommendation for avoidance of the prone position among healthy infants in the US.[63] Seven case–control studies with data for usual sleep position met their inclusion criteria and all but one had significant odds ratios over 1 (ranging from 1.3 to 11.57); seven did not meet all their criteria and of these, six had significant odds ratios over 1 (ranging from 3.76–13.91) and one did not have controls. For studies including data for position put down for last sleep, three studies met the criteria and all had significant odds ratios over 1 (ranging from 3.53–9.46), and two did not meet the criteria but had significant odds ratios over 1 (4.76 and 12.91). Mitchell *et al.* published a meta-analysis of 17 case–control studies that had been published in 1992 or earlier (no US or Scandinavian studies were included).[64] The calculated common OR was 2.8 (2.1–3.6). In 14 of the 17 studies, the association between prone position and SIDS was significant; in none of the remainder was the supine position more frequent in cases than controls.

Of studies published since 1992, in a Tasmanian study with 58 SIDS cases and 120 controls (1988–1991) usual prone position had a UOR of 4.5 (2.1–9.6).

The strength of the association was increased among infants who slept on natural-fiber mattresses, were swaddled, were recently ill with a minor illness within one day of death/interview, and slept in a heated room. In a US study of 47 infants and 142 matched controls conducted 1992–1994, comparing usual sleep position as prone with non-prone resulted in a UOR of 4.69 (2.17–10.17) and an AOR of 3.12 (1.08–9.03).[65] In another US study, routine sleep position of prone among cases was 66% and among controls 64% (*P*=0.91), AOR 1.03, (0.65–1.62). However, at the time of death, 72% were last placed and 80% were found prone; no comparable data were available for controls. Weaknesses of this study that could explain in part the lack of an association include delays in interviewing cases (6–12 months post-event) and the age disparities between cases and controls (controls were older when their parents were interviewed).[66]

As rates of SIDS have declined in countries post-intervention, odds ratios for prone sleeping have increased. In the UK, data were collected for 95 SIDS cases and 780 matched controls, 1993–1995 and results were as follows: put down for last sleep in prone position UOR 9.58 (4.86–18.87) and found prone after being placed on side UOR 21.36 (11.67–39.08).[58] In Norway, two periods were studied, 1987–1989 and 1990– 1992; the first campaign promoting avoidance of the prone sleeping position was in January 1990.[13] For the first period, the UOR for placed prone was 2.0 (0.8–4.5) and for found prone 5.2 (1.7–17.9). For the second period the UOR for placed prone was 11.3 (3.6–36.5) and for found prone 30.6 (8.1–41.1). Over the two time periods, prone sleeping among reference infants decreased from 64% (placed and found) to 11% and 12%, respectively, while for cases, prone position remained high (78% and 90% vs 57% and 81%). This indicates that studies may need to be large to disclose prone sleeping as a risk factor if prone is the predominant position in the population. In a study of the Nordic countries, including 244 SIDS cases and 869 controls (1992–1995), the following results were reported: placed in prone position UOR 13.9 (8.2–24.0) or side UOR 3.5 (2.1–5.7), and found prone UOR 14.1 (8.8–23.0) or side UOR 2.0 (1.2–3.6).[40] In Scotland, a study of 201 SIDS cases and 276 controls was conducted 1992–1995, during which time SIDS rates fell from 1.1 to 0.7/1000 live births.[17] Routine prone sleeping had an AOR of 6.96 (1.51–31.97) and side position 1.51 (0.76–2.98). In the Netherlands, where rates of SIDS are extremely low, a study was conducted in 1995–1996 with 73 SIDS cases (up to 2 years of age) and 146 controls.[67] Risks for prone and side sleeping were as follows: placed prone AOR 8.36 (2.65–26.42) or side AOR 4.03 (1.36–11.96), and found prone AOR 18.73 (6.86–51.14) or side AOR 8.27 (2.49–27.51).

Unaccustomed and secondary prone

More recently, attention has been paid to the issues of unaccustomed and secondary prone sleeping. 'Unaccustomed prone' refers to infants who are usually placed non-prone for sleep, but are placed prone for the last sleep. 'Secondary prone' refers to infants who were placed non-prone for sleep, but were found prone. In the Nordic Study, the infants who were usually placed non-prone but were placed prone for last sleep and had a higher risk (UOR 8.7 [4.1–19.0]) than infants who were placed prone usually and for last sleep (UOR

6.9 [4.6–10.0]).[40] Analyses from the New Zealand Cot Death Study found that 20% of the SIDS deaths involved lack of experience with prone sleeping and unaccustomed prone had the highest risk (AOR 19.3, 8.2–44.8) compared with the next highest risk category, usual and last prone (AOR 4.6, 3.4–6.3).[68] Twelve per cent of the SIDS cases had spontaneously turned prone during the last sleep, and a majority of these (91.5%) usually slept non-prone, indicating that they were inexperienced at prone sleeping. (No control data were available for calculation of odds ratios.) In the Netherlands, the highest risk (AOR 17.89, 5.98–53.48), was found in infants who were usually placed and found non-prone but were found prone on last occasion of sleep.[67] In the US, data were collected on 1916 SIDS deaths from 11 states, 1995–1997, of which 20.4% occurred in child care settings.[69] Comparing SIDS deaths in child care with those not in child care, the former were older more commonly and of a racial background other than African American, and their mothers were more educated. Deaths in child care were more likely to be associated with being last placed prone (P=0.004) or being found prone (P=0.011) when the usual sleep position was side or supine, implying that secondary care givers were more likely to use the prone position and this may have increased the risk for SIDS among those infants who were usually placed non-prone. Infants who have a history of spontaneously changing their position, even into prone, do not have an increased risk of SIDS,[67,68] and may even have a reduced risk.[17]

Side

In a review of side sleeping position and the risk for SIDS, Scragg and Mitchell identified nine studies reporting odds ratios for side position, of which eight were over 1.[70] The Mantel–Haenszel summary odds ratio for all studies combined was found to be 2.02 (1.68–2.43) for side vs back sleep position. They postulate that the instability associated with the side position is the likely explanation for this increased risk based on evidence that cases placed on the side have been more likely to change to the prone position than controls. As prone sleeping rates have declined following SIDS risk reduction campaigns, side sleeping has become a more critical risk factor in some locations. (See final section, Changes in SIDS epidemiology following reduction in rates, for further discussion.)

Sleeping supine is safe for infants

The evidence to support that supine sleeping is safe for infants was summarized in a review by Henderson-Smart and colleagues.[71] In Asian countries where sleeping supine has been routine, aspiration has not been found to be a problem, nor has there been an increase in aspiration deaths in the UK following back sleep recommendations. Rather, evidence shows that the risk of regurgitation and choking is highest among infants sleeping face down. Infants sleeping on their back do not have increased episodes of apnea or cyanosis. Reports of apparent life-threatening events were decreased in the UK and Norway following increased rates of supine sleeping.[71]

BED-SHARING/ROOM-SHARING

Bed-sharing

A small number of epidemiologic studies have examined the relationship between bed-sharing and SIDS risk. In seven early case–control studies, five showed an increased risk of SIDS with bed-sharing, one showed a non-significant increased risk and one showed a non-significant lower risk.[72] The latter included only 16 cases. Scragg and coauthors in New Zealand were the first to report an interaction between bed-sharing and smoking, finding that bed-sharing in last sleep was a significant risk factor for SIDS among smoking mothers (AOR 4.55, 2.63–7.88) but not among non-smokers (AOR 0.98, 0.44–2.18).[73] A later study in New Zealand, following reduction of SIDS rates after implementation of the country's SIDS risk reduction program, resulted in similar findings.[19] The AOR for maternal smoking and bed-sharing was 5.01 (2.01–12.46) and for bed-sharing without smoking 0.55 (0.17–1.78). Similarly, a study of 198 SIDS infants and 780 controls in England identified bed-sharing as a risk factor only among smoking mothers (AOR 9.25, CI 2.51–34.02) rather than non-smokers (AOR 2.27, 0.41–12.54).[58] The authors of this and other studies reported that the risk for routine bed-sharing is smaller or non-significant compared with last sleep.[74] For example, a study in Scotland reported increased risk for SIDS among routine bed-sharing infants (UOR 3.92, 1.35–11.37), but it became non-significant after adjustment (AOR 2.90, 0.75–11.26).[17] While 11 of 147 cases (7.5%) had routinely bed-shared, at death, 48 had bed-shared (32.7%), further suggesting that the sleep practices at last sleep may be a more critical factor. A study in the United States also reported odds ratios greater than one for routine daytime and night-time bed-sharing, but they were not statistically significant (AOR 1.53, 0.92–2.52 and 1.28, 0.81–2.03, respectively), and there was no interaction with parental smoking, alcohol or recreational drugs.[75] In another US study, risk from bed-sharing in the last 2 weeks was elevated for both smokers and non-smokers, and there was no interaction between the two variables (AOR 5.27, 3.90–7.11 and 1.97, 1.73–2.83, respectively).[76] Bed-sharing has been found to be particularly hazardous under certain circumstances: sleeping with other children (with or without the parents), sleeping with parents on a sofa, and for infants under the age of 4 months.[27,77]

While some authors have suggested that maternal alcohol or drug intoxication may explain the increased risk of bed-sharing through accidental overlying,[16,41,78–80] there is a paucity of evidence from published case–control studies to support this theory. Fleming and coauthors found that more of the SIDS bed-sharing mothers (44.8%) had consumed three or more units of alcohol in the preceding 24 hours than the control mothers (19.3%), but the effect of bed-sharing was still significant in mothers who did not consume alcohol (OR 2.92, 1.44–5.87).[58]

Some authors have promoted bed-sharing as a more evolutionarily sound method of infant sleeping, and propose that this may in fact confer a protective effect against SIDS through promotion of breastfeeding, maternal inspections, infant respiration, and/or arousals.[81–84] Ecological data would also lend credibility to this hypothesis, as the incidence of SIDS has been found to be lower among infants of Asian origin in whom bed-sharing is more common.[85–87] However, these populations also have a much lower rate of the known risk factors for SIDS, such as prone sleeping and maternal smoking, making it impossible to draw conclusions about the influence of bed-sharing without appropriate studies to measure the independent influence of each of these factors. To date there have been no published reports of a statistically significant protective effect from bed-sharing and, to this author's knowledge, no 'reduce the risk' campaigns are advocating bed-sharing as a preventive strategy. A multidisciplinary forum convened in Australia to review the evidence concerning risk factors for SIDS concluded that there were insufficient data to 'provide complete reassurance to non-smoking parents that bed-sharing is safe.'[71] It has been suggested that placing the infant in a crib within arm's reach of the parents is an alternative solution to those who prefer close contact.[88] Additional studies are needed to further elucidate this issue.

Room-sharing

Studies addressing room-sharing and SIDS are limited. In New Zealand, room sharing was found to confer a protective effect over sleeping in any other room (AOR for last sleep 0.35, 0.26–0.49 and for last 2 weeks, AOR 0.35, 0.25–0.48).[72] The lowest risk of SIDS was associated with being in the parents' room but not bed-sharing. In contrast, the 1993–1995 case–control study in the UK found no difference in the proportion of case and control infants who shared a room with an adult or another child usually or during the last or reference sleep.[58] Similarly, in Scotland, room-sharing was common among cases (78%) and controls (75%) and was not found to be a protective factor (UOR 1.20, 0.69–2.09).[17]

BEDDING SURFACE–SOFTNESS AND PILLOWS

Softness of the sleep surface has been found to be associated with SIDS in most studies in which this factor were examined. In the postal follow-up of cases and controls previously included in the New Zealand Cot Death Study (105 cases and 828 controls), the AOR for soft bedding compared with average was 2.36 (1.06–5.25).[89] The firmness of the mattress did not interact with the sleep position of the infant. Kemp and colleagues studied the bedding surfaces of two groups of infants, one at higher risk for SIDS ($n=29$) and the second at lower risk ($n=29$) based on demographic risk factors for SIDS.[90] The high risk group had softer bedding ($P<0.0001$) based on the amount of surface contact with a weighted mannequin head, which caused more limitation of carbon dioxide dispersal using a mechanical model ($P=0.008$). In another study conducted by Kemp *et al.*, the softness of bedding from infants who died from SIDS in a face down position ($n=14$) was compared with conventional 'firm' infant bedding (crib mattresses and hospital bassinet mattresses).[91] The first group was softer ($P\leq0.005$) and limited carbon dioxide dispersal to a greater degree ($P\leq0.009$). This finding supports the hypothesis that carbon dioxide rebreathing may be one mechanism underlying the association between certain kinds of bedding with SIDS. In Scotland,[17] use of an old mattress was associated with increased risk for SIDS (AOR 2.51, 1.39–4.52); it can be postulated that these mattresses were less firm. In this same study, routine use of a pillow was not associated with a higher risk for SIDS, but pillow use was greater at the time of death (14% and 24%, respectively). In a US study of 206 infants who died from SIDS, 29% were found with their external airways covered.[92] Comparing infants found with and without the airways covered, factors increasing the risk of death with the airways covered included using soft bedding under the infants, such as pillows (AOR 3.12, $P \leq 0.05$) and comforters (AOR 2.59, $P \leq 0.05$). In a California study, no differences between cases and controls were found in the use of baby pillows (22% vs 16%, $P = 0.29$).

ARRANGEMENT OF BEDDING–HEAD/FACE COVERING AND USE OF QUILTS (DUVETS)

As rates of SIDS have declined following reductions in prone sleeping, other risk factors related to the sleep environment have emerged, i.e. head and face covering and use of quilts, also known as comforters or duvets. In the UK, more babies who died from SIDS were found with their heads covered (19%) vs controls (2%, UOR 18.93, 8.05–44.48).[58] The effect was stronger after adjustment for other sleep environment factors (AOR 21.58, 6.21–74.99). Duvet use was more common among cases than controls (42% vs 23% or UOR 2.82, 1.95–4.08). Duvets therefore, were associated with increased risk both in themselves and through their likelihood to cover the infant's head. This study took place after the country's back sleeping campaign when most of the infants had been sleeping on their back or side.

In the New Zealand Cot Death Study, firm tucking of the covering was associated with decreased risk (AOR 0.44, 0.26–0.73) and 15.6% of the cases were found with their head covered, but comparable data for controls were not available.[93] There were no differences in the number of blanket layers, but cases were more likely to use duvets than controls (58.3% vs 45.7%, $P < 0.001$). In a case series in South Australia, 22% (44/203) of the SIDS cases were found with their head underneath or tangled up in bedding.[94] In the Tasmania case–control study of 100 SIDS and 196 controls, an adverse effect was found for quilt use only in infants whose usual sleep position was not prone (AOR 6.16, 2.01–18.87).[95] Infants 12 weeks of age and older who did not sleep prone were at higher risk from quilt use than were younger infants. Facial covering by the quilt was reported for many of the infants from the death scene reports; the higher risk for SIDS was postulated by the authors to be related to facial obstruction caused by the quilt.

In Norway, a case–control study was conducted for two periods, one before and one after a campaign to reduce SIDS risk.[13] Information on head covering was available for 56 of the SIDS victims and for 123 reference infants born in 1990; 48% of the SIDS victims were found with their head covered by a quilt, while none of the reference infants were found with the head covered. In Scotland,

24% of the SIDS cases had ever moved under the bedclothes while only 13% of controls had (AOR 2.18, 1.03–4.64).[17] On the discovery of death, 13% of cases had been found under their covers.

The increased risk from head/face covering has been postulated to be due to diminished heat loss leading to hyperthermia[96] or rebreathing of carbon dioxide.[97,98] These mechanisms have also been proposed for infants found in the prone and face down position as contributing to the increased risk of SIDS from prone sleep.[96, 99]

THERMAL ENVIRONMENT

The association between overheating and SIDS has been established for several years, and led to the hypothesis of hyperthermia as an important link in the causal pathway. Various indicators of overheating have been identified: (1) room heating[58,96,100]; (2) high body temperature, sweating or other signs of over-heating[96,101–106]; and excessive clothing and/or bedding.[58,96,102–105,107] A study in California reported no difference in the type of heating source.[66] However, this study was conducted in southern California, where temperatures throughout the year are moderate and infants were not typically bundled or exposed to excessive amounts of heating.

Interactions between overheating and sleep position have also been identified in some studies. In the Tasmania study, room heating was not associated with increased risk in non-prone sleeping infants, but was associated with a tenfold increased risk in prone infants.[56] Similarly, Williams *et al.* found that sleep position modified the relationship between excess thermal insulation and SIDS, i.e., prone infants had a higher risk from excess thermal insulation (AOR 6.07, 3.83–9.60), whereas there was no increased risk for non-prone infants.[108] The higher reductions in SIDS deaths in the colder months by reducing prone sleeping may be explained by these interactions.[56]

PACIFIERS (DUMMIES)

Pacifiers have been found to be associated with lower risk for SIDS. Investigators from England found that the odds ratio for pacifier use at last sleep was 0.62 (0.46–0.83), and after multivariate adjustment, the OR was even lower, 0.41 (0.22–0.77).[109] There were no differences between cases and controls in usual pacifier use. Researchers from New Zealand reported an odds ratio of 0.76 (0.57–1.02) for pacifier use in the past 2 weeks, and 0.44 (0.26–0.73) for last sleep, with little change after adjustment.[110] In the Netherlands, pacifiers were associated with an OR of 0.19 (0.08–0.46) after adjustment for confounders and 0.05 (0.01–0.29) in multivariate modeling including sleep position, head covered, and use of duvet or sleep sack.[67] In Norway, pacifier use was also found to be more common among controls than cases (UOR 0.27, 0.14–0.51 for night-time and UOR 0.36, 0.19–0.69 for daytime, birth to 2-month-olds; respective figures for 2 to 3-month-olds were UOR 0.17, 0.08–0.36 and UOR 0.17,

0.08–0.39).[111] In a report from the Nordic Study, highest risk was associated with partial pacifier use and lowest with daily use; compared with partial use, the UOR for non-use was 0.7 (0.4–1.0) and for daily use 0.5 (0.3–0.7).[112] A Chicago study also reported an odds ratio below one for pacifier use in last sleep (AOR 0.3, 0.17–0.55).[113] Only one published study found no protective effect for routine pacifier use (26% vs 21%, $P=0.40$).[66]

While the findings are remarkably consistent, most authors have been hesitant to recommend pacifier use as a strategy to reduce the risk of SIDS. A primary concern about recommending pacifiers is duration of breastfeeding, which has been shown to be lower among pacifier-using infants. However, since the majority of studies examining this relationship were cross-sectional, it is not known if pacifiers were a direct cause of or aid to weaning.[59,114–116] In a prospective study it was found that using pacifiers did not result in lower breastfeeding rates of infants during the first 6 months of life.[117] In focus groups conducted with mothers and health professionals in New Zealand, most participants had a negative view of pacifiers, but no mothers personally reported problems with breastfeeding due to pacifier use.[118] Other concerns that have been expressed include injuries sustained from pacifiers. However, in one year of national data (1997) from the the US National Injury Information Clearinghouse, reports of injuries from pacifiers were low: (personal communication, Hope Barrett, National Injury Information Clearinghouse, US Consumer Product Safety Commission, March 1999).

Malocclusion has been reported to not be a problem as long as pacifiers are used correctly,[119] and if malocclusion does occur, it generally spontaneously corrects after discontinuation of pacifier use.[120] While pacifiers have been found to increase the incidence of acute otitis media in day care settings, the effect was most pronounced for children over the age of 2 years.[121] The Netherlands (among non-breastfeeding infants) and Germany (among all infants) have been the first countries to recommend pacifier use in their SIDS risk reduction educational materials (personal communication, Dr Monique L'Hoir, March 1999).[122] Other countries have been cautious about recommending pacifiers until more information is known about the potential consequences of pacifier use, both harmful and beneficial, as well as the physiologic effects of pacifier use that may have bearing on SIDS risk and causation.[109,110,115,123]

Changes in SIDS epidemiology following reductions in SIDS rates

The SIDS winter excess has decreased in Australia and the UK[44] and in Sweden,[124] and has disappeared in New Zealand.[39] However, it did not change over the period 1967–1995 in Norway.[125] Among African–American infants in California, whose rates of SIDS declined only 20% for the period 1990–1995, there was no attenuation of seasonality, but there was for other infants, whose rates declined 41%.[45] In England and Wales, for the period 1987–1992, SIDS declines were greatest in the postneonatal period.[54] Other studies are needed to determine if this finding has occurred elsewhere.

In countries where prone sleeping has became very low following intervention activities, the side position, because of its greater frequency, has become more important on a population basis than prone sleeping.[69] As Scragg and Mitchell reported in their review of this issue, in England, the population attributable risk for side sleep was found to be 18.4% compared with 14.2% for prone, in Scotland, these figures were 14% and 2%, respectively, and in New Zealand they were 37% and 1%, respectively.[69] The authors further point out that side sleep position in post-intervention populations ranks second in importance only to maternal smoking. The association of side sleeping with increased risk is most likely related to it being an unstable position, resulting in a certain proportion of these infants rolling to the secondary prone position during sleep.

In Scandinavia, over the course of a 3-year case–control study during which rates of SIDS declined following risk reduction interventions, the odds ratios for usually placed prone for sleep, maternal smoking during pregnancy, and bottle-feeding increased over the study period; the latter became significant only in the last year of study.[7] Data on risk for supine sleeping were not provided. In the UK study, prone position was still associated with a ninefold increased risk for SIDS (AOR 9.00, 2.84–28.47).[58] As these studies demonstrate, prone sleep position continues to be of great importance for those infants who are placed prone, and as discussed in a preceding section, especially for those unaccustomed to prone. Every effort must be made to decrease both prone and side sleeping in countries and within communities where this is still common practice.

Preliminary reports indicate that as rates of SIDS have declined, newer cases have more complex medical histories and death scene investigation findings[126] and a higher proportion are from socially disadvantaged backgrounds.[127] As described earlier in this chapter, disparities in SIDS rates among some ethnic–racial groups are increasing, as rates decline disproportionately. Greater efforts are needed to address these emerging issues and to apply new methods to ensure that SIDS reduction education reaches all members of society.

The changing epidemiology of SIDS has resulted in parental smoking being the most important risk factor for SIDS on a population basis. Blair *et al.* calculated a population attributable risk (PAR) of 61% for smoking by at least one parent.[47] Mitchell and coauthors calculated a PAR of 44% for maternal smoking without bed-sharing, and an additional 33% for maternal smoking and bed-sharing, following New Zealand's risk reduction campaign.[19] Based on a pooled relative risk from eight studies (including the preceding two) following declines in SIDS rates, the PAR is 48%, assuming a 25% prevalence of maternal smoking.[46] As a behavior much more difficult to change than the infant's sleeping position or other sleep environment factors, challenges for the public health community will be great to motivate and educate families about modification of smoking habits.

In conclusion, the evidence linking several of the risk factors described in this chapter and SIDS is now very strong. For sleep position and parental smoking the high, consistent odds ratios from numerous studies amount to evidence of a 'causal' relationship.[15,128,129] While this does not mean that all infants who are placed prone for sleep or who are exposed to tobacco will die from SIDS, these factors act in an important way along the causal pathway. Removing these factors will have a major impact on reducing SIDS incidence around the world.[58]

Acknowledgements

The author would like to thank Ms Catherine Nealon for her excellent secretarial assistance, and gratefully acknowledges the following individuals for providing information about SIDS rates and campaigns for their countries: P Blair, H Brooke, RW Byard, J Durst, D Fischer, S Fukui, D Ghelfi, A Jenick, G Jorch, R Kerbl, K Kolodny, MP L'Hoir, T Matthews, EA Mitchell, EAS Nelson, C Poets, C Rambaud, TO Rognum, M Stramba-Bardiale, E Wilson, and AG Winge.

References

1. Dwyer T, Ponsonby A-L. The decline of SIDS: A success story for epidemiology. *Epidemiology* 1996;7:323–5.
2. Wigfield R, Gilbert R, Fleming PJ. SIDS: risk reduction measures. *Early Hum Dev* 1994;38:161–4.
3. Mitchell EA, Aley P, Eastwood J. The national cot death prevention program in New Zealand. *Aust J Public Health* 1992;16:158–61.
4. Recommendation: a scientific review of the association between prone sleeping position and the sudden infant death syndrome. *J Paediatr Child Health* 1991;27:323–4.
5. Risk factors associated with sudden infant death syndrome. October 1991. In: *Program and abstracts of the 112th Session of NHMRC Council.* Canberra, Australia.
6. Jonge GA de, Burgmeijer RJF, Engelberts AC, Hoogenboezem J, Kostense PJ, Sprij AJ. Sleeping position for infants and cot death in the Netherlands 1985–91. *Arch Dis Child* 1993;69:660–3.
7. Wennergren G, Alm B, Oyen N *et al.* on behalf of the Nordic Epidemiologic SIDS Study. The decline in the incidence of SIDS in Scandinavia and its relation to risk-intervention campaigns. *Acta Paediatr* 1997;86:963–8.
8. Willinger M, Hoffman H, Hartford RB. Infant sleep position and risk for sudden infant death syndrome: report of meeting held January 13 and 14, 1994, National Institutes of Health, Bethesda, MD. *Pediatrics* 1994;93:814–9.
9. American Academy of Pediatrics and Selected Agencies of the Federal Government. Infant sleep position and the sudden infant death syndrome (SIDS) in the United States [joint commentary]. *Pediatrics* 1994;93:820.
10. Hiley CMH, Morley CJ. Evaluation of government's campaign to reduce risk of cot death. *Br Med J* 1994;309:703–4.
11. Mitchell EA, Brunt JM, Everard C. Reduction in mortality from sudden infant death syndrome in New Zealand: 1986–1982. *Arch Dis Child* 1994;70:291–4.
12. Dwyer T, Ponsonby A-L, Blizzard L, Newman NM, Cochrane JA. The contribution of changes in the prevalence of prone sleeping position to the decline in sudden infant death syndrome in Tasmania. *JAMA* 1995;273:783–9.
13. Markestad T, Skadberg B, Hordvik E, Morild I, Irgens LM. Sleeping position and

sudden infant death syndrome (SIDS): effect of an intervention programme to avoid prone sleeping. *Acta Paediatr* 1995;84:375–8.

14. Willinger M, Hoffman HJ, Wu K-T *et al*. Factors associated with the transition to nonprone sleep positions of infants in the United States. *JAMA* 1998;280:329–35.

15. Mitchell EA, Ford RPK, Taylor BJ *et al*. Further evidence supporting a causal relationship between prone position and SIDS. *J Paediatr Child Health* 1992;28 (Suppl. 1):S9–S12.

16. Rintahaka PJ, Hirvonen J. The epidemiology of sudden infant death syndrome in Finland in 1969–1980. *Forens Sci Int* 1986;30:219–33.

17. Brooke H, Gibson A, Tappin D, Brown H. Case–control study of sudden infant death syndrome in Scotland, 1992–5. *Br Med J* 1997;314,1516–20.

18. Kraus JF, Greenland S, Bulterys M. Risk factors for sudden infant death syndrome in the US Collaborative Perinatal Project. *Int J Epidemiol* 1989;18:113–20.

19. Mitchell EA, Tuohy PG, Brunt JM *et al*. Risk factors for sudden infant death syndrome following the prevention campaign in New Zealand: A prospective study. *Pediatrics* 1997;100:835–40.

20. Dalveit AK, Irgens LM, Oyen N *et al*. Sociodemographic risk factors for sudden infant death syndrome: associations with other risk factors. *Acta Paediatr* 1998;87:284–90.

21. Hoffman HJ, Damus K, Hillman L, Krongrad E. Risk factors for SIDS: results of the National Institute of Child Health and Human Development SIDS Cooperative Epidemiological Study. *Ann NY Acad Sci* 1988;533:13–30.

22. Alessandri LM, Read AW, Burton PR, Stanley FJ. An analysis of sudden infant death syndrome in Aboriginal infants. *Early Hum Dev* 1996;45:235–44.

23. Adams MM. The descriptive epidemiology of sudden infant deaths among Natives and whites in Alaska. *Am J Epidemiol* 1985;122:637–43.

24. Oyen N, Bulterys M, Welty TK, Kraus JF. Sudden unexplained infant deaths among American Indians and whites in North and South Dakota. *Paediatr Perinatal Epidemiol* 1990;4:175–83.

25. Schoendorf KC, Kiely JL. Relationship of sudden infant death syndrome to maternal smoking during and after pregnancy. *Pediatrics* 1992;90:905–8.

26. Lozoff B, Wolf AW, Davis NS. Cosleeping in urban families with young children in the United States. *Pediatrics* 1984;74:171–82.

27. Hauck FR, Kemp JS. Bedsharing promotes breastfeeding and AAP Task Force on Infant Positioning and SIDS (Letter). *Pediatrics* 1998;102:662–3.

28. Mitchell EA, Stewart AW, Scragg R *et al*. Ethnic differences in mortality from sudden infant death syndrome in New Zealand. *Br Med J* 1993;306:13–16.

29. New Zealand Health Information Service. 1999. *Fetal and infant deaths, 1996.* Ministry of Health, Wellington, New Zealand.

30. Alessandri LM, Read AW, Burton PR, Stanley FJ. Sudden infant death syndrome in Australian Aboriginal and non-Aboriginal infants: an analytic comparison. *Paediatr Perinatal Epidemiol* 1996;10:309–18.

31. Irwin KL, Mannino S, Daling J. Sudden infant death syndrome in Washington State: Why are Native American infants at greater risk than white infants? *J Pediatr* 1992;121:242–7.

32. Honigfield LS, Kaplan DW. Native American postneonatal mortality. *Pediatrics* 1987;80:575–8.

33. Lee NNY, Chan YF, Davies DP, Lau E, Yip DCP. Sudden infant death syndrome in Hong Kong: confirmation of low incidence. *Br Med J* 1989;298:721.
34. Statistics Information Department. *Vital Statistics on General Conditions, 1997.* Ministry of Health and Welfare, Tokyo, Japan, 1998.
35. Rasmussen F, Oldenburg M, Cotton N. Ethnic differences in rates of infant mortality and sudden infant death syndrome in Sweden, 1978–1990 (Abstract). *Paediatr Perinatal Epidemiol* 1995;9:A16.
36. MacDorman MF, Atkinson JO. Infant mortality statistics from the 1996 period linked birth/infant death data set. *Month Vital Stat Report* (Suppl.) 1998;46:20.
37. Alessandri LM, Read AW, Eades S, Gurrin L, Cooke CT. Recent sudden infant syndrome rates in Aboriginal and non-Aboriginal infants. *J Sud Inf Death Synd Inf Mort* 1996;1:315–19.
38. Hoffman HJ, Hillman LS. Epidemiology of the sudden infant death syndrome: maternal, neonatal and postneonatal risk factors. *Clin Perinatol* 1992;19:717–37.
39. Mitchell EA. The changing epidemiology of SIDS following the national risk reduction campaigns. *Pediatr Pulmonol* (Suppl.) 1997;16:117–19.
40. Oyen N, Markestad T, Skjaerven R *et al.* Combined effect of sleeping position and prenatal risk factors in sudden infant death syndrome: The Nordic Epidemiological SIDS Study. *Pediatrics* 1997;100:613–21.
41. Norvenius SG. Sudden Infant Death Syndrome in Sweden in 1973–1977 and 1979. *Acta Paediatr Scand* (Suppl.) 1987;333:1–138.
42. Alessandri LM, Read AW, Stanley FJ, Burton PR, Dawes VP. Sudden infant death syndrome in Aboriginal and non-Aboriginal infants. *J Paediatr Child Health* 1994;30:234–41.
43. Beal S, Porter C. Sudden infant death syndrome related to climate. *Acta Paediatr Scand* 1991;80:278–87.
44. Douglas AS, Allan TM, Helms PJ. Seasonality and the sudden infant death syndrome during 1987–9 and 1991–3 in Australia and Britain. *Br Med J* 1996;312:1381–3.
45. Adams EJ, Chavez GF, Steen D, Shah R, Iyasu S, Krous HF. Changes in the epidemiologic profile of sudden infant death syndrome as rates decline among California infants: 1990–1995. *Pediatrics* 1998;102:1445–51.
46. Mitchell EA, Milerad J. Smoking and sudden infant death syndrome. In: *International consultation on environmental tobacco smoke (ETS) and child health.* World Health Organization, Geneva, 1999, pp. 105–29.
47. Blair PS, Fleming PJ, Bensley D *et al.* Smoking and the sudden infant death syndrome: results from 1993–5 case–control inquiry into stillbirths and deaths in infancy. *Br Med J* 1996;313:195–8.
48. Ward SLD, Bautista D, Chan L *et al.* Sudden infant death syndrome in infants of substance-abusing mothers. *J Pediatr* 1990;117:876–81.
49. Chavez CJ, Ostrea EM, Stryker JC, Smialek Z. Sudden infant death syndrome among infants of drug-dependent mothers. *J Pediatr* 1979;95:407–9.
50. Kandall SR, Gaines J, Habel L, Davidson G, Jessop D. Relationship of maternal substance abuse to subsequent sudden infant death syndrome in offspring. *J Pediatr* 1993;123:120–6.
51. Fares I, McCulloch KM, Raju TNK. Intrauterine cocaine exposure and the risk for sudden infant death syndrome: A meta-analysis. *J Perinatol* 1997;17:179–82.
52. L'Hoir MP, Engelberts AC, van Well GTHJ *et al.* Case–control study of current

validity of previously described risk factors for SIDS in the Netherlands. *Arch Dis Child* 1998;79:386–93.

53. Kleemann WJ, Hiller AS, Troger HD. Infections of the upper respiratory tract in cases of sudden infant death. *Int J Legal Med* 1995;108:85–9.

54. Gilbert R. The changing epidemiology of SIDS. *Br Med J* 1994;70:445–9.

55. Gilbert R, Rudd P, Berry PJ *et al*. Combined effect of infection and heavy wrapping on the risk of sudden unexpected infant death. *Arch Dis Child* 1992;67:171–7.

56. Ponsonby A-L, Dwyer T, Gibbons LE, Cochrane JA, Wang YG. Factors potentiating the risk of sudden infant death syndrome associated with the prone position. *N Engl J Med* 1993;329:377–82.

57. Klonoff-Cohen HS, Edelstein SL, Lefkowitz ES *et al*. The effect of passive smoking and tobacco exposure through breast milk on sudden infant death syndrome. *JAMA* 1995;273:795–8.

58. Fleming PJ, Blair PS, Bacon C *et al*. Environment of infants during sleep and the risk of sudden infant death syndrome: results of 1993–95 case–control study for confidential inquiry into stillbirths and deaths in infancy. *Br Med J* 1996;313:191–5.

59. Ford RPK, Mitchell EA, Scragg R. Stewart AW, Taylor BJ, Allen EM. Factors adversely associated with breastfeeding in New Zealand. *J Paediatr Child Health* 1994;30:483–9.

60. L'Hoir MP, Engelberts AC, van Well GTHJ *et al*. Ins and outs of dummy-use, mouth breathing and cot death. In: L'Hoir MP. *Cot Death. Risk Factors and Prevention in the Netherlands 1995–1996* (Thesis). Utrecht, the Netherlands, 1998.

61. World Health Organization. *Protecting, promoting and supporting breast-feeding. The special role of maternity services*. A Joint WHO/UNICEF Statement. World Health Organization, Geneva, 1989.

62. Beal SM, Finch CF. An overview of retrospective case–control studies investigating the relationship between prone sleeping position and SIDS. *J Paediatr Child Health* 1991;27:334–9.

63. American Academy of Pediatrics Task Force on Infant Positioning and SIDS. *Pediatrics* 1992;89:1120–6.

64. Mitchell EA. Sleeping position of infants and the sudden infant death syndrome. *Acta Paediatr* (Suppl.) 1993;389:26–30.

65. Taylor JA, Krieger JW, Reay DT, Davis RL, Harruff R, Cheney LK. Prone sleep position and the sudden infant death syndrome in King County, Washington: A case–control study. *J Pediatr* 1996;128:626–30.

66. Klonoff-Cohen HS, Edelstein SL. A case–control study of routine and death scene sleep position and sudden infant death syndrome in Southern California. *JAMA* 1995;273:790–4.

67. L'Hoir MP, Engelberts AC, van Well GTHJ *et al*. Risk and preventive factors for cot death in The Netherlands, a low-incidence county. *Eur J Pediatr* 1998;157:681–8.

68. Mitchell EA, Thach B, Thompson J, Williams S. Changing infants' sleep position increases risk of sudden infant death syndrome. *Arch Pediatr Adolescent Med* 1999;153:1136–41.

69. Moon RY, Patel K, Shaefer SJ. Sudden infant death syndrome in child care settings. *Pediatrics* 2000; 106: 295–300.

70. Scragg RKR, Mitchell EA. Side sleeping position and bed-sharing in the sudden infant death syndrome. *Ann Med* 1998;30:345–9.

71. Henderson-Smart DJ, Ponsonby A-L, Murphy E. Reducing the risk of sudden infant death syndrome: A review of the scientific literature. *J Paediatr Child Health* 1998;34:213–9.
72. Mitchell EA, Thompson JMD. Co-sleeping increases the risk of SIDS, but sleeping in the parents' bedroom lowers it. In: Rognum TO (ed.) S*udden Infant Death Syndrome, New Trends in the Nineties*. Scandinavian University Press, Oslo, 1995, pp.266–9.
73. Scragg R, Mitchell EA, Taylor BJ *et al*. Bed-sharing, smoking, and alcohol in the sudden infant death syndrome. *Br Med J* 1993;307:1312–8.
74. Blair P, Fleming P, Smith I. Case–control study of sudden infant death syndrome in Scotland. Income level or bed-sharing would confound any effect of previous use of mattress. (Letter). *Br Med J* 1997;315:812–3.
75. Klonoff-Cohen H, Edelstein SL. Bed-sharing and the sudden infant death syndrome. *Br Med J* 1995;311:1269–72.
76. Willinger M, Hoffman HJ, Wu K-T, Gloeckner CK, Hillman LS. Sleep environment: The NICHD SIDS Cooperative Epidemiologic Study (Abstract). *Fourth SIDS International Conference*. Bethesda, MD, USA,1996.
77. Blair PS, Fleming PJ, Smith IJ *et al*. Babies sleeping with parents: case–control study of factors influencing the risk of sudden infant death syndrome. *Br Med J* 1999;319: 1457–62.
78. Bourne AJ, Beal SM, Byard RW. Bed-sharing and sudden infant death syndrome. (Letter). *Br Med J* 1994;308:537–8.
79. Gilbert-Barness E, Hegstrand L, Chandra S *et al*. Hazards of mattresses, beds and bedding in deaths of infants. *Am J Forensic Med Pathol* 1991;12:27–32.
80. Luke JL. Sleeping arrangements of Sudden Infant Death Syndrome victims in the District of Columbia – A preliminary report. *J Forensic Sci* 1978;23:379–83.
81. McKenna JJ, Mosko SS, Richard CA. Bedsharing promotes breastfeeding. *Pediatrics* 1997;100:214–19.
82. McKenna JJ, Mosko S, Richard C, Drummond S, Hunt L, Cetel MB, Arpaia J. Experimental studies of infant–parent co-sleeping: mutual physiologic and behavioral influences and their relevance to SIDS (sudden infant death syndrome). *Early Hum Dev* 1994;38:187–201.
83. Mosko S, Richard C, McKenna J, Drummond S, Mukai D. Maternal proximity and infant CO_2 environment during bedsharing and possible implications for SIDS research. *Am J Phys Anthropol* 1997;103:315–28.
84. Mosko S, Richard C, McKenna J. Infant arousals during mother-infant bed-sharing: Implications for infant sleep and sudden infant death syndrome research. *Pediatrics* 1997;100:841–9.
85. Farooqi S, Perry IJ, Beevers DG. Ethnic differences in infant-rearing practices and their possible relationship to the incidence of sudden infant death syndrome (SIDS). *Paediatr Perinatal Epid* 1993;7:345–52.
86. Fukui S, Nishida H, Sawaguchi T. Child care practices in Japan: holistic care for babies. (Abstract) Fifth SIDS International Conference, Rouen, France, 50, 1998.
87. Nelson EAS, Chan PH. Child care practices and cot death in Hong Kong. *NZ Med J* 1996;109:144–6.
88. Byard RW. Is co-sleeping in infancy a desirable or dangerous practice? *J Paediatr Child Health* 1994;30:198–9.

89. Mitchell EA, Scragg L, Clements M. Soft cot mattresses and the sudden infant death syndrome. *NZ Med J* 1996;109:206–7.

90. Kemp JS, Livne M, White DK. Softness and the potential to cause rebreathing: differences in bedding used by infants at high and low risk for sudden infant death syndrome. *J Pediatr* 1998;132:234–9.

91. Kemp JS, Nelson VE, Thach BT. Physical properties of bedding that may increase risk of sudden infant death syndrome in prone-sleeping infants. *Pediatr Res* 1994;36:7–11.

92. Scheers NJ, Dayton CM, Kemp JS. Sudden infant death with external airways covered. Case–comparison study of 206 deaths in the United States. *Arch Pediatr Adolesc Med* 1998;152:540–7.

93. Wilson CA, Taylor BJ, Laing RM, Williams SM, Mitchell EA, and the New Zealand Cot Death Study Group. Clothing and bedding and its relevance to sudden infant death syndrome: Further results from the New Zealand Cot Death Study. *J Paediatr Child Health* 1994;30:506–12.

94. Beal SM, Byard RW. Accidental death or sudden infant death syndrome? *J Paediatr Child Health* 1995;31:269–71.

95. Ponsonby A-L, Dwyer T, Couper D, Cochrane J. Association between use of a quilt and sudden infant death syndrome: case–control study. *Br Med J* 1998;316:195–6.

96. Nelson EAS, Taylor BJ, Weatherall IL. Sleeping position and infant bedding may predispose to hyperthermia and the sudden infant death syndrome. *Lancet* 1989;i:199–201.

97. Skadberg BT, Markestad T. Consequences of getting the head covered during sleep in infancy. *Pediatrics* 1997;100:6.

98. Skadberg BT, Oterhals A, Finbourud K, Markestad T. CO_2 rebreathing: a possible contributory factor to some cases of sudden infant death? *Acta Paediatrica* 1995;84:988–95.

99. Kemp JS, Kowalski RM, Burch PM, Graham MA, Thach BT. Unintentional suffocation by rebreathing: A death scene and physiologic investigation of a possible cause of sudden infant death. *J Pediatr* 1993;122:874–80.

100. Ponsonby A-L, Dwyer T, Kasl SV, Cochrane JA. The Tasmanian SIDS Case–Control Study: univariate and multivariate risk factor analysis. *Paediatr Perinatal Epidemiol* 1995;9:256–72.

101. Wailoo MP, Peterson SA, Whitaker H. Disturbed nights and 3–4 month old infants: the effects of feeding and thermal environment. *Arch Dis Child* 1990;65:499–501.

102. Fleming PJ, Gilbert R, Azaz Y *et al.* Interaction between bedding and sleeping position in the sudden infant death syndrome: a population based case–control study. *Br Med J* 1990;301:85–9.

103. Ponsonby A-L, Dwyer T, Gibbons LE *et al.* Thermal environment and sudden infant death syndrome: Case control study. *Br Med J* 1992;304:277–82.

104. Stanton DJ, Scott DJ, Downham MAPS. Is overheating a factor in some unexpected infant deaths? *Lancet* 1980;i:1054–7.

105. Stanton DJ. Overheating and cot death. *Lancet* 1984;i:1199–201.

106. Kleemann WJ, Schlaud M, Poets CF, Rothamel T, Troger HD. Hyperthermia in sudden infant death. *Int J Legal Med* 1996;109:139–42.

107. Tuohy PG, Tuohy RJ. The overnight thermal environment of infants. *NZ Med J* 1990;103:36–8.

108. Williams SM, Taylor BJ, Mitchell EA. New Zealand Cot Death Study Group. Sudden infant death syndrome: Insulation from bedding and clothing and its effect modifiers. *Int J Epidemiol* 1996;25:366–75.

109. Fleming PJ, Blair PS, Pollard K *et al*. Pacifier use and sudden infant death syndrome: results from the CESDI/SUDI case control study. *Arch Dis Child* 1999;81: 112–6.

110. Mitchell EA, Taylor BJ, Ford RPK *et al*. Dummies and the sudden infant death syndrome. *Arch Dis Child* 1993;68:501–4.

111. Arnestad M, Andersen M, Rognum TO. Is the use of dummy or carry-cot of importance for sudden infant death? *Eur J Pediatr* 1997;156:968–70.

112. Alm B, Wennergren G, Norvenius G *et al*. Dummy use in the Scandinavian Countries 1992–1995. The Nordic Epidemiological SIDS Study. *Proceedings of VIIth ESPED Conference*, 1997.

113. Hauck FR. Pacifiers and SIDS: Results from the Chicago Infant Mortality Study (Abstract). *The SIDS Alliance 1999 National Conference*. Atlanta, Georgia, 1999.

114. Barros FC, Victora DG, Semer TC, Filho ST, Tomasi E, Weiderpass E. Use of pacifiers is associated with decreased breast-feeding duration. *Pediatrics* 1995;95:497–9.

115. Righard L. Sudden infant death syndrome and pacifiers: A proposed connection could be a bias. *Birth* 1998;25:128–9.

116. Victora DG, Behague DP, Barros FC, Olinto MTA, Weiderpass E. Pacifier use and short breastfeeding duration: Cause, consequence, or coincidence? *Pediatrics* 1997;99:445–53.

117. Schubiger G, Schwarz U, Tonz O for the Neonatal Study Group. UNICEF?WHO baby-friendly hospital initiative: does the use of bottles and pacifiers in the neonatal nursery prevent successful breastfeeding? *Eur J Pediatr* 1997;156:874–7.

118. Vogel A, Mitchell EA. Attitudes to the use of dummies in NZ; a qualitative study. *NZ Med J* 1997;110:395–7.

119. Larsson E. Artificial sucking habits: Etiology, prevalence and effect on occlusion. *Int J Orofacial Myol* 1994;20:10–21.

120. Larsson E. The effect of dummy-sucking on the occlusion: a review. *Eur J Orthodont* 1986;8:127–30.

121. Niemela M, Uhari M, Mottonen. A pacifier increases the risk of recurrent otitis media in children in day care centers. *Pediatrics* 1995;96:884–8.

122. Jorch H, Schleimer B. *The optimal sleep environment for your child. A guide for parents and all who want to become parents.* (Translated from German.) Johanniter-Unfall-Hilfe, Bochum, Germany, 1998.

123. American Academy of Pediatrics Task Force on Infant Sleep Position and Sudden Infant Death Syndrome. Changing concepts of Sudden Infant Death Syndrome: implications for infant sleeping environment and sleep position. *Pediatrics* 2000;105:650–6.

124. Alm B, Wennergren G, Norvenius SG *et al*. SIDS in Sweden before and after the intervention period (Abstract 27). *Fifth SIDS International Conference*, Rouen, France, 1998.

125. Baste V, Oyen N, Irgens LM, Skjaerven R. Seasonality of SIDS has not disappeared during low incidence in Norway. (Abstract 29). *Fifth SIDS International Conference*, Rouen, France, 1998.

126. Krous HR, Hauck FR, Herman SM *et al*. Laryngeal basement membrane thicken-

ing is not a reliable postmortem marker for SIDS. Results from the Chicago Infant Mortality Study. *Am J Forens Med Pathol* 1999;20:221–7.

127. Kiechl-Kohlendorfer U, Pupp U, Oberainger W, Sperl W. Changing epidemiology of sudden infant death syndrome (SIDS) before and after an intervention campaign in the Tyrol (Abstract). *Fifth SIDS International Conference*. Rouen, France, 1998.

128. Sibert J, Fleming PJ. Poisoning, accidents and sudden infant death syndrome. In: Campbell AGM, Macintosh N (eds). *Forfar and Arneil's Textbook of Paediatrics*. 5th ed., Chapter 29. Churchill Livingstone, New York, NY, 1998, pp.1705–26.

129. Mitchell EA. Smoking: the next major and modifiable risk factor. In: Rognum TO (ed.) *Sudden Infant Death Syndrome. New Trends in the Nineties*. Scandinavian University Press, Oslo, 1995, pp.114–8.

CHAPTER 4

Death scene investigation

RANDY HANZLICK

Introduction   58
Where is the scene?   59
Brief historical perspective   59
Guideline specifics   60
Critical aspects of scene investigation   61
Other considerations   64
Summary   65
References   65

Introduction

Because SIDS-like deaths are usually sudden and unexplained, most such deaths are investigated and certified by medical examiners and coroners in accordance with state death investigation statutes.[1] From the medical examiner/coroner's perspective, there are several reasons to perform death scene investigation in suspected SIDS cases. A major reason is that infant death may result from one of several causes – any of which can cause similar, or minimal autopsy findings. Only examination of the 'scene' in a planned and organized manner can provide the necessary information to:

- assess some possible causes of death
- confirm the likelihood of causes other than SIDS
- rule out the possibility of causes of death other than SIDS
- continue to consider some causes of death as possibilities
- reconstruct how injuries may have been sustained
- more closely estimate the time of death
- facilitate the interpretation of autopsy findings.

These considerations are the main reason that the definition of SIDS most commonly referred to in the United States includes a diagnostic criterion that death scene investigation has been performed and that a cause of death remains undetermined after autopsy and review of the clinical history.[2] It should be made clear, however, that not all medical examiners and coroners who certify SIDS deaths require that scene investigation be performed to make a diagnosis of SIDS.[3]

Other benefits of a scene investigation include immediate access to witnesses from whom information may be obtained; the ability to collect information of potential evidence that might assist the pathologist at postmortem examination or follow-up investigation; and the ability to provide needed services or referrals to family members.

Where is the scene?

The 'death scene' must be loosely interpreted to include the location where an infant may have been discovered unresponsive (but not dead), or where the events leading to death occurred. In some instances, such a scene may be different than the home environment where the infant spent most of its time, and 'death scene investigation' may also need to include a visit to and examination of the home environment or other place. For example, an infant may have been apparently fine at home, then taken to the doctor for immunizations, then to a day care center where it is later found unresponsive, and then to the hospital emergency room where death occurs. Each of these locations may have to be visited to conduct a 'scene investigation.' In this chapter, the word 'scene' will be used to encompass all such places as applicable in a given case.

Brief historical perspective

The importance of death scene investigation has been recognized by medical examiners, coroners, and the death investigation community for a long time. The Model Postmortem Examinations Act of 1954, however, did not address infant deaths, nor was the importance of scene investigation emphasized.[4] The importance of scene investigation to suspected SIDS cases was first formally published in 1976 in a Special Report of a working group to recommend protocol for the investigation of suspected SIDS deaths.[5] Even in that document, the importance of investigating the scene was given only cursory treatment and the bulk of the article was directed at autopsy protocol. In the late 1980s, the SIDS literature began to include articles in which it was suggested that a good portion of apparent SIDS cases were actually due to other causes that could be disclosed with adequate scene investigation. In 1989, the definition of SIDS was changed to require a scene investigation as a component in the diagnostic criteria. Only in the past decade, however, has death scene investigation become a topic of national concern and federal publications. Two sets of federal guidelines are relevant to infant death scene investigation: The Centers for Disease Control (CDC) and Prevention's Guidelines for Death Scene Investigation of Sudden, Unexplained Infant Deaths; and the National Institute of Justice's (NIJ)* National Guidelines

---

* In 1998, NIJ changed the name of its publication to *Death Investigation: A Guide for the Scene Investigator*.

for Death Investigation.[2,6] Recently, the NIJ has also published 'Crime Scene Investigation: A Guide for Law Enforcement,' but that publication is geared more toward law enforcement officers and evidence collection and is beyond the scope of this chapter.[7] The CDC guidelines were published in June 1996, three years after the first workshop to develop them was held following a congressional recommendation to do so. The details of their development have been published.[8] The NIJ death investigation guidelines were published in December 1997 and were developed through a grant issued in 1996, and details of their development are contained in the guidelines publication.[6]

Other publications also contain checklists and guidelines for investigation of infant deaths, and, although useful, have not gained widespread use or recognition.[9] They will not be further considered in this chapter.

Guideline specifics

The CDC and NIJ guidelines are different in scope, approach and focus. Both are concerned with deaths requiring medicolegal death investigation, but the CDC guidelines focus on infant deaths and the NIJ guidelines on all deaths.

The CDC guidelines consist of standard definitions and forms, named the Sudden Unexplained Infant Death Investigation Report Forms (SUIDIRF). The CDC guidelines are not a set of step-by-step 'how to' guidelines or procedural checklists. The SUIDIRF are the heart of the guidelines and are geared toward collecting a standard set of data items in a consistent format, and ensuring that investigation covers a defined set of issues and topics. The guidelines have been reproduced in Appendix II, but is worth noting the major sections of the SUIDIRF:

- Documentation of basic circumstances (dates, places, times, people).
- Basic medical information, mainly about the infant, with some questions on pregnancy and birth history.
- *Evaluation of the household environment.*
- *Information about the immediate environment in which the infant was found.*
- Tracking of investigative procedures and interviews.
- *Forms for diagramming the scene and noting bodily findings.*

The scene investigation facilitates the collection of all of the above information, but the italicized sections are the most directly linked to the need for investigating the scene.

The NIJ guidelines are more procedure-oriented than the CDC guidelines, but still fall short of being specific step-by-step instructions. They are geared toward general scene procedures such as maintaining adequate tools and supplies for the investigation, ensuring scene safety, collecting and safeguarding potential evidence, photographing the scene from afar and close up and before and after the body is moved. The guidelines have been developed with the purpose that each of the procedures should be performed at 'every scene, every time.' The major sections of the NIJ guidelines include:

- Investigative tools and equipment.
- Arriving at the scene.
- Documenting and evaluating the scene.
- Documenting and evaluating the body.
- Establishing and recording decedent profile information.
- Completing the scene investigation.

Overall, the six major sections in the NIJ Guidelines contain 29 basic procedures, each of which is based on a sound principle, the source of authority which requires or allows the procedure to be performed, a statement of specific policy regarding the procedure, a list of components of the procedure, and an overall summary of the procedure's purpose. Procedures that are especially relevant to suspected SIDS cases include:

- Performance of a scene 'walk through'.
- Photography of the scene and body.
- Collection of evidence.
- Interviewing of witnesses.
- Documentation of the discovery, terminal episode, medical, and social history.
- Assisting the family.

The CDC and NIJ guidelines have three major points in common. First (perhaps with rare exceptions in a few states), neither is required to be used by law. Use is voluntary, although professional 'peer pressure' may have some impact, as might the potential of their being used in court or legal proceedings as an alleged 'professional standard' by which to compare performance. Second, funding for training and implementation has been nil. Except in a few areas where research has been funded, use of the guidelines has depended on the interest and resources of the local authorities in charge of death investigation. Third, each is potentially useful for improving the quality of death investigations and more accurately determining the cause and manner of death. Studies are lacking, however, to document what impact, if any, use of these guidelines has had. A survey study is underway to assess the extent in which the CDC guidelines are being used, to evaluate potential problems with the guidelines, and to solicit suggestions for improvement or modification.

Critical aspects of scene investigation

There are several specific aspects of scene investigation that are worthy of mention in regard to suspected SIDS cases.

Doll re-enactment (using a life-sized doll to help demonstrate positioning of the infant when placed and when found) can be very helpful in clarifying the details of body position that can be difficult for witnesses to adequately describe in terms of where and how the infant was last placed, last known or thought to be alive, and where it was discovered unresponsive or dead. Using a life-size flexible baby doll is analogous to the old saying that a 'picture can say a thousand words.'

Many diseases that can cause death in a way that presents as possible SIDS (such as inborn errors of metabolism) may be detected through autopsy and appropriate laboratory tests done on postmortem specimens. In such cases, the scene investigation is still important, however, because the possibility of competing or contributory causes of death must still be assessed. For example, an infant may have medium chain acyl-coenzyme A dehydrogenase deficiency (MCAD), but actually die of overlaying.

There are a number of circumstances in which death may be due to external causes such as injury, environmental factors, or poisoning, which, even with a good scene investigation, may be missed because autopsy findings are minimal, nonspecific, or absent. The most probable of these are:

- Asphyxia, by a wide variety of mechanisms including: wedging between surfaces; overlaying; entrapment; rebreathing of carbon dioxide; airway obstruction by adjacent items; hanging or compression of the neck; prolonged head down position; vitiated atmosphere (oxygen depleted); and intentional suffocation, smothering or other asphyxial mechanisms.
- Intoxication/poisoning with: medications intended for the infant or others in the household; alcohol; illicit drugs; household products such as cleansers and insecticides; venoms from insects and other animals.
- Drowning.
- Electrocution.
- Environmental problems such as: hypothermia; hyperthermia; carbon monoxide poisoning; water contamination; and food poisoning.

The list above is not exhaustive, but it does cover most potential encounters, including infrequent and rare ones. Many of the causes of death listed above may occur unintentionally or be intentionally inflicted, so even if the cause of death is identified, the manner of death may remain in question (accidental drowning versus homicidal drowning, for example), and scene investigation may be helpful in clarifying the manner of death in such cases.

Regarding scene investigation, the question is: what can one do at the scene to reasonably assess which causes of death are suggested or likely? Some suggestions that may be helpful are listed below. At the outset, it must be remembered that in many, if not most cases, the infant will not be present in the same position in which it was discovered, and it is also quite possible that the scene has been altered (either intentionally or during the panic of the situation and medical response).

- Be sure it is safe to enter and work in the scene area. Obtain assistance from law enforcement or other agencies as needed to assess and ensure scene safety.
- Collect the same basic information that would be obtained during any death investigation, such as medical history and the reported sequence of events.
- Using a doll, have the placer and finder recreate exactly the position in which the infant was placed and in which it was found, making certain to document the position of the face relative to surrounding objects.

- If the infant is available for examination at the scene, document the distribution of livor mortis as precisely as possible; also document if rigor mortis is present and the position of various body parts such as arms, legs, and head.
- Assess the general appearance of the scene as to its level of tidiness, evidence of alcohol or substance abuse, and location of drugs and other potential poisonous substances.
- Determine if there is any evidence of the use of any cultural or folk remedies in the home (such as white clay ingestion, coin rubbing, cupping, etc.).
- Determine the source of drinking water.
- Measure the temperature of the infant, especially if it is still at the scene. Guidance on when and how to obtain body temperature should be provided by the medical examiner or coroner.
- Ascertain whether any heating or cooling devices were operative at the time of the incident and their type (gas, electric, kerosene, central heat, space heater, etc.) Specifically check to see if there are any likely sources of noxious gases or carbon monoxide.
- Document the thermostat temperature setting and the actual temperature in the room upon arrival.
- Attempt to assess the temperature of the area in which the infant was found. This may involve recreating the circumstances (such as closing doors that were closed at the time the infant was found; resetting a thermostat to kick on a heater, etc.) in an attempt to mimic the actual conditions.
- Determine how many layers of clothing and blankets were on/around the infant and exactly what those items were.
- If the diaper has been removed, collect it. Also collect any clothing that was worn but was removed from the infant.
- Collect a sample of the food/formula that the infant had been eating.
- Determine if there were any electrical devices or cords near the infant.
- Determine whether there is any water in the bath tub or sink; whether these fixtures are wet (recently used, and if so, by whom); whether there are any wet or damp towels in the area; whether any of the infant's clothing (either worn or nearby) is wet or damp; and whether the infant's hair or body is wet or dry.
- Inspect the toilet for any evidence of blood-tinged fluid.
- Determine if there are any plastic bags in the area or in trash/waste receptacles. If so, establish how and when they got there and collect them if needed (tests may be done for saliva or other body fluids).
- Examine the area near to where the infant was discovered for evidence of any dangling objects such as curtain cords that may pose a hazard of entanglement or neck constriction.
- Measure the distance between crib slats if the incident occurred in a crib.
- Measure the distance between the edge of the sleeping surface (such as a mattress) and adjacent objects (such as a wall or crib rail).
- Document all items on the sleeping surface or near the infant that could conceivably obstruct the nose, mouth, or airway. Collect any suspect items–especially those small enough to fit in, or of a nature that could obstruct, the nose or mouth.

- Determine whether the sleeping location was the usual one for the infant.
- Assess the softness and material components of the sleeping surface. Collect these as needed so they may be examined by the pathologist.
- Document whether there was cosleeping and, if so, with whom and the precise position and size of each person.
- Inventory any medicines being taken by members of the household, including the infant.
- Note the nature of any plants in the home.
- Note whether there is any evidence of insect infestation (cockroaches etc.).
- Document the type of pets kept in or around the home.
- Determine whether there is any evidence of very recent use of household cleansers, paint, spray preparations, or other substances that can cause toxic vapors (paint remover etc.).
- If an apnea or other monitor or medical device (such as a vaporizer) was being used, collect it so it may be examined and tested and, if applicable, so the data may be downloaded and analysed.
- Take photographs and prepare diagrams (liberally).

Going hand-in-hand with the scene investigation is the collection of several pieces of important information, which may be initially addressed at the scene but followed up subsequently if further information or confirmation is needed:

- Determine whether the police have ever been called to the home, and if so, when, and for what reasons.
- Determine if the Department of Family and Children's Services (protective services) has ever intervened or assigned a social worker to the family.
- Determine whether there has been any documented history of child abuse.
- In addition to asking about siblings, both living and deceased, obtain the mother's maiden name, county and state of birth, and county and state of other places of residence. This information may be used to link birth and death certificates and confirm whether or not the mother has had other children who have died.

Interview first responders carefully to determine exactly what was done with, and to the infant after it was found.

Other considerations

From the death investigator's standpoint, questioning of witnesses at the scene usually takes the form of an interview. However, if preliminary information suggests foul play or inflicted injury, the investigation and questioning of witnesses may tend to evolve toward an interrogation. If information is obtained improperly in such cases, prosecution may be jeopardized. Be sure to appropriately involve law enforcement so that those making statements can be legally informed of their rights, and that appropriate warrants are obtained if searches are needed that go beyond that conducted during a routine death investigation.

Summary

It is difficult to take a cookbook approach to infant death scene investigation because each case is different and the actual circumstances have bearing on how the investigation needs to be performed. This chapter has provided some general guidelines and important points to consider. The CDC Guidelines are contained in Appendix II of this book. Be familiar with any additional requirements, laws, or procedures in your jurisdiction.

References

1. Combs, DL. Parrish RG, Ing R. *Death investigation in the United States and Canada, 1996.* US Department of Health and Human Services, Public Health Service, CDC, Atlanta, 1996.
2. CDC. Guidelines for death scene investigation of sudden, unexplained infant deaths: recommendations of the Interagency Panel on Sudden Infant Death Syndrome. *MMWR* 1996;45:RR-10.
3. Kaplan JA, Hanzlick R. The diagnosis of sudden infant death syndrome: medical examiner practices and attitudes. *Proceedings of the American Academy of Forensic Sciences Annual Meeting*, Seattle, Washington, February 1995, pp. 135–6.
4. National Conference of Commissioners on Uniform State Laws. Model Postmortem Examinations Act, 1954. In: Combs, DL, Parrish RG, Ing R. *Death investigation in the United States and Canada, 1996.* US Department of Health and Human Services, Public Health Service, CDC, Atlanta, 1996.
5. Jones AM, Weston JT. Examination of the sudden infant death syndrome: investigative and autopsy protocols. *J Forensic Sci* 1976;21:833–41.
6. NIJ. *National Guidelines for Death Investigation.* National Institute of Justice, Office of Justice Programs. US Department of Justice, Washington, DC, 1997.
7. NIJ. *Crime Scene Investigation.* National Institute of Justice, Office of Justice Programs. US Department of Justice, Washington, DC, 2000.
8. Iyasu S, Hanzlick R, Rowley D, Willinger M. Proceedings of 'Workshop on Guidelines for Scene Investigation of Sudden, Unexplained Infant Deaths'. *J Forensic Sci* 1994;39:1126–36.
9. Ernst MF, Caplan YH. The Death Scene. In: Caplan YH, Frank RS (eds). *Medicolegal Death Investigation: Treatises in the Forensic Sciences,* 2nd edn. The Forensic Sciences Foundation Press, Colorado Springs, CO, 1991, pp. 7–104.

CHAPTER 5

Respiratory mechanisms and hypoxia

THOMAS G. KEENS AND SALLY L. DAVIDSON WARD

Introduction   66
Development of the infant respiratory system   66
Respiratory disorders which may cause SIDS   68
Role of hypoxia in SIDS   72
How are we to understand SIDS?   74
Summary   77
References   78

Introduction

For nearly 3000 years, it has been recognized that apparently healthy infants could die suddenly and unexpectedly during their sleep.[1] Throughout most of history, it was believed that these infants somehow suffocated, either by maternal overlaying or by strangling in bedclothes, implying that these babies died a respiratory death. While these explanations have largely been discarded, nearly one infant per thousand live births continues to die suddenly and unexpectedly from SIDS. The cause of SIDS remains unknown, but most SIDS research has focused on some failure of the respiratory system as the cause of death. This chapter will review potential respiratory mechanisms and the possible role of hypoxia in SIDS.

Development of the infant respiratory system

The ability to sustain spontaneous ventilation requires adequate function of the mechanisms which control ventilation, ventilatory muscle function, and lung mechanics. Significant dysfunction of any of these three components of the respiratory system may impair the ability to breathe spontaneously. Apnea or respiratory failure occurs when central respiratory drive and/or ventilatory muscle power are inadequate to overcome the respiratory load (Fig. 5.1).

SIDS occurs at a time when the infant respiratory system is developmentally immature and rapidly changing. From an engineering perspective, a rapidly changing system is intrinsically unstable.[2] Lung mechanics are different in infants than in older children. This makes the infant's respiratory system more vulnerable to respiratory failure in the event of lung disease. The rapid growth and development during infancy also makes the respiratory system vulnerable to the effects of lung injury. During late fetal life and early postnatal life, the lungs grow by adding alveoli. Only ten per cent of alveoli are present at birth. Thus, relatively few alveoli are available for gas exchange. In addition, the walls of alveoli contain elastic tissue. The role of elastic tissue in the lungs is to provide support for intrapulmonary structures: alveoli, airways, blood vessels and lymphatics. As lung volume increases, elastic tissue stretches, increasing the pull on the walls of these structures, increasing their caliber, and preventing collapse. The decreased number of alveoli is accompanied by decreased elastic support of intrapulmonary structures. Because of decreased chest wall stability in infants, there is a tendency for decreased lung volume. Thus, in infants undergoing any disease or stress to the lungs, this decreased elastic support causes a tendency toward atelectasis, airway obstruction, increased pulmonary vascular resistance, and increased lung water or pulmonary edema. Further, the upper airway is predisposed to collapse, causing obstructive apnea during sleep.[3,4]

The diaphragm is the major muscle of breathing. Ventilatory muscles can fatigue, resulting in respiratory failure, when either the muscle is too weak (decreased strength or endurance) and/or the respiratory load is too great. Infants have a decreased proportion of fatigue-resistant muscle fibers in their diaphragms compared with older children or adults.[5] Thus ventilatory muscle endurance is severely decreased in infants, making ventilatory muscle fatigue, and resulting

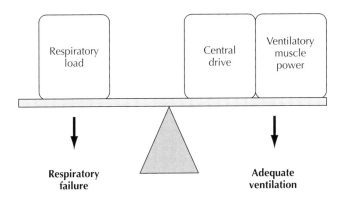

Fig. 5.1   The respiratory system balance. In order to sustain adequate spontaneous ventilation, ventilatory muscle power and central respiratory drive must be sufficient to overcome the respiratory load. Alterations in either side of the balance can tip the balance toward inadequate ventilation, or respiratory failure.

respiratory failure, more likely. Diaphragm strength is also decreased in infants compared with older children.[6]

Neurologic control of breathing must ensure adequate ventilation to meet the metabolic needs of the body during sleep, rest, and exercise.[7,8] Ventilation varies with the state of the individual. It becomes less adequate during sleep, and it is nearly unresponsive to modulation by chemoreceptor input during active sleep. It is not surprising that sleep is the most vulnerable period for the development of inadequate ventilation in disorders of respiratory control.[7,8] Even in healthy infants, neurologic control of breathing is unstable. Ventilation is depressed by hypoxia, and immature reflexes cause apnea.[7] Further, the infant spends 40–70% of sleep time in active or REM sleep, in contrast to 15–20% in the adult, and sleeps for a longer portion of the day.[9] Active sleep is associated with greater variation in respiratory timing and amplitude, resulting in periods of inadequate gas exchange.[8]

Therefore, infants and children are predisposed to apnea and respiratory dysfunction compared with adults, because of differences in the control of sleep and breathing, decreased ventilatory muscle strength and endurance, and immature lung mechanics. Even normal infants frequently have respiratory pauses during sleep, which last up to 20 seconds, and hypoxic events, which cause arterial oxygen desaturations to as low as 80%.[10] While these developmental aspects of respiratory dysfunction are present in all infants during the peak age range for SIDS, most infants survive and do not die from SIDS. Thus, it is controversial whether the respiratory dysfunction seen in all infants is enough to cause SIDS, or if SIDS infants require an additional abnormality or predisposition.

Respiratory disorders which may cause SIDS

There is a great deal of circumstantial evidence suggesting that respiratory mechanisms are important in SIDS. Cessation of breathing (apnea) can cause sudden death, which may not be detected at postmortem examination.[11] Thus, it fits the definition of SIDS. Respiratory disorders can be categorized in terms of how they affect the respiratory system.

PRIMARY LUNG DISEASE

A lung disease sufficient to cause death would likely be detectable at autopsy. Thus, SIDS is not likely due to a single lung disease. However, common postmortem findings in the SIDS victim include intrathoracic petechiae, pulmonary congestion and edema, and minor airway inflammation.[11] While not generally considered to be severe enough to have caused death, these findings raise the possibility that lung disease has a role in SIDS. Martinez hypothesized that the small airways of infants are predisposed to collapse, and that increased resistance of small airways could cause sudden death by progressive peripheral bronchial occlusion.[12] The presumed trigger for this chain of events is an acute viral lower respiratory tract illness causing inflammation.[12] Susceptible infants are believed to have decreased airway conductance (increased resistance) due to congenital and environmental factors.[12] Kao measured lung function in ten infants with unexplained apnea, a group of infants with a statistically increased risk for SIDS.[13] She found that specific airway conductance was decreased, suggesting airway obstruction, lending support to the Martinez hypothesis.

Morley and others have described surfactant abnormalities in SIDS victims, which would predispose to atelectasis.[14,15,16] If other mechanisms which maintain the functional residual capacity in babies are compromised, then larger areas of lung collapse may occur, causing hypoxia. These results would predict that lung compliance is low in SIDS victims, but Fagan and Milner found normal pressure–volume loops in SIDS victims postmortem.[17] Thus, Morley speculated that this surfactant abnormality causes physiologic lung dysfunction during life, but that the physiologic consequences of these surfactant abnormalities are difficult to measure postmortem.[14,15,18] The cause of these surfactant abnormalities in SIDS is not known. Morley speculates that it could be related to viral infections of the lung.[19] Even if surfactant abnormalities are not the sole cause for SIDS, they may be a contributor to the mechanism of death in SIDS and/or provide a mechanism whereby viral infections may be associated with SIDS.

In general, SIDS victims do not manifest symptoms of chronic lung disease prior to death. However, infants with chronic lung disease, bronchopulmonary dysplasia, do have an increased risk for SIDS,[20,21,22] suggesting that abnormal lung function may contribute to the mechanism causing SIDS.

VENTILATORY MUSCLE WEAKNESS OR FATIGUE

There has been little research on ventilatory muscles in SIDS. Keens described a 'normal' maturational pattern of increasing fatigue-resistant muscle fiber types in the human diaphragm and intercostal muscles over the first year of life.[5] However, he used autopsy samples, and nearly all infant diaphragms were derived from SIDS victims. Thus, it is not clear whether this increase in the first year of life is normal, or is aberrant and a characteristic of SIDS.[5] Scott measured maximal transdiaphragmatic pressure, as a measure of diaphragm strength, in infants with unexplained apnea.[23] He found that diaphragm strength was not decreased, but rather it was significantly increased compared with controls. This could be interpreted as representing ventilatory muscle training in response to lung disease or upper airway obstruction. However, there is no evidence supporting a primary ventilatory muscle dysfunction as the cause of SIDS.

UPPER AIRWAY OBSTRUCTION

A common autopsy finding in SIDS victims is the presence of *intra*thoracic petechiae on the thymus, lungs, pleural surfaces, and heart.[24,25] *Extra*thoracic portions of the thymus do *not* show petechiae. These intrathoracic petechiae may have been formed by the generation of highly negative intrathoracic pressures, as might occur when an infant attempts to breathe against upper airway obstruction.[25] Intrathoracic petechiae suggest that obstructive apnea may be involved in the final mechanism of SIDS deaths.[25]

The anatomy of the infant's upper airway and relatively increased amount of active sleep predisposes infants to upper airway obstruction.[3,4,7,8] Traditionally, SIDS researchers have been concerned about central apnea possibly causing death in infants.[26,27,28] However, obstructive apneas have more recently been identified in infants at increased risk for SIDS.[29,30] Kahn and coworkers examined overnight polysomnographic recordings from 30 infants who subsequently died from SIDS, and compared them with recordings from 60 matched controls infants.[29] They found significantly more and longer obstructive breathing events in the SIDS infants.[29] Obstructive events were accompanied by bradycardia and hypoxemia. Central apneas were not different between the two groups. Tishler and associates have identified an increased family history of sudden unexpected infant deaths in adults with the obstructive sleep apnea syndrome, and have hypothesized a familial association between the two.[31] In the past, recordings performed in the home on infants who subsequently died from SIDS, or who are at risk from SIDS, have not had the technical capability to detect obstructive apneas. Therefore, the question of the importance of obstructive apnea in SIDS remains unanswered.

VENTILATORY CONTROL DISORDERS

Infants with unexplained apnea have an increased risk of dying from SIDS.[26,27,28,32,33] Tissue markers of chronic hypoxia and hypoxemia have been described in many SIDS victims by some investigators.[34–40] Brainstem lesions have been seen in areas controlling ventilation and sleep/wakefulness in many SIDS victims.[41,42] Many infants at high risk for SIDS have ventilatory control disorders.[26,27,43,44] While these findings do not prove that SIDS is due to a respiratory disorder, there is considerable circumstantial evidence suggesting that SIDS may involve abnormal neurologic control of breathing.[7,8]

The circumstantial evidence in favor of respiratory causes for SIDS prompted many investigators to formulate *the apnea hypothesis of SIDS*. The simplistic version of this hypothesis says: (1) SIDS occurs when infants stop breathing during sleep.[7,26,27,28,32,33,43] (2) One can test infants to see if they have apneas. (3) Infants with increased apnea during sleep are at high risk for SIDS and should be treated or protected.[26,27] Home apnea–bradycardia monitoring, which sounds an alarm to summon trained parents when an infant has a prolonged apnea or bradycardia, has been advocated as the preferred method to protect these infants.[27] However, relatively few SIDS victims had any previous apneas observed prior to death.[45] Prospective studies of the sleeping ventilatory pattern do not predict SIDS or death in infants.[22,33,46] Home apnea–bradycardia monitoring and infant apnea evaluations have not substantially decreased the SIDS rates for the general population.[45] Thus, the simplistic approach to treating apnea in infants has not resulted in decreases in SIDS. However, it is still possible that SIDS involves a respiratory disorder.

Kinney and others have found gliosis and subtle changes in brainstem centers responsible for control of breathing and control of sleep/wakefulness.[37,41,42] More recently, she has found a decrease in muscarinic cholinergic receptors in the arcuate nucleus of the brainstem in SIDS victims.[42] This area of the brainstem is thought to be related to the physiologic responsivity to increased CO_2. These findings suggest that the origins of SIDS may lie in abnormal control of breathing or abnormalities in regulation of sleep/wakefulness.[7,8,42] However, these theories remain unproven.

The study of genes which may affect control of breathing could improve our understanding of SIDS. Brain-derived neurotrophic factor (BDNF) may be important in determining the development of control of breathing.[47] Infant mice which lack the gene for BDNF have a loss of neurons responsible for normal ventilatory control. These mice appear to demonstrate an abnormality in carotid body, or peripheral chemoreceptor, function which provides a chronic stimulus to breathing, and is the body's primary sensor of low oxygen. Infant mice without the BDNF gene breathe slower and shallower, and do not respond to hypoxia.[47] BDNF-deficient mice showed a normal response to elevated CO_2, suggesting that the BDNF gene is not active in the CO_2 response. Thus, the BDNF gene may control the development and/or survival of nerve cells in the carotid body, which affect an infant's protective response to low oxygen.[47] It is unclear how this may relate to SIDS, and studies have not been performed in SIDS victims. In the near future, it is likely that other genes will be described which affect control of breathing. While it is tempting to postulate a genetic etiology to SIDS,[31] studies in twins[48,49] and in SIDS siblings[33,50,51,52,53] do not convincingly suggest that SIDS is hereditary.

AROUSAL RESPONSES TO RESPIRATORY STIMULI

Arousal from sleep is an important defense mechanism against danger-signalling stimuli during sleep. All infants have frequent breathing pauses during sleep. The inability to arouse from sleep in response to an apnea or hypoxia could prevent an infant from terminating an apnea, resulting in death.[44,54,55,56] The process of changing from sleep to wakefulness (arousal) is associated with many changes in the respiratory system which improve breathing.[8] Thus, arousal is a logical defense mechanism to protect breathing during sleep.

Preliminary evidence suggested that infants at high risk for SIDS had abnormal arousal responses to hypoxia.[44,55,57,58,59] These same infants also had alterations in circulating catecholamine levels.[55,60] However, normal control infants also often fail to arouse in response to hypoxia.[56,61] Normal infants arouse frequently under 9-weeks of age, but not between 9-weeks and 6-months of age.[56] This corresponds to the peak age distribution for SIDS. It is possible that infants are born with a protective brainstem-mediated hypoxic arousal response, which is inhibited by increasing cortical development after 2-months of age. However, this is quite preliminary, and not proven. Other factors also affect arousal. For example, repetitive hypoxic events depress the arousal response to hypoxia.[55,62] Thus, infants with frequent hypoxic events, may depress their protective arousal responses and increase their risk of death.[44,56] A great deal more work is required to establish a link between these altered arousal patterns and SIDS.[44,54-58]

McNamara and coworkers tested the arousal response of 10 healthy infants to tactile stimuli.[63] Arousal could be abolished by repeated exposure (habituation).[63] While brainstem and spinal mediated responses were more resistant to habituation than cortically mediated responses, even they were eventually inhibited. As mentioned, repeated exposure to hypoxia blunted hypoxic arousal responses.[55,62] Thus, habituation of the infant arousal response to repeated stimuli, especially hypoxia, hypercapnia, or airway occlusion, may be relevant to SIDS.[55,62,63]

Prenatal and postnatal exposure to cigarette smoking are now recognized as significant risk factors for SIDS.[64] Infants born to cigarette-smoking mothers have higher arousal thresholds to auditory stimuli than infants not so exposed.[65] Thus, decreased arousal is associated with an important risk factor for SIDS.

Role of hypoxia in SIDS

Tissue markers of chronic hypoxia and hypoxamia have been described in many SIDS victims by some investigators.[34-40] While some of these findings are controversial, the search for evidence of chronic hypoxia as a cause of SIDS is an active area of research.

Neonates tolerate acute hypoxia or oxygen deprivation better than adults.[66,67] Ninety-five per cent of neonatal rats survived anoxia for 50 minutes, while all adults died within 4 minutes.[68] This is not surprising since neonates have just come from an intrauterine environment where the mean oxygen tension is 26–30 torr. They have several adaptations to this hypoxic state, such as increased fetal hemoglobin. An important neonatal adaptation is that they have the ability to decrease oxygen consumption during hypoxia.[69,70] Adults will increase ventilation in response to hypoxia (fight). However, neonates decrease their oxygen requirement in response to decreased oxygen substrate (accommodate), rather than try to increase available oxygen. Further, this decrease in oxygen consumption is not accompanied by an increase in anaerobic metabolism.[71,72] Thus, oxygen consumption is decreased in response to the hypoxic state, and may not be simply a consequence of failure to supply enough oxygen for aerobic metabolism.

Although neonates tolerate hypoxia better than older children or adults, there is evidence that this tolerance is rapidly lost in infancy, when the incidence of SIDS increases. Infants have decreased tolerance for hypoxia compared with neonates. Infants have decreased ability to autoresuscitate (gasp) in response to anoxia than neonates or older children.[73] Infants also have a shorter time to last gasp than neonates or adults.[74] Infants have less ability to continue mitochondrial function during hypoxia than neonates or adults.[75] Finally, peripheral chemoreceptor denervation is better tolerated by neonates and adults than by infants.[76] Thus, the infant period, after the neonatal period, is associated with an increased vulnerability to hypoxia or anoxia and with an increased risk for SIDS.

Repeated exposure to hypoxia in infancy may be even more deleterious. Repeated exposure to hypoxia depresses the arousal response to hypoxia during sleep.[55,62] Repeated exposure of newborn piglets to hypoxia also decreases their hypoxic ventilatory response compared to piglets exposed to continuous hypoxia.[77] Repeated hypoxic exposure also decreases cardiac glycogen levels.[78] Thus, repeated exposure to hypoxic events inhibits protective physiologic responses to hypoxia, making infants more vulnerable to the effects of a hypoxic event.[55,62,77,78] Even normal infants have frequent hypoxic episodes during sleep, which may predispose them to the consequences of these repetitive hypoxic stresses.[10] Infants with bronchopulmonary dysplasia are at increased risk for SIDS,[20,21,22] and have frequent spontaneous hypoxic events.[79] Although these infants have an intact hypoxic arousal response at term, they have an abnormal response to hypoxia after arousal leading to apnea and bradycardia.[80] Thus, even when repeated hypoxia does not depress arousal responses, it may be associated with an inability to rescue oneself from hypoxia-induced apnea and bradycardia.[79,80]

Compared with neonates on the one hand, and older children and adults on the other, infants have inadequate physiologic responses to protect against hypoxia, which may cause the infant to enter a physiologic pattern leading to death. Repeated exposure to short hypoxic events makes this even worse.

The studies described suggest a mechanism where hypoxia can lead to death in any infant (Fig. 5.2). Hypoxia occurs commonly in infants.[10] The infant responds to hypoxia by decreasing oxygen consumption and metabolic rate.[69–72] Decreased metabolic rate decreases CO_2 production, and thus decreases central

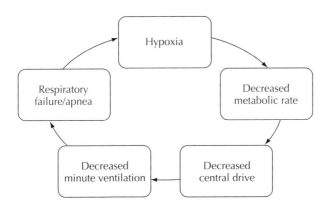

Fig. 5.2 Mechanism by which hypoxia can cause infant death. Hypoxia occurs commonly in infants. The infant responds to hypoxia by decreasing oxygen consumption and metabolic rate, which decreases CO_2 production, which decreases central ventilatory drive, which decreases minute ventilation, which causes apnea or respiratory failure, which causes more hypoxia, which perpetuates the cycle. Thus, hypoxia may cause infants to enter a pattern of maladaptive physiologic responses which can result in death.

ventilatory drive. Decreased central ventilatory drive decreases minute ventilation. Decreased minute ventilation may result in apnea or respiratory failure. Decreased minute ventilation, apnea, and respiratory failure can all cause more hypoxia, which perpetuates the cycle.[81] Thus, hypoxia may cause infants to enter a pattern of maladaptive physiologic responses which can result in death.

How are we to understand SIDS?

Much of SIDS research has searched for a single abnormality or disorder in a single physiologic system. The idea that some infants might be vulnerable to SIDS, and others not, based on a pre-existing abnormality, has not been a productive research strategy. If SIDS were as simple as one abnormality in one physiologic system, the major research thrust directed toward solving the mystery of SIDS would likely be closer to answering the question by now. Thus, SIDS must be more complex than a single abnormality in a single physiologic system. Further, there is no evidence of serious disease or injury found at autopsy in SIDS victims, suggesting that these infants have an increased vulnerability to phenomena which occur frequently in normal infants.

In order to better focus SIDS research, Mortola suggested we imagine a car attempting to drive up a steep mountain road.[81] The car has stopped, and cannot go up the hill. Perhaps all four tires are flat. If one changes the tires, the car could continue to go up the hill. This is the traditional medical model of disease. One identifies a problem and finds a solution. SIDS research has followed this model for the past 2–3 decades, yet this approach has not identified the cause of SIDS. Another possibility is that the car does not go up the hill, yet the tires are inflated, the engine is running, and there are no apparent problems with the car. Perhaps the car does not go up the hill because there are too many passengers, the engine is not powerful enough, the road is too rocky, or the road is too steep. In this view, the car does not go up the hill because of intrinsic characteristics of the car and/or circumstances, not because of a problem which can be fixed. It is, perhaps, this second view which will more accurately reflect the nature of SIDS.

SIDS may be an interaction between intrinsic characteristics of the infant and circumstances. This does not necessarily imply that a distinct *abnormality* exists in SIDS infants. Rather, SIDS may occur in infants without definitive abnormalities, due to intrinsic characteristics of infant physiology, developmental influences, and circumstance. SIDS is more properly viewed as a dynamic interaction of many factors, which are constantly changing, and which together dictate the infant's chances of dying from SIDS. This fundamentally changes the way we view SIDS, and what now becomes important is the interaction of at least three factors (Fig. 5.3).

that SIDS can occur, especially if it occurs during the 2–4 month age in an infant with more 'vulnerable' physiologic responsivity. For other infants, prone sleeping may pose little danger, especially over 6 months of age. Respiratory infections, overheating, cigarette smoke, soft bedding, and other stresses are variable environmental challenges which may trigger SIDS in some infants, but not in others.

Thus, SIDS is likely to be a multifactorial problem requiring the dynamic interaction of many components to cause death. For example, SIDS may start with a more vulnerable infant with subtle decreases in physiologic responses. Then, the infant may need to be at an age when infants are increasingly vulnerable, such as 3 months of age when the respiratory system is unstable in all infants. Then, SIDS may require an environmental trigger, such as an upper respiratory infection. Sleeping position may be an additional contributing factor to such an infant, even if it makes no difference to breathing in an otherwise healthy infant at a younger or older age.

If SIDS causes death through respiratory mechanisms in infants with robust physiology, who breathe regularly and control oxygenation precisely, then SIDS would have to be a catastrophic event to move from regular respirations and consistent oxygenation to death. Results from home recordings of respiratory inductance plethysmography, ECG, and pulse oximetry suggest that the normal infant's control of ventilation and oxygenation is not precise.[10] Normal infants commonly have prolonged central, obstructive, or mixed apneas up to 20 seconds duration in the home. In addition, normal infants commonly have spontaneous arterial oxygen desaturations during periodic breathing to the low 80 per cent range, and occasional infants will spontaneously desaturate to the low 70 per cent range.[10] Prolonged obstructive apneas were recorded in a few normal infants with a simple upper respiratory infection. If infants have such spontaneous events frequently, then SIDS may not have to be such a catastrophic event. A less severe event might be sufficient to cause death in an infant who already has frequent apneas and/or desaturations during sleep.

It is likely that SIDS represents a series of events, modified by the above factors, which are initiated by common events (Fig. 5.4).[81,82] All infants sleep. However, sleep is associated with respiratory abnormalities, even in normal infants. These respiratory abnormalities are modified by developmental immaturity of the respiratory system in infants; and they include irregular breathing (central respiratory pauses), obstructive apneas, and resultant hypoxia and CO_2 retention. The infant responds to hypoxia by decreasing its oxygen requirement or metabolic rate. When the oxygen demand is decreased, the central drive to breathe also decreases. Therefore, ventilation decreases in response to hypoxia, which results in worse hypoxia, which eventually causes cessation of breathing (apnea) or respiratory failure. In order to prevent death, the infant must rescue himself from these hypoxic respiratory sequelae. Arousal from sleep is one protective physiologic response to hypoxia. However, recurrent hypoxia blunts this arousal response.[55,62] Further, the hypoxic arousal response naturally decreases at 2 months of age,[56] which begins the peak incidence of SIDS. Thus, infants in the peak age range for SIDS, and those exposed to repetitive hypoxia, may have blunted arousal responses to hypoxia.[44,55,56,62] If arousal fails to revive the infant, then gasping (auto-resuscitation) must be used. Gasping is the last

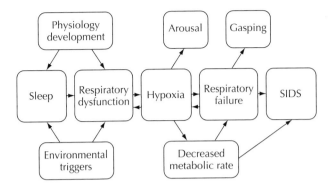

Fig. 5.4 A conceptual model of the mechanism of SIDS death. The origins of SIDS lie in common events. All infants sleep, which disturbs respiration, which causes hypoxia, which produces apnea, which can result in death. Infants may escape this path by arousal, or later by gasping. The amount of respiratory disturbance caused by sleep is modified by development, intrinsic physiologic responsivity of the infant, and environmental triggers.

protective response to reinstate breathing.[73,74] However, gasping is also inhibited in infants. Infants with hypoxia or respiratory failure, without effective arousal or gasping responses, may die from SIDS.

Summary

There is a great deal of evidence pointing to respiratory dysfunction and hypoxia as important mechanisms of death in SIDS. The search for specific abnormalities in the respiratory system, which might cause SIDS, has not been fruitful. However, all infants have vulnerability to hypoxia and respiratory dysfunction, and have inadequate protective physiologic responses to defend against common stresses. Thus, all infants may share vulnerability for SIDS, and there are numerous respiratory and hypoxic mechanisms of SIDS which can occur in nearly every infant. The current conceptual model of SIDS is not a single abnormality in a single physiologic system, but rather a dynamic interaction of factors which come together to cause SIDS.

SIDS may be initiated by common events, such as respiratory dysfunction during sleep. Normal infants have had prolonged apneas and desaturations recorded at home. Infants may not have to be *abnormal* to initiate SIDS. Respiratory dysfunction leads to hypoxia. Hypoxia decreases metabolic rate in infants which, in turn, depresses ventilation, causing more hypoxia. Repetitive hypoxia and age may inhibit protective physiologic responses, such as arousal or gasping. Hypoxic depression of ventilation worsens hypoxia, which may proceed to apnea, respiratory failure, and death. The hypoxic depression of metabolic rate may prevent resuscitation of SIDS infants, even if ventilation and circulation are transiently restored.

This chapter has focused on respiratory mechanisms and hypoxic responses, present in every infant, which can proceed to SIDS. But, we must return to the fact that 999 out of 1000 infants survive these maladaptive mechanisms. Future research must attempt to understand why only a few infants die from these mechanisms while most survive.

References

1. The Bible. 1 Kings, 3:19,900 BC.
2. Fleming PJ, Levine MR, Long AM, Cleave JP. Postnatal development of respiratory oscillations. *Ann NY Acad Sci* 1988;533:305–13.
3. Brouillette RT, Thach BT. A neuromuscular mechanism maintaining extrathoracic airway patency. *J App Physiol* 1979;46:772–9.
4. Wilson SL, Thach BT, Brouillette RT, Abu-Osba YK. Upper airway patency in the human infant: Influence of airway pressure and posture. *J Appl Physiol* 1980; 48:500–4.
5. Keens TG, Bryan AC, Levison H, Ianuzzo CD. Developmental pattern of muscle fiber types in human ventilatory muscles. *J Appl Physiol Respirat Environ Exer Physiol* 1978;44:909–13.
6. Scott CB, Nickerson BG, Sargent CW, Platzker ACG, Warburton D, Keens TG. Developmental pattern of maximal transdiaphragmatic pressure in infants during crying. *Pediatr Res* 1983;17:707–9.
7. Bryan AC, Bowes G, Maloney JE. Control of breathing in the fetus and the new-born. *The Handbook of Physiology: Section 3: The Respiratory System.* Volume II, Part 2. American Physiological Society, Baltimore, Maryland, 1986, pp. 621–48.
8. Phillipson EA, Bowes G. Control of breathing during sleep. *The Handbook of Physiology: Section 3: The Respiratory System.* Volume II, Part 2. American Physiological Society, Baltimore, Maryland, 1986, pp. 649–90.
9. Roffwarg HP, Muzio JN, Dement WC. Ontogenetic development of the human sleep-dream cycle. *Science* 1966;152:604–19.
10. Hunt CE, Corwin MJ, Peucker M *et al.* Longitudinal assessment of oxygen saturation and sleep position in healthy term infants during the first 6 months of life. *Pediatr Res* 1997;41:199A.
11. Krous HF. The international standardized autopsy protocol for sudden unexpected infant death. In: Rognum TO (ed.) *Sudden Infant Death Syndrome. New Trends in the Nineties.* Scandinavian University Press, Oslo, 1995, pp. 81–95.
12. Martinez FD. Sudden infant death syndrome and small airway occlusion: Facts and a hypothesis. *Pediatrics* 1991;87:190–8.
13. Kao LC, Keens TG. Decreased specific airway conductance in infant apnoea. *Pediatrics* 1985;76:232–5.
14. Morley CJ, Hill CM, Brown BD, Barson AJ, Davis JA. Surfactant abnormalities in babies dying from sudden infant death syndrome. *Lancet* 1982;1:1320–32.
15. Hill CM, Brown BD, Morley CJ, Davis JA, Barson A. Pulmonary surfactant 2: In sudden infant death syndrome. *Early Hum Devel* 1988;16:153–62.
16. Gibson RA, McMurchie EJ. Changes in lung surfactant lipids associated with the sudden infant death syndrome. *Aust Paediatr J* 1986;22:77–80.

17. Fagan DG, Milner AD. Pressure volume characteristics of lungs of sudden infant death syndrome. *Arch Dis Child* 1985;60:471–85.

18. Talbert DG, Southall DP. Spherical alveoli and sudden infant lung collapse syndrome. *Lancet* 1985;2:217–8.

19. Loosl CG, Stinson SF, Ryan DP, Hertweck MS, Hardy JD, Serebrin R. The destruction of type 2 pneumocytes by airborne influenza PR8–A virus: its effect on surfactant and lecithin content of the pneumonic lesions of mice. *Chest* 1975;67:7S–14S.

20. Werthammer J, Brown ER, Neff RK, Taeusch Jr HW. Sudden infant death syndrome in infants with bronchopulmonary dysplasia. *Pediatrics* 1982;69:301–4.

21. Kulkarni P, Hall RT, Rhodes PG, Sheehan MB. Postneonatal infant mortality in infants admitted to a neonatal intensive care unit. *Pediatrics* 1978;62:178–83.

22. Southall DP, Richards JM, Rhoden KJ *et al*. Prolonged apnea and cardiac arrhythmias in infants discharged from neonatal intensive care units: failure to predict an increased risk for sudden infant death syndrome. *Pediatrics* 1982;70:844–51.

23. Scott CB, Nickerson BG, Sargent CW, Dennies PC, Platzker ACG, Keens TG. Diaphragm strength in near-miss sudden infant death syndrome. *Pediatrics* 1982;69:782–4.

24. Krous HF, Jordan J. A necropsy study of distribution of petechiae in non-sudden infant death syndrome. *Arch Pathol Lab Med* 1984;108:75–6.

25. Krous HF, Catron AC, Farber JP. Norepinephrine-induced pulmonary petechiae in the rat: an experimental model with potential implications for sudden infant death syndrome. *Pediatr Pathol* 1984;2:115–22.

26. Steinschneider A. Prolonged apnea and the sudden infant death syndrome: clinical and laboratory observations. *Pediatrics* 1972;50:646–54.

27. Kelly DH, Shannon DC, O'Connell K. Care of infants with near-miss sudden infant death syndrome. *Pediatrics* 1978;61:511–4.

28. Oren J, Kelly D, Shannon DC. Identification of a high-risk group for sudden infant death syndrome among infants who were resuscitated for sleep apnea. *Pediatrics* 1986;77:495–9.

29. Kahn A, Groswasser J, Rebuffat E *et al*. Sleep and cardiorespiratory characteristics of infant victims of sudden death: A prospective case–control study. *Sleep* 1992;15:287–92.

30. Ramanathan R, Corwin MJ, Hunt CE *et al*. Preterm infants have prolonged apneas with obstruction and associated oxygen desaturation at home. *Pediatr Res* 1997;41:71A.

31. Tishler PV, Redline S, Ferrette V, Hans MG, Altose MD. The association of sudden unexpected infant death with obstructive sleep apnea. *Am J Respir Crit Care Med* 1996;153:1857–63.

32. Duffty P, Bryan MH. Home monitoring in 'near-miss' sudden infant death syndrome (SIDS) and in siblings of SIDS victims. *Pediatrics* 1982;70:69–74.

33. Davidson Ward SL, Keens TG, Chan LS *et al*. Sudden infant death syndrome in infants evaluated by apnea programs in California. *Pediatrics* 1986;77:451–5.

34. Naeye RL. Pulmonary artery abnormalities in sudden infant death syndrome. *N Eng J Med* 1973;289:1167–70.

35. Naeye RL, Whalen P, Ryser R, Fisher R. Cardiac and other abnormalities in sudden infant death syndrome. *Am J Pathol* 1976;82:1–8.

36. Valdes-Dapena M, Gillane MM, Catherman R. Brown fat retention in sudden infant death syndrome. *Arch Pathol Lab Med* 1976;100:547–9.
37. Naeye RL. Brainstem and adrenal abnormalities in the sudden infant death syndrome. *Am J Clin Pathol* 1976;66:526–30.
38. Naeye RL, Fisher RM, Ryser M, Whalen P. Carotid body in sudden infant death syndrome. *Science* 1976;191:567–9.
39. Williams A, Vawter G, Reid L. Increased muscularity of the pulmonary circulation in victims of sudden infant death syndrome. *Pediatrics* 1979;63:18–24.
40. Rognum TO, Saugstad OD. Hypoxanthine levels in vitreous humor: Postmortem evidence of hypoxia. *Pediatrics* 1991;87:306–10.
41. Kinney HC, Burger PC, Harrell FE, Hudson RP. 'Reactive gliosis' in the medulla oblongata of victims of the sudden infant death syndrome. *Pediatrics* 1983;72: 181–7.
42. Kinney HC, Filiano JJ, Sleeper LA, Mandell F, Valdes-Dapena M, Frost White W. Decreased muscarinic receptor binding in the arcuate nucleus in sudden infant death syndrome. *Science* 1995;269:1446–50.
43. Steinschneider A, Weinstein SL, Diamond E. The sudden infant death syndrome and apnea/obstruction during neonatal sleep and feeding. *Pediatrics* 1982;70:858–63.
44. van der Hal AL, Rodriguez AM, Sargent CW, Platzker ACG, Keens TG. Hypoxic and hypercapneic arousal responses and prediction of subsequent apnea in apnea of infancy. *Pediatrics* 1985;75:848–54.
45. National Institutes of Health Consensus Development Conference on Infantile Apnea and Home Monitoring. *Pediatrics* 1987;79:292–9.
46. Southall DP, Richards JM, deSwiet M *et al.* Identification of infants destined to die unexpectedly during infancy: Evaluation of predictive importance of prolonged apnea and disorders of cardiac rhythm or condition. *Br Med J* 1983;286:1091–6.
47. Erickson JT, Conover JC, Borday V *et al.* Mice lacking brain-derived neurotrophic factor exhibit visceral sensory neuron losses distinct from mice lacking NT4 and display a severe developmental deficit in control of breathing. *J Neuroscience* 1996;16:5361–71.
48. Spears PS. Estimated rates of concordancy for the sudden infant death syndrome in twins. *Am J Epidemiol* 1974;100:1.
49. Beal S. Sudden infant death syndrome in twins. *Pediatrics* 1989;84:1038–44.
50. Irgens LM, Skjaerven R, Peterson DR. Prospective assessment of recurrence risk in sudden infant death syndrome siblings. *J Pediatr* 1984;104:349–51.
51. Peterson DR, Sabotta EE, Dalling JR. Infant mortality among subsequent siblings of infants who died of sudden infant death syndrome. *J Pediatr* 1986;108:911–4.
52. Beal S. Recurrence incidence of sudden infant death syndrome. *Arch Dis Child* 1988;63:924–30.
53. Guntheroth WG, Lohmann R, Spiers PS. Risk of sudden infant death syndrome in subsequent siblings. *J Pediatr* 1990;116:520–4.
54. Walker AM, Johnston RV, Grant DA, Wilkinson MH. Repetitive hypoxia abolishes arousal from sleep in newborn lambs. In: Rognum TO (ed.) *Sudden Infant Death Syndrome. New Trends in the Nineties.* Scandinavian University Press, Oslo, 1995, pp. 238–41.
55. Rodriguez AM, Warburton D, Keens TG. Elevated catecholamines and abnormal hypoxic arousal in apnea of infancy. *Pediatrics* 1987;79:269–74.

56. Davidson Ward SL, Bautista DB, Keens TG. Hypoxic arousal responses in normal infants. *Pediatrics* 1992;89:860–4.
57. Hunt CE. Abnormal hypercapnic and hypoxic arousal responses in near-miss SIDS infants. *Pediatr Res* 1981;15:1462–4.
58. McCulloch K, Brouillette RT, Guzetta AJ, Hunt CE. Arousal responses in near-miss sudden infant death syndrome and in normal infants. *J Pediatr* 1982;101:911–7.
59. Davidson Ward SL, Bautista DB, Woo MS *et al.* Responses to hypoxia and hypercapnia in infants of substance-abusing mothers. *J Pediatr* 1992;121:704–9.
60. Davidson Ward SL, Bautista DB, Buckley S *et al.* Elevated circulating norepinephrine in infants of substance abusing mothers. *Am J Dis Child* 1991;145:44–8.
61. Milerad J, Hertzberg T, Wennergren G, Lagercrantz H. Respiratory and arousal responses to hypoxia in apnoeic infants revisited. *Eur J Pediatr* 1989;148:565–70.
62. Fewell JE, Konduri GG. Influence of repeated exposure to rapidly developing hypoxaemia on the arousal and cardiorespiratory response to rapidly developing hypoxaemia in lambs. *J Dev Physiol* 1989;11:77–82.
63. McNamara F, Wulbrand H, Thach BT. Habituation of the infant arousal response. *Pediatr Pulmonol* 1996;22:45.
64. Blair PS, Fleming PJ, Bensley D *et al.* Smoking and the sudden infant death syndrome: results from the 1993–95 case–control study for confidential inquiry into stillbirths and deaths in infancy. *Br Med J* 1996;313:195–8.
65. Franco P, Hainautm M, Pardou A, Groswasser J, Kahn A. Prenatal exposure to cigarette smoke increases auditory arousal thresholds in infants *Pediatr Pulmonol* 1996;22:426.
66. Duffy TE, Kohle SJ, Vannucci RC. Carbohydrate and energy metabolism in perinatal rat brain: relation to anoxia and survival. *J Neurochem* 1974;24:271–6.
67. Glass HG, Snyder FF, Webster E. The rate of decline in resistance to anoxia of rabbits, dogs, and guinea pigs from the onset of viability to adult life. *Am J Physiol* 1944;140:609–15.
68. Winn K. Similarities between lethal asphyxia in postneonatal rats and the terminal episode in SIDS. *Pediatr Pathol* 1986;5:325–35.
69. Mortola JP, Rezzonico R. Metabolic and ventilatory rates in newborn kittens during hypoxia. *Respir Physiol* 1988;73:55–68.
70. Mortola JP, Rezzonico R, Lanthier C. Ventilation and oxygen consumption during acute hypoxia in newborn mammals: a comparative analysis. *Respir Physiol* 1989;78:31–43.
71. Sidi D, Puipers JRG, Heymann MA, Rudolph AM. Developmental changes in oxygenation and circulatory response to hypoxemia in lambs. *Am J Physiol* 1983;245:H674–H682.
72. Moss M, Moreau G, Lister G. Oxygen transport and metabolism in the conscious lamb: the effect of hypoxemia. *Pediatr Res* 1987;22:177–83.
73. Jacobi MS, Thach BT. Effect of maturation on spontaneous recovery from hypoxia apnea by gasping. *J Appl Physiol* 1989;66:2384–90.
74. Thach BT, Lawson EE. Death from upper airway obstruction: Decreased survival time in 33 day old rabbits. *Pediatr Res* 1979;135–42.
75. Niola S, Smith DS, Mayevsky A, Dobson GP, Veech RL, Chance B. Age dependency of steady state mitochondrial oxidative metabolism in the in vivo hypoxic dog brain. *Neurol Res* 1991;13:25–32.

76. Coté A, Porras H, Meehan B. Age-dependent vulnerability to carotid chemodenervation in piglets. *J Appl Physiol* 1996;80:323–31.
77. Waters K, Beardsmore CS, Paquette, Meehan JB, Coté A, Moss IR. Respiratory responses to rapid-onset, repetitive vs continuous hypoxia in piglets. *Respir Physiol* 1996;105:135–42.
78. Stafford A, Weatherall JAC. The survival of young rats in nitrogen. *J Physiol* 1960;153:457–72.
79. Garg M, Kurzner SI, Bautista DB, Keens TG. Clinically unsuspected hypoxia during sleep and feeding in bronchopulmonary dysplasia. *Pediatrics* 1988;81:635–42.
80. Garg M, Kurzner SI, Bautista DB, Keens TG. Hypoxic arousal responses in bronchopulmonary dysplasia. *Pediatrics* 1988;82:59–63.
81. Mortola JP. *Proceedings of the Fourth SIDS International Conference*. Bethesda, Maryland, 1996.
82. Walker, A. *Proceedings of the Fourth SIDS International Conference*. Bethesda, Maryland, 1996.

CHAPTER 6

QT prolongation and SIDS – from theory to evidence

PETER J. SCHWARTZ

Introduction   83
The QT hypothesis   83
Arguments against the QT hypothesis   88
The molecular link   90
References   93

Introduction

The suggestions over the years that cardiac mechanisms and specifically life-threatening arrhythmias[1,2] might account for a significant portion of cases of SIDS have been controversial.

This chapter describes the rationale and origin of the cardiac hypothesis that some SIDS cases are due to ventricular fibrillation associated with prolongation of the QT interval, summarizes the results of our almost 20 years prospective study by recording an ECG in 34,000 infants,[3] and presents our new finding[4] which provides for the first time the molecular evidence linking SIDS to the long QT syndrome (LQTS).

The QT hypothesis

Many hypotheses have been proposed to explain SIDS but none has yet been proven. There is a consensus that SIDS is multifactorial,[2,5] a concept implying that a sudden and unexpected death in infancy may be due to different causes. A logical corollary is that the validity of one mechanism is not negated by the validity of another. What really matters is to dissect out those mechanisms accounting for the larger portion of those deaths that are currently labeled as SIDS, largely because of our inability to identify a more specific disease or cause. It should be remembered that SIDS is a diagnosis of exclusion: when we cannot explain, on the basis of current knowledge and after a thorough and expert postmortem examination, why an apparently healthy infant has been found dead then the diagnosis becomes that of SIDS.

Most SIDS cases probably result from an abnormality in either respiratory or cardiac function,[5,6] or in their neural control, that may be transient in nature but sufficient to initiate a lethal sequence of events. In my original reasoning, shared by Peter Froggatt, a pioneer in the role of cardiac mechanisms in infant deaths,[7] I gave weight to the fact that in the Western world the leading cause of mortality in age 20–65 is sudden cardiac death,[8] and the mechanism involved is almost always a lethal arrhythmia, ventricular fibrillation. It would be quite strange if sudden cardiac death, and therefore lethal arrhythmias, would not contribute at all to some infant sudden deaths.

It was thus that in 1974, in a funded NIH grant application,[9] and in 1976,[1] I proposed that some cases of SIDS might have been due to a mechanism similar to that responsible for the sudden death of the patients affected by LQTS, the leading cause of sudden death below age 20.[10,11] One such mechanism might have been a developmental abnormality in cardiac sympathetic innervation predisposing some infants to lethal arrhythmias in the first year of life.[1] Another likely mechanism might have been the same genetic alterations that only very recently have been shown to cause the LQTS.[10,11] The only clinically detectable marker for these mechanisms is a QT interval prolongation on the electrocardiogram (ECG).

Following my 1976 editorial,[1] the hypothesis that QT interval prolongation may play a role in the genesis of SIDS received considerable attention but it was rapidly, and perhaps prematurely, discarded on the basis of a series of apparently negative results.[12–16] The arguments against the role of prolonged QT in SIDS had weaknesses previously discussed in detail, and the interested reader is referred to these publications.[2,17]

Most of these 'so-called' negative studies were performed in populations of very small size or in infants defined as 'at increased risk for SIDS', like the siblings of SIDS victims[13,15] or the so-called 'near-miss' or aborted SIDS[12,14] who were not found to have QT prolongation. Conclusions drawn from these studies are quite unlikely to be relevant to the assessment of the risk for SIDS associated with QT interval prolongation. It is essential to remember that for diseases characterized by a very low incidence, such as SIDS, any risk factor will yield a high number of false positives. In the case of SIDS, even assuming a risk as high as two per thousand, a factor that increases the risk by five times will still leave 99% of false positives! This means that whenever investigators study 100 of these infants, they can expect only one to subsequently die of SIDS; the fact that this one SIDS victim does not show a proposed marker of risk has no implications whatsoever for the relevance of that marker. It follows that the absence of a given marker, prolonged QT interval in our case, among subjects 'at high risk for SIDS' only indicates that this factor is not important in the specific patients under study; moreover, extrapolation to the general population and to the true SIDS victims is simply unwarranted. These considerations seemed to escape many SIDS investigators.

THE ITALIAN STUDY ON NEONATAL ELECTROCARDIOGRAPHY AND SIDS

To test the hypothesis of a relationship between QT interval prolongation and SIDS, in 1976 we designed a prospective study based on the recording of a standard ECG in 3–4 day old infants. Given the low incidence of SIDS (0.5–1.5 per 1000 live births), we had to prospectively collect neonatal ECGs in a very large population and to subsequently follow these infants for one year to assess the occurrence of SIDS or deaths for other causes. The results of this study were published in 1998[3] and, partly because of the accompanying editorial[18] and partly because of the media attention, were widely publicized. For this reason, here we will simply summarize the main facts and findings. Details on the methodology and on the discussion of the results can be easily obtained through the original publication.

Twelve lead ECGs were recorded in 34,442 neonates born in nine maternity hospitals. The QT interval was measured on the ECGs of all infants that died and on the ECGs of a random sample of 9725 infants taken from the entire study population. All measurements were performed by investigators blind to the survival status of the infant. The study lasted 19 years.

Of the 34,442 infants enrolled, 33,034 (96%) completed the one-year follow-up. The lost-to-follow-up were due to change of residence. The mean QTc (QT interval corrected for heart rate) was 400±20 msec and it did not differ between males and females (401±19 vs 400±20 msec). The normal and symmetrical distribution of the QTc in our population made the 97.5th percentile value of QTc correspond to 440 msec, two standard deviations above the mean. Consequently, we considered a value greater than 440 msec as a prolonged QTc.

During the one-year follow-up there have been 34 deaths: 24 due to SIDS and 10 due to other causes. All postmortem examinations of SIDS victims were negative and failed to document an adequate cause of death. No SIDS victim had a family history of LQTS or sudden death.

The mean QTc was 435±45 msec in the SIDS group, significantly longer than that of the non-SIDS victims (392±26 msec, $P<0.05$) and of that of healthy controls (400±20 msec, $P<0.01$, Fig. 6.1). More importantly, the analysis of the individual values of QTc in the two groups of victims (Fig. 6.1) showed that 12/24 (50%) infants who died for SIDS had a QTc greater than 440 msec, whereas all the infants who died for other causes had a QTc shorter than 440 msec.

Since heart rate in the neonatal period is relatively high, the Bazett's formula might not be appropriate to correct QT interval for short cycle lengths. Accordingly, we also divided the RR intervals in 17 classes with progressively increasing values (20 msec stepwise) and for each class we calculated the percentile distribution of the corresponding absolute values of QT interval (from the 2.5th to the 97.5th). Figure 6.2 shows that the individual values of 12/24 (50%) SIDS victims were located above the 97.5th percentile, whereas all the values of the non-SIDS victims were below the 90th percentile.

On the basis of our results the absolute risk of SIDS in infants with a normal QTc is 0.37 per thousand, while that of infants with a QTc $\geq$ 440 msec is 15 per thousand. The odds ratio for SIDS associated with a prolonged QTc (>440

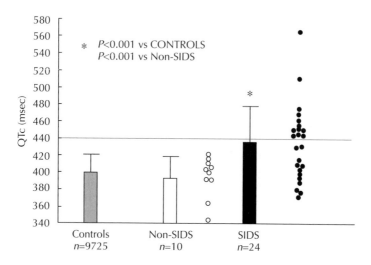

Fig. 6.1   Mean QT interval corrected for heart rate (QTc) in control infants, in sudden infant death syndrome victims (SIDS) and in victims for other causes (non-SIDS). The line represents the 97.5th value of QTc in the whole population and corresponds to 440 msec, 2 standard deviations above the mean. The filled and the open circles represent the individual values of QTc of the SIDS victims and of the non-SIDS victims, respectively. (From Ref. 3.)

msec) is 41.3 (95% CI 17.3–98.4), significantly greater than that of infants with a normal QTc.

This large prospective study based on more than 34,000 infants provided the demonstration that QT interval prolongation, on the standard ECG recorded on the 3rd–4th day of life, is a major risk factor for SIDS.

QT PROLONGATION AND LIFE-THREATENING ARRHYTHMIAS

The evidence for a strong association between SIDS and QT interval prolongation, a marker of reduced cardiac electrical stability, suggests that in some infants there may be an increased susceptibility to life-threatening arrhythmias.

Experimental and clinical studies have shown that QT interval prolongation favors the occurrence of lethal arrhythmias and is associated with increased risk for sudden death in several clinical conditions[19,20] and also in apparently healthy individuals.[21] Among these conditions the most relevant to SIDS undoubtedly is the LQTS.[10,11]

The presence of false positives (2.5%), i.e. infants with prolonged QT interval who did not die of SIDS, indicates that – besides the high probability of cases of 'spurious QT prolongation' (i.e. an infant with a normal QT interval who on day 3–4 has a measurement just above the cut-off point and who on subsequent measurements would show normal values) – other factors in the post-natal

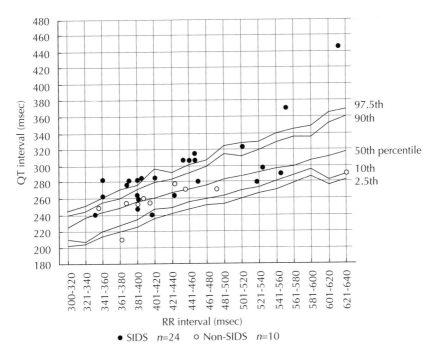

Fig. 6.2 Relation between QT interval and cardiac cycle length. Each line represents the percentile values of uncorrected QT intervals at the corresponding range of RR intervals. The filled and the open circles represent the individual values of QTc of the SIDS victims and of the non-SIDS victims, respectively. (From Ref. 3.)

period contribute to the lethal event. This is consistent with the concept of QT prolongation acting as an arrhythmogenic 'substrate' which requires a 'trigger' for the occurrence of life-threatening arrhythmias. The best known 'triggers' for lethal arrhythmias in the setting of QT prolongation are represented by release of catecholamines secondary to activation of the sympathetic nervous system and by factors (e.g. hypokalemia or drugs that block the I_{Kr} current, as many antibiotics, antihistaminic, and prokinetics such as cisapride) that further prolong the QT interval.[10,22] It is interesting to note, and we do that here for the first time, that the prone sleeping position may be one of these triggers. Indeed, this recently discovered risk factor for SIDS[23] is associated with signs of increased sympathetic and decreased vagal activity to the heart – an established risk factor for arrhythmic death.[24]

CLINICAL IMPLICATIONS

Our article[3] ended by mentioning two rather obvious, but nonetheless troublesome, clinical implications. One was that the highly significant association between QT prolongation and occurrence of SIDS unavoidably raises the issue of the potential value of a routine neonatal ECG screening. The low incidence of SIDS in the general population (<0.1%) forces a low predictive value for any factor associated with the event, and QT prolongation (1.5%) is no exception even though its relative risk of 41 is strikingly higher than any previously reported. Despite this limitation, a simple electrocardiographic screening might contribute to identify a portion of the infants at high risk for SIDS.

The second big issue is the management of the infants found to have a prolonged QTc. Our study contained no data to justify new therapeutic recommendations; however, the association between prolonged QT interval and SIDS should allow some cautious speculation. The lethal arrhythmias favored by QT prolongation are usually triggered by sudden increases in sympathetic activity. In the first year of life this may be often elicited by multiple conditions[2] including sudden noise, exposure to cold, REM sleep, apnea leading to a chemoreceptive reflex, arousals, and probably the prone position. In LQTS antiadrenergic interventions are quite successful.[10] Data from almost 1000 LQTS families indicate that treatment with beta-blockers has reduced mortality below 3%.[10] This information is relevant to the prevention of SIDS in newborns with a prolonged QT interval. It also provides a ready therapy for those infants serendipitously identified, by neonatal ECG screening, as definitely affected by the LQTS and offers a valid option for the yet unproven but reasonable possibility of reducing risk in all neonates with a prolonged QT interval.

Practically, whenever infants at risk because of QT prolongation are identified early on, preventive therapy could be considered and then instituted for a few months. Normalization of the QT interval during development will allow rapid withdrawal of therapy in the unavoidably large number of false positives, but will allow also the continuation of therapy in the minority of infants with a persistent QT prolongation in whom beta-blockers are likely to be life-saving.

Arguments against the QT hypothesis

There are several ways to discuss one's own data. A difficult one, but probably the best in the long term, is to take into account the points of view reflecting the most common criticism.

One frequently made statement is the following: 'There is no evidence for lethal arrhythmias as precipitating events in infants who have died of SIDS while on cardiorespiratory monitors.'[25]

The issue of 'no evidence for arrhythmias' calls into question the mechanisms underlying arrhythmic sudden death and the implications of SIDS being a multifactorial disease. The infants who are on cardiorespiratory monitors represent a population with a specific selection bias; namely, to have been discovered by the parents during an apparently life-threatening event. As carefully discussed almost 20 years ago,[6] most 'near miss' infants enter in this category because of an episode of apnea. A respiratory death is slow and allows time for struggle and cyanosis, whereas death by ventricular fibrillation is fast and silent. There are simply more statistical chances that a mother will find her baby dying a respiratory than a cardiac death, and this will allow her to interrupt the deadly process and the end-result will be a new 'near miss'. Thus, it is likely that most true 'near misses' would have died a respiratory death, and it is expected that these infants would show some respiratory abnormality. The fact that an infant considered at increased risk because an apneic episode does not have ventricular arrhythmias should not surprise a competent clinician; why should he have cardiac arrhythmias if his risk comes from a respiratory abnormality?

Another common criticism is the following: 'Ventricular arrhythmias have not been described in patients who have been evaluated after survival of an acute life-threatening event'.[25]

This comment calls into question the understanding of lethal arrhythmias and, specifically, of the arrhythmias associated with a prolonged QT interval. These arrhythmias, mostly Torsade-de-Pointes ventricular tachycardia degenerating into ventricular fibrillation, are of very short duration. They either convert spontaneously to sinus rhythm within 20–30 seconds or proceed toward ventricular fibrillation leading to loss of consciousness and sudden death within a few minutes. In the first case, if the patient is an adult he/she will have syncope and faint and this will not escape attention; however, if the patient is an infant lying in his crib where he is going to fall? A transient, non-fatal episode will almost always go unnoticed. In the second case, only a fortuitous set of circumstances may allow the parents to observe and attempt to interrupt a lethal episode that would be over in 3–5 minutes; the point here is that when prolonged ventricular tachycardia deteriorates into ventricular fibrillation the infants almost never survive and would not be available for further monitoring. Those more likely to survive are the infants who have life-threatening episodes for respiratory abnormalities and in the subsequent monitoring there is no reason to expect ventricular tachyarrhythmias. Finally, it is extremely unusual for patients affected by LQTS to have ventricular arrhythmias outside their life-threatening episodes; they are almost always in sinus rhythm and then, all of a sudden, they may have a run of Torsade-de-Pointes and faint or die.

Another critique is that 'the most damning problem is the lack of independent confirmation in the past 22 years. In fact, there have been four prospective studies[16,26–28] that have contradicted the Italian data.'[29] This is simply not correct, as shown by the following review of the four studies mentioned above.

Southall *et al.*[16] studied 7254 infants, 15 of whom subsequently died of SIDS. Even though they concluded for no difference between SIDS victims and controls, six of the 15 (40%) infants who died of SIDS had a QTc equal or greater than the value corresponding to the 90th percentile of their own population. This incidence is four times higher than expected and implies an odds ratio for SIDS of 6, significantly greater than that of infants with a QTc below the 90th percentile. The erroneous conclusion was reached because the authors compared the means of the two groups (victims and survivors), an analysis appropriate if SIDS had one cause only and quite wrong when dealing with multifactorial diseases. The detailed arguments for the methodologically correct approach to Southall's data have been presented elsewhere.[17] Another significant problem lies in the fact that his study was performed on day 2 when the physiologic fluctuation in the QT is still high and when many infants who 1–2 days later will have a normal QT may still show a prolonged QT interval.[30] This results in a spuriously high number of infants with QT prolongation which of course reduces the power of the study and the possibility of correctly assessing the relative risk associated with a prolonged QT interval.

The other three studies[26–28] are simply not relevant. The study by Weinstein and Steinschneider,[26] was a retrospective analysis of eight SIDS victims studied as part of an investigation on apnea and whose QT interval was found similar to that of other infants. It is critical to note that these infants were studied at a temperature of 90°F. Heating modifies sympathetic activity and may revert to normal a neurally mediated QT prolongation. The study by Schaffer *et al.*[27] is based on one SIDS victim with a normal QT. The study by Gillette and Garson[28] is on three SIDS victims with a normal QT and one of them is the single victim described by Schaffer.

This brief overview shows how the validity of the QT hypothesis is not affected by the arguments commonly used in the literature.

The molecular link

POTENTIAL CAUSES FOR QT PROLONGATION IN INFANTS

We have provided considerable evidence that a prolonged QT interval increases the risk of SIDS.[3] A major question, however, remains. Why should an infant have a QT prolongation? Which mechanisms would be involved? It is clear that inability to provide rational explanations to these questions would weaken the QT hypothesis.

We have proposed three different mechanisms that might be involved in the genesis of QT interval prolongation in some newborns. The first is a developmental abnormality in cardiac sympathetic innervation.[1] The second is a *de novo* mutation in one of the LQTS genes. The third involves cases of LQTS with low penetrance.[31]

The first is partly based on the fact that an imbalance in cardiac sympathetic innervation with left dominance, experimentally produced by removing the right stellate ganglion, prolongs the QT interval and increases susceptibility to ventricular fibrillation in several conditions, including 3-week-old puppies with normal hearts.[32] The sympathetic innervation of the heart continues to develop after birth and becomes functionally complete by approximately the sixth month of life.[33] The right and left sympathetic nerves may occasionally develop at different rates and lead temporarily to a harmful imbalance. A sudden increase in sympathetic activity might easily trigger a lethal arrhythmia in these electrically unstable hearts. Infants with these characteristics would be more vulnerable during the first few months of life and the higher risk for SIDS could be identified by the observation of a prolonged QT interval.

As the other two possibilities, that actually are more easily testable, involve LQTS and some related concepts of genetics it becomes necessary to summarize here some critical points concerning the information available on the genetics of LQTS. LQTS is a familial disease, which may nonetheless present also 'sporadic'

cases (no apparent familial involvement) and is characterized by QT prolongation and high risk for sudden death, usually under stressful conditions but also
during sleep.[34] LQTS has genetic heterogeneity and genes located on chromo-
somes 3, 7, 11 and 21 have been identified.[11] A potential difficulty for linking
LQTS to SIDS is that the latter is not a familial disease. Two important concepts
are highly relevant here. The first is that among 'sporadic' cases of LQTS *de novo*
(spontaneous) mutations have been found in the two genes, *HERG* and
KvLQT1, which encode the potassium channels for I_{Kr} and I_{Ks}, two of the major
repolarizing currents.[11] A *de novo* mutation, by definition, is not found among
the parents. The second is represented by the demonstration of 'low penetrance'
in LQTS.[31] Penetrance is defined as the ratio between gene-carriers and individuals showing the full phenotype of the disease. A low penetrance implies that
clinical diagnosis is often inadequate and that many affected individuals may
appear completely normal at clinical examination. We have just obtained the
evidence that the second of these three possibilities may indeed account for
some cases of SIDS and thus explain prolongation of the QT interval in some
SIDS victims with parents who have a completely normal QT interval.

MOLECULAR EVIDENCE

We have very recently reported a case which demonstrates that *de novo* mutations in LQTS genes may manifest as, and be indistinguishable from, classic
cases of 'near-miss' for SIDS or as SIDS itself.[4] A 7-week-old infant was found
cyanotic, apneic, and pulseless by his parents. He was rushed to a nearby hospital while his father was attempting CPR; in the emergency room an ECG
showed ventricular fibrillation (Fig. 6.3). Thus, this infant presented as typical
'near-miss' for SIDS. After defibrillation, the ECG revealed a major QT prolongation (QTc 648 msec), LQTS was diagnosed and effective therapy was instituted by combining beta-blockade and the sodium channel blocker mexiletine.
Four years later the little boy was doing well and remained asymptomatic; his
QTc shortened considerably but remained prolonged with a value of 500 msec.
The QT interval of both parents was normal and paternity was confirmed.
Molecular screening identified a mutation on *SCN5A*, the cardiac sodium channel gene responsible for the LQT3 subtype of LQTS.[12] This disease-carrying
mutation was not present in the mother nor in the father, thus establishing that
this is a *de novo* mutation (Fig. 6.4).

The documentation of ventricular fibrillation at arrival in the emergency
room is quite important given the frequent statements such as 'no one has
recorded ventricular arrhythmias in infants at risk for SIDS'.[29] Had the infant
died, a certainty without cardioversion, the absence of an ECG, the normal QT
of both parents would have ruled out any suspicions of LQTS and would have
prompted the classic diagnosis of SIDS. Thus, infants who have similar *de novo*
mutations, involving one of the ionic channels controlling ventricular repolarization, may have a prolonged QT interval at birth. Some of them may die
because of ventricular fibrillation already *in utero*, and thus become stillbirths,
or during the first few months of life and without an available ECG they would

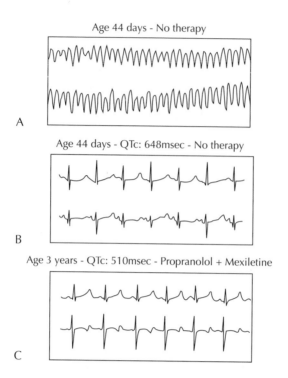

Age 44 days - No therapy

A

Age 44 days - QTc: 648msec - No therapy

B

Age 3 years - QTc: 510msec - Propranolol + Mexiletine

C

Fig. 6.3 ECG leads DII and V2, showing ventricular fibrillation at hospital admission (panel A); QT interval prolongation observed the same day after restoration of sinus rhythm (panel B); and ECG recorded at the last follow-up visit (panel C). (Modified from Ref. 4.)

be labeled as SIDS victims. Others would probably begin to have syncopal episodes or non-fatal cardiac arrests during their childhood and would then be diagnosed as sporadic cases of LQTS.

The significance of this finding exceeds by far that commonly associated with a single case report because it represents 'proof of concept' for the link between LQTS and SIDS. It does indeed provide the first unequivocal demonstration that a life-threatening event in infancy, with all the characteristics for SIDS or for 'near miss' for SIDS, can depend on a *de novo* mutation in one of the LQTS genes thus escaping recognition in the parents and lead to sudden death due to ventricular fibrillation.

The major difference between negative and positive findings is not always fully appreciated. A very large number of negative findings is required in order to dismiss the possible involvement of a given mechanism. By contrast, a single positive finding is sufficient to demonstrate that a given mechanism *can* be operant; what then remains to be assessed is the frequency with which this mechanism is operant. In the case of prolonged QT interval and SIDS, this

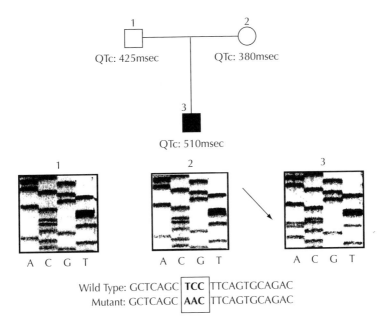

Fig. 6.4 Family tree and results of the molecular screening. DNA sequences of the exon 16 of *SCN5A* gene demonstrate the presence of two abnormal bands (arrow), determining a heterozygous mutation in the proband, absent in the parents. (Modified from Ref. 4.)

quantitative information has already been suggested by our large prospective study showing that 50% of SIDS victims had a prolonged QT interval in the first few days of life. Even with very conservative estimates, it is difficult to imagine that in larger populations this figure would be below 20–30%.

This case provides definitive evidence for one of the mechanisms involved in SIDS, it supports the concept of widespread neonatal ECG screening, and it indicates that at least this subset of infants at high risk for sudden infant death can be diagnosed early on and that their impending death can probably be prevented.

Addendum

Our group has just identified, from the cardiac tissue of a 4-month-old SIDS victim, a mutation on *KvLQT1*, the LQTS gene encoding the potassium current I_{Ks}. No ECG is available for this infant and this is another *de novo* mutation (Priori & Schwartz, manuscript in preparation).

Acknowledgements

This study was partially supported by the following grants:
CEE BMH4-CT96-0028;
Telethon N° 1058;
I am grateful to Pinuccia De Tomasi for expert editorial support.

References

1. Schwartz PJ. Cardiac sympathetic innervation and the sudden infant death syndrome. A possible pathogenetic link. *Am J Med* 1976;60:167–72.
2. Schwartz PJ. The quest for the mechanism of the sudden infant death syndrome. Doubts and progress. *Circulation* 1987;75:677–83.
3. Schwartz PJ, Stramba-Badiale M, Segantini A *et al.* Prolongation of the QT interval and the sudden infant death syndrome. *N Engl J Med* 1998;338:1709–14.
4. Schwartz PJ, Priori SG, Dumaine R *et al.* A molecular link between the sudden infant death syndrome and the long QT syndrome. *N Engl J Med* 2000;343:262–7.
5. Schwartz PJ, Southall DP, Valdes-Dapena M (eds). The sudden infant death syndrome. Cardiac and respiratory mechanisms and interventions. *Ann NY Acad Sci*, 1988; 533:474 pp.
6. Schwartz PJ. The sudden infant death syndrome. In: Scarpelli EM, Cosmi EV (eds). *Reviews in Perinatal Medicine.* Raven Press, New York, 4:475–524, 1981.
7. Froggatt P. A cardiac cause in cot death: a discarded hypothesis? *Ir Med J* 1977;70: 408–14.
8. Lown B. Sudden cardiac death: the major challenge confronting contemporary cardiology. *Am J Cardiol* 1979;43:313–28.
9. NIH Grant HDO8796 1975/1978. Experimental reproduction of long QT syndrome and SIDS.
10. Schwartz PJ, Priori SG, Napolitano C. The long QT syndrome. In: Zipes DP, Jalife J (eds). *Cardiac Electrophysiology. From Cell to Bedside.* 3rd edn. WB Saunders, Philadelphia, 2000, pp. 597–615.
11. Priori SG, Barhanin J, Hauer RNW *et al.* Genetic and molecular basis of cardiac arrhythmias: impact on clinical management. Part I and II. *Circulation* 1999;99: 518–28, and Part III *Circulation* 1999;99:674–81, and *Eur Heart J* 1999;20:174–95.
12. Kelly DH, Shannon DC, Liberthson RR. The role of the QT interval in the Sudden Infant Death Syndrome. *Circulation* 1977;55:633–5.
13. Steinschneider A. Sudden infant death syndrome and prolongation of the QT interval. *Am J Dis Child* 1978;132:688–91.
14. Haddad GG, Epstein MAF, Epstein RA, Mazza NM, Mellins RB, Krongrad E. The QT interval in aborted sudden infant death syndrome infants. *Pediatr Res* 1979;13: 136–8.
15. Montague TJ, Finley JP, Mukelabai K *et al.* Cardiac rhythm, rate and ventricular repolarization properties in infants at risk for Sudden Infant Death Syndrome: comparison with age- and sex-matched control infants. *Am J Cardiol* 1984;54:301–7.
16. Southall DP, Arrowsmith WA, Stebbens V, Alexander JR. QT interval measurements before sudden infant death syndrome. *Arch Dis Child* 1986;61:327–33.

17. Schwartz PJ, Segantini A. Cardiac innervation, neonatal electrocardiography and SIDS. A key for a novel preventive strategy? *Ann N Y Acad Sci* 1988;533:210–20.
18. Towbin JA, Friedman RA. Prolongation of the QT interval and the sudden infant death syndrome. *N Engl J Med* 1998;338:1760–1.
19. Schwartz PJ, Wolf S. QT interval prolongation as predictor of sudden death in patients with myocardial infarction. *Circulation* 1978;57:1074–7.
20. Algra A, Tijssen JGP, Roelandt JRTC, Pool J, Lubsen J. QTc prolongation measured by standard 12–lead electrocardiography is an independent risk factor for sudden death due to cardiac arrest. *Circulation* 1991;83:1888–94.
21. Schouten EG, Dekker JM, Meppelink P, Kok FJ, Vandenbroucke JP, Pool J. QT interval prolongation predicts cardiovascular mortality in an apparently healthy population. *Circulation* 1991;84:1516–23.
22. Napolitano C, Schwartz PJ, Brown AM *et al.* Evidence for a cardiac ion channel mutation underlying drug-induced QT prolongation and life-threatening arrhythmias. *J Cardiovasc Electrophysiol* 2000;1:691–6.
23. Dwyer T, Ponsonby AL, Blizzard L, Newman NM, Cochrane JA. The contribution in the prevalence of prone sleeping position to the decline in Sudden Infant Death Syndrome in Tasmania. *JAMA* 1995;273:783–9.
24. Schwartz PJ, La Rovere MT, Vanoli E. Autonomic nervous system and sudden cardiac death. Experimental basis and clinical observations for post-myocardial infarction risk stratification. *Circulation* 1992;85(Suppl. I):77–91.
25. Martin RJ, Miller MJ, Redline S. Screening for SIDS: a neonatal perspective. *Pediatrics* 1999;103:812–13.
26. Weinstein SL, Steinschneider A: QTc and R-R intervals in victims of the sudden infant death syndrome. *Am J Dis Child* 1985;139:987–90.
27. Schaffer MS, Trippel DL, Buckles DS, Young RH, Dolan PL, Gillette PC. The longitudinal time course of QTc in early infancy. Preliminary results of a prospective sudden infant death syndrome surveillance program. *J Perinatol* 1991;11:57–62.
28. Gillette PC, Garson A Jr. Sudden cardiac death in the pediatric population. *Circulation* 1992;85(Suppl. I):64–9.
29. Guntheroth WG, Spiers PS. Prolongation of the QT interval and the sudden infant death syndrome. *Pediatrics* 1999;103:813–14.
30. Walsh ZS. Electrocardiographic intervals during the first week of life. *Am Heart J* 1963;66:36–43.
31. Priori SG, Napolitano C, Schwartz PJ. Low penetrance in the long QT syndrome. Clinical impact. *Circulation* 1999;99:529–33.
32. Stramba-Badiale M, Lazzarotti M, Schwartz PJ. Development of cardiac innervation, ventricular fibrillation and Sudden Infant Death Syndrome. *Am J Physiol* 1992;263:H1514–22.
33. Gootman PM (ed.) *Developmental Neurobiology of the Autonomic Nervous System.* Humana Press, Clifton, NJ, 1986.
34. Schwartz PJ, Priori SG, Spazzolini C *et al.* Genotype-phenotype correlation in the long QT syndrome. Gene-specific triggers for life-threatening arrhythmias. *Circulation* 2001;103:89–95.

CHAPTER 7

Arousal and brain homeostatic control

RONALD L. ARIAGNO AND MAJID MIRMIRAN

Introduction   96
Sleep, arousal and circadian rhythms   98
Influence of sleeping position on sleep   103
Respiratory and cardiac mechanisms during sleep in SIDS   104
Thermoregulatory control   108
Summary   111
Acknowledgements   112
References   112

Introduction

The purpose of this chapter is to review SIDS research from the perspective of sleep. We believe that the etiology of SIDS lies in understanding brain mechanisms controlling sleep, arousal, circadian rhythms, body temperature and breathing during development. There are strong interactions between these homeostatic mechanisms and the strengths of those interactions are changing during the critical period of brain development at 2–4 months of age when the risk for SIDS is greatest. We share the view of Filliano and Kinney[1] of a triple-risk model of SIDS; i.e. death results from the coincidence of three factors: a vulnerable infant, a critical developmental period in homeostatic control, and an exogenous stressor or event.

The *vulnerability* to SIDS is in part due to transient imbalances in development of neuronal mechanisms underlying sleep depth, arousal, and cardiorespiratory control. These imbalances may be due to variability in normal development or can be exacerbated by *in utero* and/or postnatal exposure to nicotine; in the case of nicotine there may be an association with prolonged effects on the neuronal mechanisms controlling sleep and arousal. The *critical developmental period* is the period in which the brain mechanisms controlling depth of sleep and arousal threshold are emerging. The *exogenous stressors* that precipitate SIDS are factors such as environmental temperature that work through normal interactions with the homeostatic thermoregulatory system to alter sleep, arousability and cardiorespiratory control.

At the 4th International SIDS Conference in 1996 in Washington, DC, keynote speakers J.P. Mortola, and A.M. Walker presented their views on mechanisms of SIDS: 'Hypoxia and Neonatal Respiration' and 'Potential Neural Mechanisms in SIDS', respectively. Mortola presented the view that neonatal mammals were relatively resistant to hypoxia and utilized a thermoregulatory mechanism to reduce core temperature and metabolic demand in response to hypoxia. Although less oxygen was available to the organism, less was required at a lower core temperature. He also offered the analogy of a car which may fail to successfully travel up a mountainous road. He suggested that there may be less wrong with the car than what the car was expected to do under the conditions prevailing at altitude on a dirt road in the mountains. It is generally accepted that SIDS is caused by multiple factors. It is significant that the overwhelming majority of SIDS occurs in apparently healthy full-term infants. There are some cases in which a neuropathologic deficit may be present, e.g. diminished muscarinic receptor development in the arcuate nucleus or decrease in kainate receptor binding in the neuropathologic specimens of infants who have succumbed to SIDS.[2] There may also be specific neuropathology associated with fetal and postnatal nicotine/cigarette smoke exposure which may explain the 4–5 times[3] higher incidence of SIDS in this population. Since the introduction of the 'Back to Sleep' campaigns for healthy infants, the risk for SIDS and the incidence have dramatically decreased by 50%. The effect of sleep position on sleep/arousal and modification of the infant's interaction with the environment is a fascinating and important area for research which will inform us about infant development and adaptational boundaries or limits. The common lay public point of view is that infants are physiologically robust if they are 'healthy' and in a 'routine' community environment. The 'car' analogy and the success of supine sleep position raise serious questions about what the physiological boundaries are for the average healthy infant who may be confronted with a variety of exogenous stressors (e.g. increased heating and upper respiratory tract infection) at a critical time in development.

Dr Walker's review primarily addressed issues of apnea, arousal, and respiratory control. There is still considerable emphasis on the apnea hypothesis and SIDS (Fig. 7.1) even though the general professional consensus is that the incidence of SIDS will not be reduced by apnea detection and monitoring. Nevertheless, in this paradigm the mechanism of SIDS lies in a series of events, e.g. respiratory arrest (apnea) which leads to hypoxia, hypercarbia and eventually death. In the text to follow, we will focus primarily on sleep, arousal, circadian rhythms and thermoregulatory factors and their integration or interactions to maintain vital homeostatic function and the physiologic adjustments required with endogenous and exogenous environmental stressors (Fig. 7.2).

Because most SIDS deaths occur during periods of presumed sleep or may result from a failure to arouse from sleep, it is necessary to understand the brain mechanisms that modify sleep and arousal during development and the manner

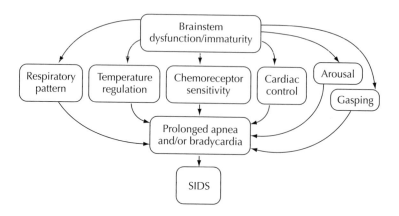

Fig. 7.1   Cardiorespiratory control hypothesis for SIDS.

in which such modulators of sleep architecture influence cardiorespiratory control. In addition to the temporal association of the SIDS event with sleep, any theory of SIDS must explain the fact that the majority of deaths occur during a relatively narrow developmental window at 1–3 months postnatal age. An important epidemiologic finding in SIDS which draws attention to the specific developmental period of infants' vulnerability is that, in addition to the peak of SIDS between 1–3 months of age, the median postnatal age (PNA) at death increases with decreasing gestational age (GA) and birth weight (BW).[4] Infants >2500 g BW had a peak age of SIDS at 83 days PNA; those with BW between 1500 and 2500 g at 92 days PNA, and those with BW ≤1500 g at 127 days PNA. It appears that when a correction is made for prematurity, the time of death occurs at similar postconceptional age. In California, although the risk of SIDS is less than 1 per 1000 for full-term babies, the incidence increases sharply in preterm infants; to 3.8 for 2000 to 2500 g BW; to 6.4 for 1500 to 2000 g BW, and to 7.5 for less than 1500 g BW babies. The incidence of SIDS in low birth weight infants with other medical problems such as bronchopulmonary dysplasia may be even greater. However, in the published reports there has often been an underemphasis on the role of chronic lung failure or dysfunction and an overemphasis on the SIDS diagnosis.

Sleep, arousal and circadian rhythms

The close temporal association between SIDS and sleep suggests that wakefulness or arousal provides protective mechanisms for survival. Arousal thresholds for respiratory, tactile, thermal and visual stimuli during sleep in infants presumably at risk for SIDS are raised. In addition spontaneous arousal from sleep to waking, or the ability to make a transition from one sleep state to another in these infants when confronted with a life-threatening challenge, is deficient. At

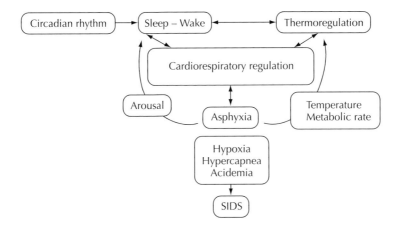

Fig. 7.2 Arousal and brain homeostatic control (hypothesis for SIDS).

1–3 months postnatal age significant changes occur in sleep organization, thermoregulation, circadian rhythms, and in the modulation of brainstem centers involved in cardiorespiratory and arousal state control. Furthermore, there is a circadian rhythm in the occurrence of SIDS and SIDS infants show a higher threshold for arousal between 3 and 7 a.m. compared with controls.[5-7]

The most notable changes in the early neonatal period (between 1 and 3 months of age) include a decrease in the percentage and bout length of active sleep (AS) (or rapid eye movement [REM] sleep), a switch from neonatal sleep onset REM to adult-like quiet sleep (QS) (or non-REM [NREM]) sleep onset, an increase in the percentage and episode length of quiet sleep, an increase in quiet sleep EEG slow wave activity, a drop of body temperature during sleep at night and an emergence of a day/night rhythm of sleep–wake with increased longest sleep and waking episodes. The development of circadian rhythms takes place during the peak incidence of SIDS, at 1–3 months of age. Our longitudinal studies in full-term infants showed a significant increase of circadian rhythm of body temperature in this period (Fig. 7.3). We are currently examining the maturation of circadian rhythm of body temperature in our preterm infant population. Although we have not yet completed the analysis of development of circadian rhythms in these infants longitudinally, at approximately 36 weeks postconceptional age (Fig. 7.3) and at 1 month corrected age (Fig. 7.4) these infants had not established a circadian rhythm of body temperature with a night-time trough to the degree found in term infants. Preterm infants recorded for three consecutive days at 36 weeks postconceptional and at 3 months corrected ages had established sleep consolidation (i.e. circadian rhythm of sleep–wake) at night by 3 months of age (Table 7.1).

Beginning at 2 months of age normal infants show a significant decline in slow wave (delta) EEG power across the night similar to that seen in adults.[8]

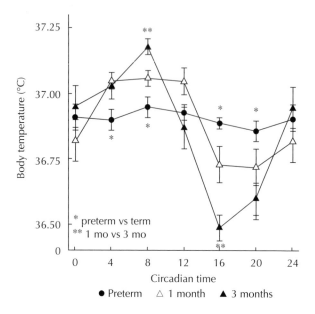

Fig. 7.3 Mean rectal temperature circadian waveforms observed in preterm (35 weeks postconceptional age), 1 month full-term, and 3 months full-term infants. Data are shown as mean values ± SEM in 4-hour bins. Circadian Time 0 = 8 a.m. Note the significant increase in rhythm amplitude in the full-term infants during both the subjective day and subjective night, and the pronounced body temperature trough at night in the nadir at 3 months of age.

Differences in temporal patterning of EEG delta power indicates differences in the depth of sleep at particular times of the night and may provide objective measures for the 'failure to arouse' hypothesis of SIDS deaths during sleep. Arousal threshold is higher during deep quiet sleep (high EEG delta power) than during REM sleep or remaining quiet sleep.[9] Preterm infants, at corrected age, had fewer and shorter duration of arousals during 12 hour night-time sleep compared with full-term infants.[10,11] In a recent study by Schechtman *et al.*[5] it was shown that siblings of SIDS show higher amount of delta EEG activity during night-time sleep at 2–4 months of age. Another developmental change during this critical period is the drop of body temperature during the night sleep.[12–14] No systematic study has been carried out to evaluate the time and rate of body temperature decline during sleep in high-versus low-risk infants, although it is known from adult studies that body temperature decline determines the depth of sleep and the level of arousal.[15] It is important to stress that the effectiveness of any life-threatening stimulus to induce arousal may depend not only on sleep state, but also on age, prior amount of sleep, circadian rhythm of body temperature, EEG delta power density, time of the day and sleeping environment.[16]

Although it is generally agreed that SIDS typically occurs during sleep, it is unclear whether SIDS occurs during sleep itself, within transitions between sleep and waking, or between sleep states. Nevertheless, the links between the peak occurrence of SIDS (1–3 months of age) and circadian rhythm, sleep, and body temperature regulation development suggest that SIDS is state-related and involves abnormal interactions between state-modulated arousability, central regulatory systems, and peripheral cardioventilatory mechanisms.[17] It is also generally agreed that infants who are at risk for SIDS may have CNS abnormalities at birth that may be too subtle to detect clinically; nevertheless, most of the SIDS pathologic data show abnormalities in the brainstem and hypothalamus, areas involved in sleep, arousal, thermoregulation, circadian rhythms, and central cardiorespiratory control.[2,18–22] Some studies have found abnormalities in sleep characteristics of infants who die of SIDS and siblings of SIDS infants.[16] These studies have led some to propose that the arousal threshold in the sleep of SIDS infants is higher than normal, and such infants may fail to arouse when a prolonged apneic event occurs.

SIDS infants may have difficulty in making the transition from sleep to wakefulness and between sleep stages, which could suggest that they would have more difficulty arousing from sleep. Furthermore, the finding[23,24] that differences in sleep organization exist as early as the first week of life suggests that prenatal factors may be important determinants in the development of sleep in these infant groups. Moreover, studied infants who later died of SIDS had more waking in the period immediately following sleep onset and much less waking during the end of the sleep period (between 3 and 7 a.m.). This is the converse of what is expected if a normal circadian body temperature (night-time body temperature trough and delta power) were normally developed. The important finding of fewer waking epochs during sleep, a characteristic of state organization in infants at risk, has been replicated by other laboratories. For complete references see Glotzbach, Ariagno, and Harper.[16]

Challamel and colleagues[25] found that sleep of high-risk infants, relative to controls, had (a) more total sleep time (TST) at 1.5, 4.5 and 6 months of age; (b) fewer awakenings (longer than one minute epochs) at 1.5 and 3 months; (c) more REM at 3 months; and (d) similar to the Guilleminault and colleagues data a decrease in deep NREM at 6 months of age.[26,27] The authors view the increased REM at 3 months in SIDS infants as secondary to the decrease in awakenings seen at this age. The hypothesis of a long-standing deficit in arousal mechanisms in SIDS infants is supported by the finding that some high-risk infants that were studied at 9 and 12 months of age still had fewer awakenings than controls. Similarly, Navelet et al.[28] studied sleep organization in control and high-risk infants using overnight polysomnography and found that high-risk infants less than 3 months of age had less wakefulness, in agreement with the findings of Harper et al.[29] High-risk infants also had more AS and longer QS and AS bout lengths, resulting in an increase in sleep cycle duration. The authors concluded that the sleep patterns of high-risk infants indicate a disturbance of sleep/wake organization, and that a decrease in wakefulness or an increase in the arousal threshold contributes to an increase in the risk for SIDS. All of these studies suggest that there is a disturbance in state organization and an apparent dampening of arousal mechanisms, which support the hypothesis that a failure of neural mechanisms regulating sleep and arousal is a key factor in SIDS. Reduced cardiorespiratory control responsivity in SIDS infants is suggested by fewer sustained interbeat heart rate changes in infants who later died of SIDS. Additionally, obstruction of the upper airway is normally terminated by an arousal, with restoration of upper airway muscle tone. When arousal fails, the SIDS mechanism can be viewed primarily as an impaired ability to make the transition to wakefulness, even though the event may have been *initiated* by an obstructed upper airway. Of particular interest is the fact that short-term sleep deprivation caused a pronounced increase in the number and duration of obstructive apneas during active sleep.[30] Because of the prominent effects of temperature on sleep and breathing, it will be important to investigate any possible synergistic effects of temperature and sleep depth on oxygen saturation, apnea, bradycardia, and arousal.

Although it is tempting to argue that the assessment of state organization in infants should have the potential to be a clinical diagnostic test for risk of SIDS, it is important to emphasize that these are group differences, and that there is exceptionally high variability in individual state measures.[31] *Intragroup* variability may result from environmental and infant factors, or from the instability of recording measures collected on only one night at any given developmental age. *Intergroup* variability may also be influenced by homogeneity of infant groups; for example, siblings of SIDS victims have been considered to be at 4–10 fold higher risk for SIDS than control infants. Even allowing for the high end of this spectrum, (i.e. a 2% vs 0.2% incidence of SIDS in siblings), a practical question is whether (and when) a consistent disorder or abnormality occurs in all siblings, or, considering the other extreme, whether 98% of SIDS siblings do not differ from controls.

Influence of sleeping position on sleep

Kahn and coworkers[32] have reported that prone sleeping position can increase total sleep time and NREM sleep and decrease arousal in term infants during the first 3 months of life. Our own studies of healthy preterm infants approaching discharge from the hospital, in which we examined the effect of sleep position on sleep organization, showed no significant differences in total sleep time or any significant change in sleep state distribution. However the number of awakenings were always greater in supine position (Table 7.2). Furthermore, when the sleep characteristics between supine and prone position during the first sleep cycle following a feeding were compared, the length of the first quiet sleep bout was significantly longer in prone (20 vs 15 minutes; Table 7.3).[33]

Table 7.2 Comparison of sleep characteristics between supine and prone position throughout the recording[†]

	Supine	Prone	*P*-value
AS (%)	70.2±6.8	68.8±6.9	0.52[S]
IS (%)	5.7±2.9	5.2±2.5	0.65[S]
QS (%)	24.1±7.3	25.9±2.5	0.36[S]
No. awakening in (AS+IS) /100 min	11.2±8.1	6.7±4.2	0.02[W]*
No. awakening in QS /100 min	5.8±12.1	0.8±3.1	0.01[W]*

Values are mean ± SD. Group differences were evaluated with paired t-test ([s]) or Wilcoxon signed-rank test ([W]). **P*-value < 0.05.
[†] Modified from Goto *et al.*, 1999.

Table 7.3 Comparison of sleep characteristics (minutes) between supine and prone position during first sleep cycle[†]

	Supine	Prone	*P*-value
Length of 1st AS	24.1±20.0	24.3±13.0	0.84
Length of 1st QS	15.0±5.8	20.1±6.3	0.02*
Length of 2nd AS	60.5±25.8	60.6±19.3	0.93
No. awakening in 1st AS/100 min	6.8±9.3	1.8±3.0	0.09
No. awakening in 1st QS/100 min	4.5±8.4	1.0±3.2	0.04*
No. awakening in 2nd AS/100 min	9.4±5.9	6.9±5.0	0.07
No. arousal in 1st AS/100 min	14.3±11.8	20.5±16.5	0.26
No. arousal in 1st QS/100 min	9.2±11.6	5.8±6.5	0.27
No. arousal in 2nd AS/100 min	21.5±11.7	18.5±8.8	0.30
Longest bout of AS in first 'AS'	14.6±10.8	21.8±9.3	0.06
Longest bout of QS in first 'QS'	14.7±6.4	18.9±6.7	0.02*
Longest bout of AS in second 'AS'	19.0±13.8	29.9±20.5	0.04*

Values are mean ± SD. Group differences were evaluated with Wilcoxon signed-rank test. **P*-value < 0.05.
[†] Modified from Goto *et al.*, 1999.

Respiratory and cardiac mechanisms during sleep in SIDS

RESPIRATORY CONTROL

A potential fatal scenario in a SIDS event includes *upper airway obstruction*, presumably during sleep. This hypothesis is supported by the frequent finding of intrathoracic petechiae at autopsy in SIDS victims (85%).[34] Petechiae are found in a variety of other circumstances; however, the particular distribution within the thorax in SIDS victims argues strongly for substantial negative thoracic pressure generating this sign. Few studies indeed measure upper airway pressure and diaphragmatic movements during sleep to detect obstructed events.

Two major characteristics of respiratory control during sleep may contribute to the potential for airway obstruction. First, although respiratory patterning is regular during QS, inspiratory time and negative thoracic pressures are enhanced. Excessive negative pressures accompanied by upper airway obstruction may lead to further airway collapse from the Venturi effect. Second, together with extreme variation in respiratory patterning during REM sleep, a substantial loss of upper airway and thoracic wall muscle tone develops; the decrease in tone is so marked as to cause paradoxical rib cage movements in young infants and a concomitant fall in vital capacity.[35] Atonia in upper airway muscles during active sleep may contribute to obstruction by increasing compliance in the pharyngeal airway. Investigations which have partitioned upper air flow and diaphragmatic activity suggest that there may be a propensity for obstructive apnea during AS.[36] Siblings of SIDS infants may breathe faster,[37] and infants who later succumb to SIDS have fewer short central apnea in both QS and REM at ages near the peak incidence of SIDS.[23] These data suggest that respiratory patterning in these infants is less responsive to other physiologic influences (respiratory, baroreceptor, or other somatic input) which normally influence breathing rate. No differences in *overall* respiratory rate or variability have been noted in infants who later die.

Normally, obstructions of the upper airway are successfully terminated by an arousal, with restoration of upper airway muscle tone by so-called 'wakefulness stimuli'.[38] One might argue that the 'cause' of the fatal event is initiated by an obstructed upper airway, but that the mechanism for failure is an inability to make the transition to the waking state, a transition which a normally adapting infant should accomplish. Within the context of 'failure to arouse', the relative propensities for arousal from different states is an issue. Responses to nasal obstruction appear to be more frequent in AS compared to QS,[39] but the effectiveness of stimuli to induce arousal may differ by state and age.[9,40] For example, the percentages of failures to arouse in response to a vibrotactile stimulus remained consistently higher in QS than AS over the first 6 months of life in normal infants.[9] However, a significant increase in the percentage of failure to arouse in AS occurred at 3 months of age. Read and colleagues have recently shown consistently higher arousal threshold during QS vs AS in infants studied at 2–3 weeks and again at 2–3 months.[41] Moreover, arousal threshold was higher in the second vs first QS period. Regression analysis showed no correlation between the length of time the infant had been in a particular sleep state and the arousal threshold in either state in 2–3 weeks of age or in AS for 2–3 months of age; however the arousal threshold increased significantly with time in QS in 2–3 month-old infants.

Walker *et al.*[42] point out that latencies to arousal in response to acute reductions in blood pressure in lambs are longer in REM than in NREM sleep, and that arousal is impaired in both sleep states compared to wakefulness. In a newborn lamb study by the Harding group,[43] obstruction of respiratory airflow by face mask occlusion induced arousal more rapidly and with less oxygen desaturation and cardiac deceleration during NREM vs REM. Repeated episodes of airflow obstruction led to reduced arousability only in REM sleep. They concluded that arousal from REM, but not NREM, sleep in response to obstruction of respiratory airflow is transiently depressed during early development and repeated obstructions and arousals also lead to a further depression of arousal response from REM sleep. In another study in infant lambs it was shown that upper airway obstruction triggers complex and coordinated laryngeal and abdominal muscle responses during wakefulness and NREM sleep; these compensatory responses are largely absent in REM sleep.[44] One should be careful in applying data from newborn lambs, which are more mature at birth, to the human infant. Nevertheless, these results are interesting in the light of the increased vulnerability to upper airway obstruction during sleep. Another perspective is that endogenous/exogenous stressors in certain infants during a narrow critical developmental period may *actively inhibit* respiratory and arousal responses by virtue of defective maturation of the brain arousal system *per se*.[45]

CARDIAC PATTERNING

The normal development of heart rate and its variability does not follow simple linear trends from birth; moreover, the trends markedly differ by state.[46] The developmental period near 1 month of age is of particular interest because of a peak in heart rate, a trough in heart rate variation values for QS, and the beginning of disparate trends in variation in other states during that time. The non-uniform overall patterns of heart rate variation direct attention to the different sources of instantaneous variation contributing to moment-to-moment changes in heart rate. It is now apparent that sources of heart rate changes differ radically with sleep state, and that different components of the autonomic nervous system are recruited to mediate these changes.

Studies of cardiac rate mean and variability have established that infants who later succumb to SIDS have higher heart rates in all states[47,48] and diminished heart rate variation in waking, particularly by variation induced by breathing.[48,49] Siblings of SIDS victims also have higher heart rates, especially in QS.[50] Recent evidence of prolongation of interval in the first week of life associated with SIDS is very interesting[51] but the potential clinical applicability of this finding is very controversial. The infants in this study were most likely recorded in a supine position during a relatively quiet, motionless period. Our own studies support that, although heart rate variability may be influenced by sleep position, and state these factors do not appear to influence the $Q-T_c$ interval. Thus the ion channel in the heart and the $Q-T_c$ are more dependent on inherent cardiac and other metabolic factors.

Examination of cardiac interbeat variability provides insights into the nature of physiological responsivity underlying autonomic control in the developing infant, and has the potential for identifying characteristics of infants at risk for SIDS. This utility stems from the exquisite sensitivity of cardiac interval patterning to sympathetic and parasympathetic activity of the autonomic nervous system, and the recognition that components of heart rate variation can be analysed to determine the sources of the underlying variation. Dynamic procedures reveal cardiac interval dispersion differences during sleep states in infants who later succumbed to SIDS.

SIDS infants show a distribution of cardiac interbeat dispersion with changing heart rate similar to that seen for infants with congenital central hypoventilation syndrome[24,52]; however, the pattern is much less pronounced. Although heart rate showed considerable variation, one interval to next interval dispersion differed from control infants in that it did not increase as rate decreased. Moreover, cardiac rate appeared to be 'clamped' around central values; i.e. a change in interval was more frequently followed by a change in the opposite direction in SIDS victims, relative to controls. These findings suggest more rigid control of cardiac variation in SIDS victims, although *overall* variation is only minimally restricted.

The *loss of change* in one cardiac interval to next interval variation at different heart rates suggests that the cardiovascular system is less responsive to modulation by other physiologic systems in those infants who succumb. The other physiologic systems may be somatomotor (respiratory influences perhaps being one source), temperature, or even baroreceptor. The interpretation of reduced responsivity is reinforced by examining patterns of heart rate changes. Infants who later succumb to SIDS show fewer sustained interbeat changes than controls. Thus, the development of sources contributing to cardiac variability appears to differ in infants at risk.

Other lines of evidence suggest some alteration of the autonomic nervous system in infants who later succumb to SIDS. Both parasympathetic and sympathetic components appear to be subtly modified; the evidence for sympathetic activation derives from findings of enhanced sweating in SIDS victims,[53] while the altered variation in heart rate intervals described earlier, including the diminished respiratory influences on heart rate variation, suggests altered vagal outflow.

In a recent study of low-risk preterm infants[33] we found that spontaneous heart rate variability was less in prone vs supine position during QS (Table 7.4). Spontaneous heart rate variability at any given time represents the net effect of the parasympathetic and sympathetic influences. Since vagal tone may be a significant contributor to resting heart rate, we speculate that the balance of

Table 7.4. Comparison of heart rate (HR) mean and heart variability (mean of SD of HR) between the supine and prone position the 1st active and quiet periods[†]

	Supine	Prone	*P*-value
AS			
Mean HR	156.2±9.4	152.2±13.3	0.02[M]
Mean of SD of HR	5.4±3.2	5.8± 2.7	0.09[M]
QS			
Mean HR	149.2±11.3	146.1±13.4	0.06[S]
Mean of SD of HR	4.0±2.3	2.8±1.5	<0.001[M]*

Values are mean ± SD. Group differences were evaluated with paired *t*-test ([S]) or Mann–Whitney U test ([M]).**P*-value < 0.05.
[†] Modified from Goto *et al.*, 1999.

sympathetic and parasympathetic tone, both of which are influenced by numerous physiologic factors, and circadian rhythm, is also affected by sleep position in early infancy. In a recent study Galland *et al.* also found less heart rate variability in the prone position in 2–4 month-old term infants.[54] They also found that full awakening to tilting was common in active sleep but significantly less in the prone position. They concluded blunted arousal responses and/or altered autonomic function are a feature of the prone sleeping position. In accordance with these results Franco *et al.*[55,56] showed that prone sleeping was associated with a decrease in cardiac responses to auditory stimulation and a possible increase in orthosympathetic activity in full-term infants with a median age of 1 week. Although these studies were not carried out in infants at risk for SIDS they may explain the mechanism by which the 'Back to Sleep' campaign may have reduced the rate of SIDS.

Thermoregulatory control

Ambient temperature has marked effects on the distribution of arousal states.[36,57,58] At the onset of sleep the circadian regulated decline in body temperature is preceded by decreases in hypothalamic thresholds for heat loss and heat production responses. In an over-bundled infant in warm surroundings where passive heat loss is at a minimum, the core temperature may not be able to follow the fall in the set points for thermoregulatory responses at sleep onset. In terms of the thermoregulatory system, this situation would be interpreted as hyperthermia even though actual core temperature is normal. An immediate consequence would be vasodilation, thus warming the skin. The combination of warm skin and high core temperature (relative to set points) would reduce the incidence of spontaneous arousals.

Environmental and core temperatures may play a direct role in SIDS mechanisms through their specific influences on sleep architecture, heart rate, respiration, and arousal. Warm ambient temperatures could: decrease arousal, increase bradycardia and/or apnea, decrease thermoregulatory and cardiorespiratory homeostatic mechanisms,[59] and lead to a reduction in upper airway patency, particularly in high-risk babies. We predict, based on recent studies,[5,11,60] that higher delta power and the circadian body temperature trough will counteract arousability. Infants who later died of SIDS had more waking in the period immediately following sleep onset and much less waking during the end of the sleep period (between 3 and 7 a.m.),[7,23] opposite to what normal sleep propensity (measured by delta power density) and circadian body temperature would predict and contrary to what is found in normal low-risk, full-term infants.

Several groups have reported an association between cold outdoor temperatures or excessive warming of infants and increased rates of SIDS.[61-63] Seasonal variation in SIDS with a peak in winter is in accordance with this. In some infants there may be an intrinsic problem of body temperature regulation and elevation of body temperature beyond the capacity of the infant's regulatory range. Stanton[64] found 'higher-than-expected' body temperatures in SIDS victims postmortem. Naeye[65] found that some SIDS victims had experienced more bouts of hypothermia and hyperthermia compared with control infants, and Kahn and colleagues[66] noted that many infants considered to be at higher risk for SIDS are observed to sweat more than normal infants. Temperature can modulate sleep state distribution, with decreased sleep and a relatively lower percentage of REM sleep as ambient temperature deviates from thermoneutrality.[15] Warm temperatures in the upper thermoneutral zone enhance sleep, and also result in more apneic periods and in reduced upper airway patency.[67–70] Many SIDS victims are reported to have had a mild illness just prior to their death; fever or the sleep disruption resulting from the illness could increase the number of obstructive apneic events,[30] and could result in the depth and duration of recovery sleep with an increased arousal threshold. Thus, temperature could influence SIDS risk by multiple routes via an interaction with sleep, respiratory control, and arousal mechanisms.

In the normal infant, thermoregulatory effector mechanisms (i.e. evaporative water loss; metabolic heat production) are operating soon after birth. Unfortunately, little data are available on the development in these effector systems during sleep state transitions, or on how the system response characteristics in REM sleep compare with those in NREM sleep. Our data from 27 healthy full-term infants (two were siblings of SIDS) during the first 6 months of life demonstrated robust increases (except for one) in evaporative water loss (EWL) to a warm environment (warming was stopped if rectal temperature exceeded 37.6°C) during sleep (REM and QS). Total sleep time and REM sleep increased significantly during warming. During warming the number of short arousals during REM increased but did not lead to awakening. None of these infants had pathologic apneas and the duration and frequency of clinically insignificant short central apneas was similar in the warm vs the control study periods. Azaz and coworkers[71] also found similar EWL responses to an increase in environmental temperature during QS and REM sleep in 22 healthy infants during the first 3 months of life. Furthermore, an increase in metabolic rate was seen in response to a mild decrease in environmental temperature during both sleep states. Bach and coworkers[72] studied 10 healthy newborns at 35–39 weeks postconceptional age and also found no impairment in the thermoregulatory response to warm and cool environments during active sleep. These studies support that sweating and active thermoregulation is not inhibited during REM or active sleep in the first 6 months of life in infants. These findings are in contrast to reports on adults in whom thermoregulation responses are markedly inhibited and who instead respond by arousal/awakening. The limits of the healthy infant's thermoregulatory capacity and arousal during sleep have not been tested. Heavy clothing in a warm environment may be more than the average infant can tolerate. Finally, the temperature effects on breathing may be independent from the influence of temperature on sleep and arousal.[73]

Additionally, Wailoo et al.[74] found that over 75% of infants 3–4 months of age aroused the parents at least once during the night and that this pattern was related to the thermal environment of the infant: the higher the room temperature or the greater the amount of bedclothes, the more often babies awoke their parents, and the majority of the infants who aroused their parents were found sweating. If an infant is unable to arouse in response to a high environmental temperature (or if a parent is unable to respond), then the infant may be at higher risk for SIDS.

Prone sleeping position has been associated with increased SIDS risk.[75–78] Ponsonby *et al.*[79] concluded that the association between prone sleeping position and elevated risk of SIDS is increased by four independent factors: (a) the use of natural-fiber mattresses; (b) swaddling; (c) recent illness; and (d) the use of heating in bedrooms. Guntheroth and Spiers[80] reviewed seven studies on sleeping position and SIDS, and calculated that the relative risk for SIDS is increased by 3.5 to 9.3 fold in the prone sleeping position, and recommended that infants avoid the prone sleeping position during the first six months of life. Similarly, the American Academy of Pediatrics, based on a review of the available literature, recommended that healthy infants be positioned on their side or back when being put down for sleep.[81,82] Some investigators have postulated that the mechanisms underlying the association between sleeping position and SIDS involve increase in body temperature due to decreases in heat loss through the face[60] and from the convex surface of the trunk of the body and potential additional heat loss surface from unencumbered extremities. However, Petersen *et al.*[14] found that the prone sleeping position was associated with only a small decrease in the effectiveness of heat loss in low-risk full-term infants. Since core body temperature vs time of night did not differ in infants sleeping prone vs supine, these authors concluded that during the first 6 months of life, normal infants can thermoregulate effectively in a variety of thermal environments independent of sleeping position.

A number of recent studies suggest that lethal rebreathing and accidental suffocation may occur in conjunction with the prone sleeping position in specific sleep environments. After examination of the death scene, Kemp and Thach[83,84] used a rabbit model, in which rabbits breathed into bedding materials through the airway of an infant mannequin, to simulate an infant's respiratory microenvironment. They concluded that accidental suffocation by rebreathing was the most likely cause of death in infants who were found face down, and certain types of cushions may hamper an infant's ability to turn their head to avoid excessive CO_2 accumulation. Therefore, there may be a need to reassess the cause of death in the victims of SIDS who are found with their faces straight down (approximately 25–50%), and the potential for lethal rebreathing needs to be established for conventional infant mattresses, bedding, and sheepskins.[83,84] Even infants with a head position of 45° relative to the bedding may experience a rapid buildup of CO_2 and depletion of O_2, posing a hazard especially in infants less than 3 months of age, at which time controlling lifting of the head is still maturing.[85] Actual measurements of environmental CO_2 levels in normal infants in a head covered or face down orientation[86] show significantly higher maximum CO_2 environmental concentrations when the head was covered at 2.5 months (median values 1.8% vs 1.4% prone) and 5 months of age (median values 1.7% vs 0.8% prone). However, transcutaneous CO_2 levels in the infants were all in the physiologic range (e.g. for the 2.5-month-old infant; 40.3, 41.1 mmHg covered and not covered when prone vs 39.9, 40 mmHg covered and not covered when supine). Comparable values were seen in the 5-month-old infants.

Thach and coworkers[87] have reported increased sequential arousal and airway defensive behavior for healthy infants 0.5 to 6 months of age in a prone face down asphyxial sleep environment by covering the head with a blanket. Increased sighs, startles and full arousals were seen as the inspired CO_2 increased (maximum value about 3%). Recent studies of head position during sleep in prone preterm infants supports that the side head position remains unchanged during sleep. Their data also point to a disturbance in respiratory pattern, and possibly a failure which includes upper airway obstruction in the terminal event; the event may become catastrophic as a result of the depressed arousal mechanisms described earlier.

We hypothesize that delayed/disturbed circadian rhythm of body temperature and/or disturbances in coupling between delta EEG power ('process S'– sleep propensity) and body temperature ('process C' – circadian-dependent changes in body temperature) put babies at high risk for disruption of homeostatic brain control of cardiorespiratory adaptation and can lead to sudden death. Understanding the maturation and interaction of sleep, arousability, circadian rhythm, and thermoregulation at different stages of development is essential to appreciate normal brain homeostatic control and abnormalities which may predispose infants to SIDS.

Summary

Throughout the fetal, neonatal and infant development period, the maturation of physiologic homeostatic regulatory systems show considerable overlap. Of particular relevance to SIDS are systems controlling sleep states, arousal states, circadian rhythms, body temperature, breathing, and cardiac control. In the adult, profound interactions occur between these regulatory systems; dependencies occur between physiologic systems in the developing infant, but the description of these interactions is still unfolding. Sleep states, which are also undergoing development, provide overriding switches which change interactions between different physiologic systems. At present, it is not possible to conclude which sleep state, AS or QS, represents a more inherently vulnerable period for the infant. Higher arousal thresholds have been demonstrated in both AS and QS. It is quite probable that *each* sleep state may provide periods of vulnerability depending on both the nature of the infant and of environmental events, and upon sleep history.

The available evidence suggests that some infants who succumb to SIDS manifest signs of physiologic and state disturbance from the first week of life. Together with epidemiologic evidence demonstrating that maternal smoking, inadequate prenatal medical care, and maternal anemia are associated with increased risk for SIDS, these signs underscore the importance of clarifying the importance of prenatal events in SIDS etiology. The physiologic evidence strongly suggests some alteration in state and circadian rhythms organization that depresses arousal mechanisms in SIDS victims. Evidence exists that autonomic influences controlling temperature, or some failure of temperature regulation, may be associated with the fatal event. Since the final event in SIDS appears to be intimately involved with sleep and in the interaction of sleep with cardiorespiratory control systems, it is imperative to analyse and understand the role of sleep state, circadian and thermoregulatory effects to clarify mechanisms leading to SIDS.

Acknowledgements

This work was supported by NIH Grants HD29732 and HD35754–01A1, by the Bloomingdale's Fund, by The Pediatric SIDS Research Fund of Stanford University School of Medicine, Christina Delmonico Memorial Fund, and by NWO, the Netherlands.

References

1. Filiano JJ, Kinney HC. A perspective on neuropathologic findings in victims of the sudden infant death syndrome: the triple-risk model. *Biol Neonate* 1994;65:194–7.
2. Kinney HC, Filiano JJ, Sleeper LA, Mandell F, Valdes-Dapena M, White WF. Decreased muscarinic receptor binding in the arcuate nucleus in sudden infant death syndrome. *Science* 1995;269:1446–50.
3. Mitchell E, Ford R, Stewart A *et al.* Smoking and the sudden infant death syndrome. *Pediatrics* 1993;91:893–6.
4. Grether JK, Schulman J. Sudden infant death syndrome and birth weight. *J Pediatr* 1989;114:561–7.
5. Schechtman VL, Harper RK, Harper RM. Aberrant temporal patterning of slow-wave sleep in siblings of SIDS victims [published erratum appears in *Electroencephalogr Clin Neurophysiol* 1995 Jun;94(6):473]. *Electroencephalogr Clin Neurophysiol* 1995;94:95–102.
6. Schechtman VL, Harper RM. Time of night effects on heart rate variation in normal neonates. *J Dev Physiol* 1991;16:349–53.
7. Schechtman VL, Harper RM, Wilson AJ, Southall DP. Sleep state organization in normal infants and victims of the sudden infant death syndrome. *Pediatrics* 1992;865–70.
8. Scher MS. A developmental marker of central nervous system maturation: Part I. *Pediatr Neurol* 1988;4:265–73.
9. Newman NM, Trinder JA, Phillips KA, Jordan K, Cruickshank J. Arousal deficit: mechanism of the sudden infant death syndrome? *Aust Paediatr J* 1989;25:196–201.
10. Scher MS, Steppe DA, Dahl RE, Asthana S, Guthrie RD. Comparison of EEG sleep measures in healthy full-term and preterm infants at matched conceptional ages. *Sleep* 1992;15:442–8.
11. Scher MS, Sun M, Steppe DA, Banks DL, Guthrie RD, Sclabassi RJ. Comparisons of EEG sleep state-specific spectral values between healthy full-term and preterm infants at comparable postconceptional ages. *Sleep* 1994;17:47–51.
12. Glotzbach S, Edgar D, Boeddiker M, Ariagno R. Biological rhythmicity in normal infants during the first three months of life. *Pediatrics* 1994;94:482–8.

13. Glotzbach SF, Edgar DM, Ariagno RL. Biological rhythmicity in preterm infants prior to discharge from neonatal intensive care. *Pediatrics* 1995;95:231–7.

14. Petersen SA, Anderson ES, Lodemore M, Rawson D, Wailoo MP. Sleeping position and rectal temperature. *Arch Dis Child* 1991;66:976–9.

15. Glotzbach SF, Heller HC. Temperature Regulation. In: Kryger MH, Roth T, Dement WC (eds). *Principles and Practice of Sleep Medicine*, 2nd edn. W.B. Saunders, Philadelphia, 1994, pp. 260–75.

16. Glotzbach SF, Ariagno RL, Harper RM. Sleep and the sudden infant death syndrome. In: Ferber R, Kryger MH (eds). *Principles and Practice of Sleep Medicine in the Child*. W.B. Saunders, Philadelphia, 1995, pp. 231–44.

17. Kinney H. Brain research in sudden infant death syndrome. In: Walker A, McMillen C (eds.) *Second SIDS International Conference*. Perinatology Press, Ithaca, 1993, pp. 13–23.

18. Kopp N, Denoroy L, Saint-Pierre G, Jordan D. [Abnormalities of the nervous system in sudden infant death syndrome.] *Pediatrie* 1992;47:429–39.

19. Kinney H, Brody B, Finkelstein D, Vawter G, Mandell F, Giles F. Delayed central nervous system myelination in the sudden infant death syndrome. *J Neuropath Exp Neurol* 1991;50:29–48.

20. Kinney HC, Filiano JJ, Harper RM. The neuropathology of the sudden infant death syndrome. A review. *J Neuropathol Exp Neurol* 1992;51:115–26.

21. Gilson TP, Balko MG, Blisard KS, Taylor KL. Morphologic variations of the external arcuate nucleus in infants dying of SIDS: a preliminary report [see comments]. *J Forensic Sci* 1994;39:1076–83.

22. Byard RW, Carmichael E, Beal S. How useful is postmortem examination in sudden infant death syndrome? *Pediatr Pathol* 1994;14:817–22.

23. Schechtman VL, Harper RM, Wilson AJ, Southall DP. Sleep apnea in infants who succumb to the sudden infant death syndrome. *Pediatrics* 1991;87:841–6.

24. Schechtman VL, Raetz SL, Harper RK *et al*. Dynamic analysis of cardiac R-R intervals in normal infants and in infants who subsequently succumbed to the sudden infant death syndrome. *Pediatr Res* 1992;31:606–12.

25. Challamel MJ, Debilly G, Leszczynski MC, Revol M. Sleep state development in near-miss sudden infant death infants. In: Harper RM, Hoffman HJ (eds). *Sudden Infant Death Syndrome: Risk Factors and Basic Mechanisms*. PMA Publishing Corp., New York, 1988, pp. 423–34.

26. Guilleminault C, Ariagno R, Korobkin R, Coons S, Owen BM, Baldwin R. Sleep parameters and respiratory variables in 'near miss' sudden infant death syndrome infants. *Pediatrics* 1981;68:354–60.

27. Guilleminault C, Coons S. Sleep states and maturation of sleep: A comparative study between full-term normal controls and near-miss SIDS infants. In: Tildon JT, Roeder LM, Steinschneider A (eds). *Sudden Infant Death Syndrome*. Academic Press, New York, 1983, pp. 401–11.

28. Navelet Y, Payan C, Guilhaume A, Benoit O. Nocturnal sleep organization in infants 'at risk' for sudden infant death syndrome. *Pediatr Res* 1984;18:654–7.

29. Harper RM, Leake B, Hoffman H *et al*. Periodicity of sleep states is altered in infants at risk for the sudden infant death syndrome. *Science* 1981;213:1030–2.

30. Canet E, Gaultier C, D'Allest AM, Dehan M. Effects of sleep deprivation on respiratory events during sleep in healthy infants. *J Appl Physiol* 1989;66:1158–63.

31. Hoppenbrouwers T, Hodgman J, Arakawa K, Sterman MB. Polysomnographic sleep and waking states are similar in subsequent siblings of SIDS and control infants during the first six months of life. *Sleep* 1989;12:265–76.

32. Kahn A, Groswasser J, Sottiaux M, Rebuffat E, Franco P, Dramaix M. Prone or supine body position and sleep characteristics in infants. *Pediatrics* 1993;91:1112–5.

33. Goto K, Mirmiran M, Adams MM *et al.* More awakenings and heart rate variability during supine sleep in preterm infants. *Pediatrics* 1999;103:603–9.

34. Krous HF, Jordan J. A necropsy study of distribution of petechiae in non-sudden infant death syndrome. *Arch Pathol Lab Med* 1984;108:75–6.

35. Henderson-Smart DJ, Read DJC. Reduced lung volume during behavioral active sleep in the newborn. *J Appl Physiol* 1979;46:1081–5.

36. Kahn A, Wachholder A, Winkler M, Rebuffat E. Prospective study on the prevalence of sudden infant death and possible risk factors in Brussels: preliminary results (1987–1988). *Eur J Pediatr* 1990;149:284–6.

37. Hoppenbrouwers T, Hodgman JE, McGinty D, Harper RM, Sterman MB. Sudden infant death syndrome: sleep apnea and respiration in subsequent siblings. *Pediatrics* 1980;66:205–14.

38. Orem J. Neural basis of behavior and state-dependent control of breathing. In: Lydic R, Biebuyck JF (eds). *Clinical Physiology of Sleep.* American Physiological Society, Bethesda, 1988, pp. 79–96.

39. Newman NM, Frost JK, Bury L, Jordan K, Phillips K. Responses to partial nasal obstruction in sleeping infants. *Aust Paediatr J* 1986;22:111–6.

40. Igras D, Fewell JE. Arousal response to upper airway obstruction in young lambs: Comparison of nasal and tracheal occlusion. *J Devel Physiol* 1991;15:215–20

41. Read PA, Horne RSC, Cranage SM, Walker AM, Walker DW, Adamson TM. Dynamic changes in arousal threshold during sleep in the human infant. *Pediatr Res* 1998;43:697–703.

42. Walker AM, Horne RS, Bowes G, Berger P. The circulation in sleep in newborn lambs. *Aust Paediatr J* 1986;22:71–4.

43. Harding R, Jakubowska AE, McCrabb GJ. Arousal and cardiorespiratory responses to airflow obstruction in sleeping lambs: effects of sleep state, age, and repeated obstruction. *Sleep* 1997;20:693–701.

44. Kianicka I, Praud JP. Influence of sleep states on laryngeal and abdominal muscle response to upper airway occlusion in lambs. *Pediatr Res* 1997;4:862–71.

45. Morrison AR. Sleep, arousal, and motor control. In: Harper RM, Hoffman HJ (eds). *Sudden Infant Death Syndrome: Risk Factors and Basic Mechanisms.* PMA Publishing Corp., New York, 1988, pp. 347–59.

46. Harper RM, Hoppenbrouwers T, Sterman MB, McGinty DJ, Hodgman J. Polygraphic studies of normal infants during the first 6 months of life. I. Heart rate and variability as a function of state. *Pediatric Res* 1976;10:945–51.

47. Wilson AJ, Stevens V, Franks CI, Alexander J, Southall DP. Respiratory and heart rate patterns in infants destined to be victims of the sudden infant death syndrome: average rates and their variability measured over 24 hours. *Br Med J (Clin Res)* 1985;290:497–501.

48. Schechtman VL, Harper RM, Kluge KA, Wilson AJ, Hoffman HJ, Southall DP. Cardiac and respiratory patterns in normal infants and victims of the sudden infant death syndrome. *Sleep* 1988;11:413–24.

49. Kluge KA, Harper RM, Schechtman VL, Wilson AJ, Hoffman HJ, Southall DP. Spectral analysis assessment of respiratory sinus arrhythmia in normal infants and infants who subsequently died of sudden infant death syndrome. *Pediatr Res* 1988;24:677–82.

50. Harper RM, Leake B, Hodgman JE, Hoppenbrouwers T. Developmental patterns of heart rate and heart rate variability during sleep and waking in normal infants and infants at risk for the sudden infant death syndrome. *Sleep* 1982;5:28–38.

51. Schwartz PJ, Stramba-Badiale M, Segantini A *et al.* Prolongation of the QT interval and the sudden infant death syndrome. *N Engl J Med* 1998;338:1709–14.

52. Woo MA, Stevenson WG, Moser DK, Trelease RB, Harper RM. Patterns of beat-to-beat heart variability in advanced heart failure. *Am Heart J* 1992;123:704–10.

53. Kahn A, Groswasser J, Rebuffat E *et al.* Sleep and cardiorespiratory characteristics of infant victims of sudden death: a prospective case-control study. *Sleep* 1992;15:287–92.

54. Galland BC, Reeves G, Taylor BJ, Bolton DPG. Sleep position, autonomic function, and arousal. *Arch Dis Child* 1998;78:F189–F194.

55. Franco P, Groswasser J, Sottiaux M, Broadfield E, Kahn A. Decreased cardiac responses to auditory stimulation during prone sleep. *Pediatrics* 1996;97:174–8.

56. Franco P, Pardou A, Hassid S, Lurquin P, Grosswasser J, Kahn A. Auditory arousal thresholds are higher when infants sleep in the prone position. *J Pediatr* 1998;132:240–3.

57. Wellby ML, Farror CJ, Pannall PR. Importance of postmortem changes in measurements of thyroid function in studies of sudden infant death syndrome. *J Clin Pathol* 1987;40:631–2.

58. Southall DP. Role of apnea in the sudden infant death syndrome: a personal view. *Pediatrics* 1988;8:73–84.

59. Read DJC and Jeffries H. Many paths to asphyxial death in SIDS: A search for underlying defects. In: Tildon JT, Roeder LM, Steinschneider A (eds). *Sudden Infant Death Syndrome.* Academic Press, New York, 1983, pp.183–200.

60. Nelson EA, Taylor BJ, Weatherall IL. Sleeping position and infant bedding may predispose to hyperthermia and the sudden infant death syndrome. *Lancet* 1989;1:199–201.

61. Anderson SC, Murrell WG, O'Neill CC, Rahilly PM. Effect of ambient temperature on SIDS rate. *Med J Aust* 1993;158:703–4.

62. Ponsonby AL, Jones ME, Lumley J, Dwyer T, Gilbert N. Climatic temperature and variation in the incidence of sudden infant death syndrome between the Australian states. *Med J Aust* 1992;156:246–8, 51.

63. Mitchell EA, Stewart AW, Cowan SF. Sudden infant death syndrome and weather temperature. *Paediatr Perinat Epidemiol* 1992;6:19–28.

64. Stanton AN. Sudden infant death. Overheating and cot death. *Lancet* 1984;2:1199–201.

65. Naeye RL, Ladis B, Drage JS. Sudden infant death syndrome. A prospective study. *Am J Dis Child* 1976;130:1207–10.

66. Kahn A, Van DMC, Dramaix M *et al.* Transepidermal water loss during sleep in infants at risk for sudden death. *Pediatrics* 1987;80:245–50.

67. Berterottiere D, D'Allest AM, Dehan M, Gaultier C. Effects of increase in body temperature on the breathing pattern in premature infants. *J Devel Physiol* 1990;13:303–8.

68. Daily WJR, Klaus M, Meyer HBP. Apnea in premature infants: Monitoring, incidence, heart rate changes, and an effect of environmental temperature. *Pediatrics* 1969;43:510–18.

69. Haraguchi S, Fung RQ, Sasaki CT. Effect of hyperthermia on the laryngeal closure reflex. Implications in the sudden infant death syndrome. *Ann Otol Rhinol Laryngol* 1983;92:24–8.

70. Perlstein PH, Edwards NK, Sutherland JM. Apnea in premature infants and incubator-air-temperature changes. *N Engl J Med* 1970;282:461–6.

71. Azaz Y, Fleming PJ, Levine M, McCabe R, Stewart A, Johnson P. The relationship between environmental temperature, metabolic rate, sleep state, and evaporative water loss in infants from birth to three months. *Pediatr Res* 1992;32:417–23.

72. Bach V, Bouferrache B, Kremp O, Maingourd Y, Libert JP. Regulation of sleep and body temperature in response to exposure to cool and warm environments in neonates. *Pediatrics* 1994;93:789–96.

73. Cooper KE, Veale WL. Effects of temperature on breathing. In: Cherniack NS, Widdicombe JG (eds). *The Respiratory System*. Williams and Wilkins, Bethesda, 1986.

74. Wailoo MP, Petersen SA, Whitaker H. Disturbed nights and 3–4 month old infants: the effects of feeding and thermal environment. *Arch Dis Child* 1990;65: 499–501.

75. Engelberts AC, De Jong GA. Choice of sleeping position for infants: possible association with cot death *Arch Dis Child* 1990;65:462–7.

76. Mitchell EA, Scragg R, Stewart AW *et al.* Results from the first year of the New Zealand cot death study. *NZ J Med* 1991;104:71–6.

77. Willinger M, Hoffman HJ, Hartford RB. Infant sleep position and risk for sudden infant death syndrome: report of meeting held January 13 and 14, 1994, National Institutes of Health, Bethesda, MD [see comments]. *Pediatrics* 1994;93:814–19.

78. Willinger M, Hoffman HJ, Wu KT *et al.* Factors associated with the transition to non-prone sleep position of infants in the United States. *JAMA* 1998;280:329–35.

79. Ponsonby AL, Dwyer T, Gibbons LE, Cochrane JA, Wang YG. Factors potentiating the risk of sudden infant death syndrome associated with the prone position [see comments]. *N Engl J Med* 1993;329:377–82.

80. Guntheroth WG, Spiers PS. Sleeping prone and the risk of sudden infant death syndrome. *JAMA* 1992;267:2359–62.

81. American Academy of Pediatrics Task Force on Infant Positioning and SIDS: Positioning and SIDS. *Pediatrics* 1992;1120–6.

82. American Academy of Pediatrics Task Force on Infant Positioning and SIDS; Positioning and sudden infant death syndrome (SIDS): update. *Pediatrics* 1996;98: 1216–18.

83. Kemp JS, Thach BT. A sleep position-dependent mechanism for infant death on sheepskins [published erratum appears in *Am J Dis Child* 1993 Aug;147(8):810]. *Am J Dis Child* 1993;147:642–6.

84. Kemp JS, Kowalski RM, Burch PM, Graham MA, Thach BT. Unintentional suffocation by rebreathing: a death scene and physiologic investigation of a possible cause of sudden infant death. *J Pediatr* 1993;122:874–80.

85. Bolton DP, Taylor BJ, Campbell AJ, Galland BC, Cresswell C. Rebreathing expired gases from bedding: a cause of cot death? *Arch Dis Child.* 1993;69:187–90.

86. Skadberg BT and Markestad T. Consequences of getting the head covered during sleep in infancy. *Pediatrics* 1997;100:6.
87. Lijowska AS, Reed NW, Chiodini BA, Thach BT. Sequential arousal and airway-defensive behavior of infants in asphyxial sleep environments. *J Appl Physiol* 1997;83:219–28.

CHAPTER 8

Brain research in sudden infant death syndrome

HANNAH C. KINNEY AND JAMES J. FILIANO

Introduction   118
Brainstem findings in SIDS victims   119
Brain findings in sites rostral to the brainstem   119
The medullary serotonergic network in SIDS victims   125
Neuropathologic findings and epidemiology of SIDS victims   130
References   132

Introduction

The most significant advance in SIDS research is the discovery of the relationship between prone sleeping position and increased risk for sudden death.[1–3] In countries with national campaigns to promote supine sleeping position, the SIDS rate has fallen by as much as one-half.[4] The mechanism of the relationship of the prone position to increased risk for SIDS is unexplained, but raises questions about the role of airway obstruction,[5] asphyxial rebreathing,[6–9] altered thermoregulation,[9] and the failure of arousal and protective reflexes[9–11] in the pathogenesis of sudden death. In light of the link between prone sleeping position and SIDS, it is not only appropriate, but also essential, to review the brain findings in SIDS infants published to date, and to rethink brain hypotheses in general in SIDS research.

With conventional neuropathologic techniques at autopsy, the brains of SIDS victims look 'normal' or, at the very most, contain inconsistent, non-specific, and 'minor' findings, such as subtle brainstem gliosis. Thus, we have learned that, if there is a critical brain abnormality in SIDS victims, it requires quantitative cellular, myelin, neurochemical, or molecular tools to uncover. Research analysis of the brain in SIDS victims has been guided by two main hypotheses: (1) the cardioventilatory/arousal hypothesis; and (2) the developmental hypothesis. According to the cardioventilatory/arousal hypothesis, SIDS is due to an abnormality in brain circuits that regulate respiration and/or autonomic activity during sleep, or that stimulate normal protective arousal during life-threatening events (apnea, bradycardia, hypotension, hypercapnia, hypoxia, or asphyxia), which occur in all infants from time to time during sleep. According to the developmental hypothesis, SIDS victims are physiologically immature, and this immaturity is reflected in delayed brain development. The two hypotheses are not mutually exclusive.

Brainstem findings in SIDS victims

The most intense interest in SIDS victims' brain research has focused upon the brainstem, as it is the major site of the neural regulation and integration of respiration, autonomic activity, sleep, and arousal. The major positive and negative findings in the brains of SIDS victims are listed in Table 8.1.[12–70] The basic pathologic processes that have been reported in the brainstem include subtle gliosis (scarring), hypomyelination, increased dendritic spine density, increased synaptic density, and neurotransmitter abnormalities (Table 8.1). These findings have been reported in nuclei related to cardioventilatory control, but are not necessarily restricted to them. Nevertheless, brainstem findings in regions involved in cardioventilatory control implicate them as part of the problem.

In some instances, the results of studies by different investigators are contradictory (Table 8.1). Consider brainstem gliosis, by definition the increase in number of reactive astrocytes, a marker, albeit non-specific, of CNS tissue injury. There are six studies that claim gliosis is present,[15–21] and three studies that refute its presence.[49–51] These studies analyse different regions that are not always precisely defined, nor rigorously matched at comparable levels, and they employ different stains, different quantitative methods, and non-comparable controls. Methodologies are also questioned, specifically, the lack of volumetric sampling in almost all of the brainstem gliosis studies. The one volumetric cell counting study of reactive astrocytes in SIDS victims reported gliosis as a positive finding in the nucleus of the solitary tract and dorsal motor nucleus of the vagus.[18] It has been questioned if subtle brainstem gliosis is a 'normal' finding in infant brainstems: in our opinion, 'gliosis' is not present in all fetal and infant cases, making it less likely to be an obligate developmental phenomenon. Yet, it is noteworthy that in many of the brainstem studies, gliosis is present in at least some SIDS cases as outliers compared to controls, suggesting that the finding may be present in at least a subset of SIDS cases (Figs 8.1 and 8.2).

Brain findings in sites rostral to the brainstem

Sites rostral to the brainstem have been analysed in SIDS victims, including the cerebellum, hypothalamus, hippocampus, and cerebrum (Table 8.1), with both the cardioventilatory/arousal and developmental hypotheses in mind. Sites rostral to the brainstem are known to be involved in respiratory and cardiovascular control, sleep, and arousal, including the basal forebrain, amygdala, hypothalamus, and

Table 8.1   Neuropathologic findings in SIDS infants

Brain Weight
Positive findings:
- Increased[12–14]

Brainstem
Positive findings:
- Subtle gliosis of nuclei related and unrelated to cardioventilatory control[15–21]
- Hypomyelination of intrinsic and extrinsic pathways[14,22]
- Decreased neurons in the hypoglossal nucleus[22]
- Morphological abnormalities of the arcuate nucleus of ventral medulla[23–28]
- Decreased muscarinic, kainate, and serotonergic receptor binding in the arcuate nucleus[29–31]
- Decreased serotonergic receptor binding in a medullary network[31]
- Elevated spine density in selected pontine and medullary reticular neurons, including the ventrolateral medulla[32–35]
- Increased number of synapses in the hypoglossal nucleus[36]
- Increased volume of the hypoglossal nucleus[39]
- Increased synaptic density in the central reticular nucleus of medulla[38]
- Postnatal changes in the volumes of pons, medulla, and cervical spinal cord[39]
- Decreased activity of adrenaline synthesizing enzyme, phenyl-ethanolamine-N-methyltransferase in punch biopsies of selected medullary regions[40,41]
- Absence of adrenergic neurons in the dorsal nucleus of the solitary tract[42,43]
- Increased substance P in homogenates of the medulla[44]
- Increased receptor binding of neurotensin in the nucleus of the solitary tract[45]
- Increase in substance P in trigeminal fibers in pons[33]
- Increased ALZ-50 immunoreactivity in the nucleus of the solitary tract, nucleus ambiguus, and nucleus centralis[46]
- Decreased serotonin and serotonin metabolites in n. raphé obscurus[47]
- Apoptosis in select nuclei (trigeminal n., vestibular n.)[48]

Negative findings:
- No gliosis[49–51]
- Normal neuronal number in the hypoglossal nucleus[37]
- Normal spine density in the hypoglossal nucleus and cervical anterior horn[52]
- Normal volumes, neuronal numbers and positions in the hypoglossal nucleus, dorsal motor nucleus of the vagus, nucleus ambiguus, and nucleus retroambiguus[53]
- No elevation of opioids in homogenates of medulla[47]
- No abnormal opioid, nicotine, and alpha-2 receptor binding in nuclei related and unrelated to cardiorespiratory control and arousal[55–57]
- No decrease in muscarinic-m2 immunostaining in arcuate nucleus[27]

Cerebellum
Positive findings:
- White matter gliosis[58]
- Hypomyelination[14]
- Delayed maturation of the external granular layer[59]

Table 8.1. Continued

Hypothalamus
Positive findings:
● Altered aminergic-cholinergic synaptic markers[60]

Hippocampus
Positive findings:
● Increased ALZ-50 immunoreactivity[46]
● Apoptosis[48]

Basal ganglia
Positive findings:
● Decreased dopamine and increased homovanillic acid/dopamine ratios in putamen[61]

Cerebrum
Positive findings:
● White matter gliosis[14]
● Hypomyelination of multiple regions and pathways[14,62]
● Lipid-laden macrophages in white matter[63,64]
● Periventricular leukomalacia[14,65]
● Ependymal changes in the lateral ventricle[66]

Negative findings:
● Normal myelination of selected white matter sites with postmortem MRI imaging[67]

Cerebrospinal Fluid
Positive Findings:
● Altered neurotransmitter levels[68,69]
● Decreased melatonin levels[70]

insular cortex. Except for the hypothalamus, these gray matter sites, albeit unremarkable by conventional histopathology (personal observations), have received little or no attention in SIDS research. Heavy brain weight (Fig. 8.3), cerebral white matter gliosis (Fig. 8.4), hypomyelination (Fig. 8.5), delayed neuronal migration (Fig. 8.6), and neurotransmitter abnormalities have all been reported in selected forebrain and/or cerebellar regions of SIDS victims (Table 8.1).

Of all neuropathologic findings, heavy brain weight is perhaps the best established (Table 8.1); (Fig. 8.3), because of the simplicity and reproducibility of the method of measurement, i.e. weighing the unfixed brain at autopsy. Heavy brain weight has been confirmed by different investigators in different SIDS and control populations since it was first emphasized by Shaw *et al.*[12] The differential diagnosis of heavy brain weight in SIDS includes cerebral edema, due either to agonal hypoxia–ischemia or other toxic/metabolic factors yet to be identified; agonal vascular congestion; and megalencephaly. Other than heavy brain weight, neuropathologic findings in the forebrain and cerebellum have not been established. Again, results are contradictory (e.g. delayed forebrain myelination[14] versus normal myelination[67]), without independent confirmation, and/or the methodology has been challenged. Nevertheless, these forebrain studies are valuable in emphasizing that an underlying failure of cardioventilatory/arousal

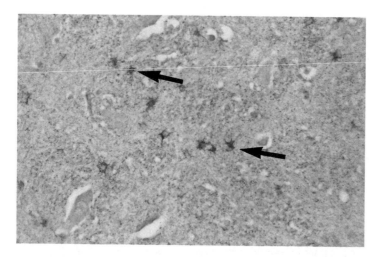

Fig. 8.1 Reactive astrocytes (arrows) in the medullary reticular formation (nucleus centralis) of a SIDS victim are highlighted by immunostaining for an astrocytic marker, glial fibrillary acidic protein (GFAP). ×10, GFAP immunostain (see also colour plate section.

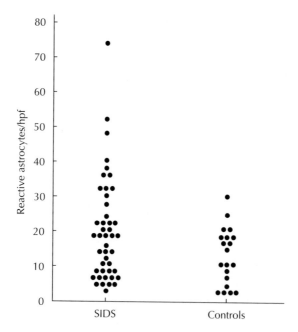

Fig. 8.2 The median reactive astrocyte counts/per high power field (hpf) are given for six regions of the medulla combined in SIDS victims and control infants. There were 11 SIDS victims in whom the total count was greater than that of the highest control infant (>30 reactive astrocytes/hpf). Reprinted with permission of *Pediatrics*.

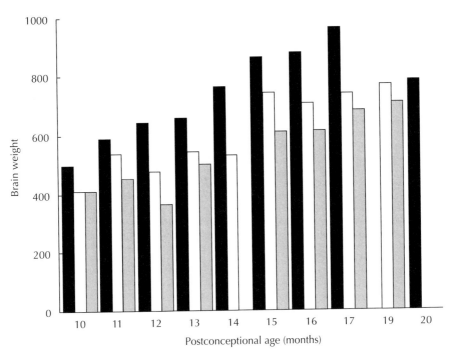

Fig. 8.3 Mean brain weight at death for SIDS (black), control (white), and infants with congenital heart disease (shaded) groups at increasing age-intervals. There were no SIDS cases at 18 postconceptional months and thus control and congenital heart disease cases were excluded from analysis at this age interval. The brain weight of SIDS victims, adjusted for postconceptional month at death, was significantly greater than that of infants dying with control causes or congenital heart disease ($P=0.0001$).[14] Reprinted with permission of the *Journal of Neuropathology and Experimental Neurology*.

mechanisms or a defect in maturation in SIDS victims may not be restricted to the brainstem, the major focus of neuropathologic studies to date, but rather, may be more widespread.

Reported brain findings in SIDS victims, including in the brainstem, are non-specific, and it is not clear which, if any, are directly related to the pathogenesis of sudden death. Several of these findings (cerebral white matter gliosis, periventricular leukomalacia, brainstem gliosis, and apoptosis in the hippocampus and brainstem) are considered, for example, to be secondary to hypoxia–schemia and implicate hypoxia–ischemia in the pathogenesis of SIDS. Other findings (delayed myelination, delayed cerebellar granule cell migration, altered dendritic spine development, and arcuate nucleus hypoplasia [see below]) suggest abnormalities in developmental programs involving neurons and oligodendrocytes. Abnormalities in neurotransmitters and gliosis in cardiorespiratory-related nuclei suggest acquired (pre-, peri-, and/or postnatal) defects specific to the

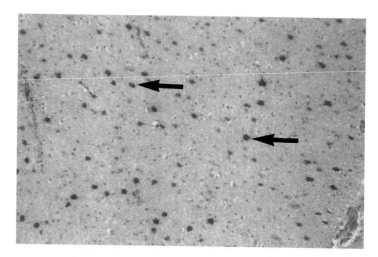

Fig. 8.4 Reactive astrocytes (arrows) in the cerebral white matter of a SIDS victim are highlighted by immunostaining for GFAP. ×10, GFAP immunostain (see also colour plate section).

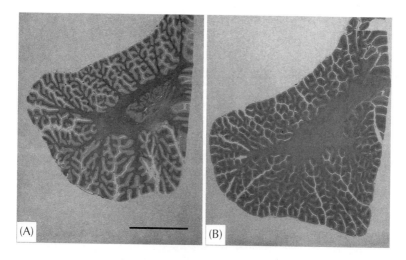

Fig. 8.5 Myelin-stained sections of the white matter of the lateral cerebellar hemisphere between an infant dying of congenital heart disease (A) and SIDS victim (B) at 16 postconceptional months. Myelin degree is 0 in the SIDS victim, compared with degree 3 ('mature') in the control. Myelin was graded in each against an internal standard of degree 3 (inferior cerebellar peduncle). Hematoxylin and eosin/Luxol fast blue. Bar: 1 cm. Reprinted with permission from the *Journal of Neuropathology and Experimental Neurology* (see also colour plate section).

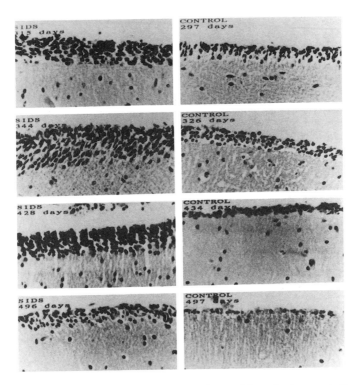

Fig. 8.6 Histologic pattern of the migration of neuroblasts in the cerebellar external granular layer in SIDS victims at different postconceptional days compared with age-related controls. Hematoxylin and eosin, × 400. Reprinted with permission from the *Journal of Neuropathology and Experimental Neurology.*

cardiorespiratory hypothesis. It is not clear how all these findings relate to one another because they have been analysed in separate studies and not within the same brains. Any of these abnormalities may represent the neuropathology of an underlying metabolic defect that results in sudden death and coincident subtle brain pathology.

The medullary serotonergic network in SIDS victims

Driven by the cardioventilatory/arousal hypothesis, work in our laboratory was originally focused upon the role of the ventral medulla in the pathogenesis of SIDS. By 'ventral medulla', we mean a complex of neuronal populations along the ventral and ventrolateral rim of the medulla that affect chemoreception to carbon dioxide (CO_2), provide tonic influence to prevent apnea, and modulate respiratory and blood pressure responses.[71] The ventral medulla is poorly characterized in humans: the arcuate nucleus along the ventral medullary surface is postulated to be homologous to widespread surface chemoreceptor regions in experimental animals.[72] The arcuate nucleus is the only distinct neuronal population along the human ventral medullary surface (Fig. 8.7). Historically it has been considered a relay nucleus from the cerebral cortex to the cerebellum via the external arcuate fibers and inferior cerebellar peduncle, and to represent downwardly displaced neurons of the basis pontis. In a comparative anatomic study between the human infant and cat ventral medullary surface, we found that the arcuate nucleus, n. conterminalis, and foci of thickened marginal glia in the human are anatomically homologous to the cat respiratory chemosensitive fields.[72] This homology is based upon cytoarchitectonic criteria (including cell size, shape, and distance from the surface) as defined by the combined anatomic and physiologic studies of the cat respiratory chemosensitive fields,[72] and upon 3–dimensional cell distributions, as determined with the aid of three-dimensional computer reconstructions.[72]

In a separate study, we applied crystals of DiI, a lipophilic dye which labels cells and cell processes by lateral diffusion along cell membranes, to 23 paraformaldehyde-fixed human fetal brainstems at 19–20 postconceptional weeks.[73] DiI diffusion from the arcuate nucleus labeled fibers and cell bodies in

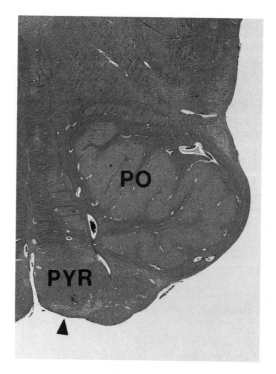

Fig. 8.7 The arcuate nucleus (arrow) is located on the ventral surface of the medulla in a human infant. Hematoxylin and eosin/Luxol fast blue. Abbreviations: PO, principal inferior olive; PYR, pyramid (see also colour plate section).

the medullary raphé complex. DiI diffusion from the medullary raphé complex, on the other hand, labeled the arcuate nucleus, nucleus of the solitary tract, and subnuclei of the reticular formation. DiI placed in the pyramid and basis pontis (negative control) labeled the corticospinal tract, with no labeling of the medullary raphé or arcuate nucleus. The results suggest the existence of cellular connections between the arcuate nucleus and the caudal raphé, the latter which is known to be involved in respiratory and blood pressure control, as well as chemoreception in experimental animals.[73] A role for the arcuate nucleus in human ventilatory control is supported by the report of its absence in an autopsied 5-month-old infant with clinical insensitivity to carbon dioxide and sudden death.[74] The idea that ventral medullary surface cell populations are involved in the response to hypercapnia in humans is supported by functional magnetic resonance imaging in adults exposed to a hypercapnic challenge in which CO_2 responsiveness is localized to the region of the arcuate nucleus, as well as to other regions.[75]

Having identified the arcuate nucleus as a putative component of the ventral medullary surface populations related to central chemoreception in humans, we then studied this nucleus with anatomic techniques. In a database of 41 SIDS victims and 27 controls, we found two SIDS cases in which the arcuate nucleus was almost totally absent (hypoplastic) by histopathologic criteria in serially or extensively sectioned medullae.[23] There were no other brainstem anomalies, nor was there gliosis or apparent neuronal atrophy within the arcuate nucleus that would suggest a destructive or degenerative process. Given that the arcuate nucleus is derived from the rhombic lip, we speculate that the hypoplasia is restricted to rhombic lip precursors.

To address the possibility of a neurochemical deficiency in the arcuate nucleus of SIDS victims, we examined six different radioligands to neurotransmitter receptor binding with quantitative tissue receptor autoradiography in alternate sections of the same data set.[76] We found a significant decrease in ^{3}H-quinuclidinyl benzilate binding to muscarinic cholinergic receptors[29] and in ^{3}H-kainate binding to kainate receptors[30] (Figs 8.8 and 8.9) in the arcuate nucleus in SIDS victims, compared to infants dying acutely of known causes. Differences in mean binding were not present in 18 other brainstem nuclei related and unrelated to cardioventilatory control and arousal. Both muscarinic and kainate receptors at the ventral medullary surface are thought to be directly involved in CO_2 responsiveness,[29,30] and thus the dual deficiency in receptor binding is likely to be disastrous in the face of hypercapnia or asphyxia. In both the muscarinic and kainate studies, mean receptor binding was analyzed in an 'acute' group ($n=15$) and a 'chronic' group ($n=18$) compared with the SIDS group ($n=52$). The acute controls were infants who died suddenly and unexpectedly, and in whom a complete autopsy established a cause of death. The chronic group was composed of infants with a history of chronic or repetitive hypoxemia from cardiac, pulmonary, or central breathing disorders. The chronic group with oxygenation or breathing disorders was included in the study in order to address the possibility that the putative neurotransmitter receptor binding deficits in the arcuate nucleus are not specific to SIDS, but rather reflect an effect of hypoxia–ischemia. The association between muscarinic and kainate binding

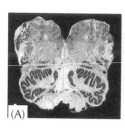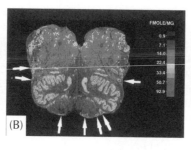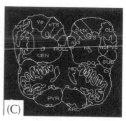

Fig. 8.8 (A) Autoradiogram of representative level of the human infant medulla for 3H-kainate binding to kainate receptors. The arcuate nucleus is located along the ventral surface, superficial to the pyramid. (B) Color-coded image of specific activity (fmol/mg tissue) in the same section. The white arrows point to the arcuate nucleus. (C) Anatomic boundaries of nuclei. Abbreviations: ARC, arcuate nucleus; CEN, n. centralis; CUL, n. cuneatus lateralis; DMX, dorsal motor nucleus of the vagus; DO, dorsal accessory olive; ICP, inferior cerebellar peduncle; MO, medial accessory olive; nXII, hypoglossal nucleus; nSPVc, nucleus of the spinal trigeminal nerve, pars caudalis; nTS, nucleus of the solitary tract; PO, principal inferior olive; PYR, pyramid; ROLL, nucleus of Roller; SUB, nucleus subtrigeminalis; VE, vestibular nucleus. Reprinted with permission of *Neuroscience* (see also colour plate section).

densities was examined in the cases in which both measurements were available. There was a positive correlation between the density of the muscarinic and kainate binding in the SIDS cases ($R=0.460$, $P=0.003$) (Fig. 8.10).[30]

Binding to nicotinic,[56] opioid,[55] and alpha-2-adrenergic[57] binding was not detected in the arcuate nucleus or controls, precluding testing of the ventral medullary/arcuate nucleus hypothesis with these receptors. There was no difference in binding between the SIDS cases and controls in any of the 18 other brainstem nuclei analysed, thus arguing against a role for nicotinic, opioid, and alpha-2-adrenergic brainstem receptor abnormalities in SIDS. Of note, however, when a post-hoc analysis of the nicotine dataset was performed in a small subset of cases with available clinical information was stratified by the history of the presence or absence of maternal cigarette smoking during pregnancy, we found there was no expected increase (upregulation) of nicotinic receptor binding in SIDS cases exposed to cigarette smoke *in utero* in three pontine nuclei related to arousal or cardiorespiratory control (n. parabrachialis lateralis, locus coeruleus, n. pontis oralis).[56] This very preliminary finding raises the possibility that altered development of nicotinic receptors in brainstem cardiorespiratory and/or arousal circuits puts at least some infants, i.e. those exposed to cigarette smoke *in utero*, at risk for SIDS, and underscores the need for further research into brainstem nicotinic receptors in SIDS victims in larger sample sizes and in which detailed correlations with smoking history (quantity and duration of exposure) can be made.

Perhaps most significantly, the brainstem receptor binding studies in the single data set demonstrated serotonergic binding deficiencies in SIDS cases compared with acute and chronic controls in the caudal raphé (n. raphé obscurus)

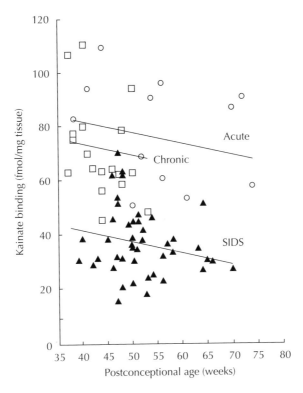

Fig. 8.9 Scatterplot of raw data and estimated regression lines (model R^2 50.606; acute controls intercept = 96.91, chronic group intercept = 88.71; SIDS intercept = 57.07, age slope = −0.391 fmol/mg tissue/week) of mean 3H-kainate binding to kainate receptors in the arcuate nucleus for SIDS cases (solid triangles), acute controls (open circles), and chronic controls (open squares) by postconceptional age. Each symbol represents one case. The age-adjusted mean binding level of the SIDS group is significantly lower than that of acute controls. The age-adjusted mean binding levels of the acute controls did not differ from the chronic group. Reprinted with permission of the *Neuroscience*.

and five other functionally and developmentally related components of the medulla (including the arcuate nucleus, n. paragigantocellularis lateralis, n. gigantocellularis, lateral reticular zone [homologous to 'gasping center' in experimental animals], and inferior olive). These are all regions involved in chemoreception, respiratory drive, blood pressure responses, upper airway reflexes, and/or thermoregulation.[76] Four of the six regions are considered derivatives of a common embryonic anlage, the rhombic lip, and five of the six regions contain serotonergic neurons in the developing human brainstem. Taken together, these findings suggest a primary defect in serotonergic neurons, derived at least in part from the rhombic lip, in SIDS cases, resulting from a failure of cell division,

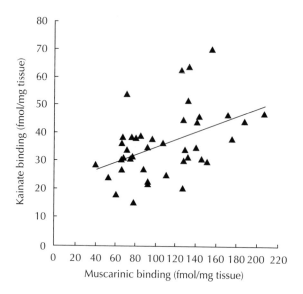

Fig. 8.10 Scatterplot of raw data for SIDS cases and estimated regression line (model $R = 0.460$; intercept $= 21.12$, muscarinic binding slope $= 0.138$) of mean 3H-kainate binding in the arcuate nucleus by muscarinic binding. Each symbol represents one case. There is a significant positive correlation between kainate and muscarinic binding density in the arcuate nucleus of SIDS cases ($P = 0.003$). Reprinted with permission of *Neuroscience.*

migration, and/or differentiation. These studies have led us to an expanded hypothesis concerning the role of the ventral medulla in SIDS: SIDS, or more likely, a subset of SIDS, is due to a developmental abnormality of a medullary network composed at least in part of rhombic-lip-derived, serotonergic neurons, including within the ventral medulla, and this abnormality results in a failure of protective responses to life-threatening challenges during sleep, as the infant passes through a critical period in homeostatic control.

Neuropathologic findings and epidemiology of SIDS victims

The question arises, how do we link the neuropathologic findings in SIDS brains with the epidemiology of SIDS, particularly with the risk factor of prone sleeping position? We propose that the neuropathologic findings and epidemiology of SIDS be considered together in the triple-risk model.[77] According to this model, SIDS results from the impingement upon the infant of three factors: (1) an underlying vulnerability; (2) a critical period in development (the major time-period of risk, the first 6 months of life); and (3) an exogenous stressor(s) (Fig. 8.11).[77] Death occurs only if all three factors intersect and only if the exogenous

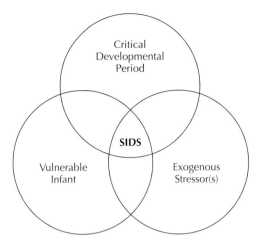

Fig. 8.11 Venn diagram of the triple-risk model. According to this model, SIDS results from the intersection of: (1) a vulnerable infant who possesses some underlying abnormality; (2) a critical period in development; and (3) an exogenous stressor(s). Reprinted with permission from *Biology of the Neonate*.

stressor matches the specific vulnerability of the individual infant. According to this model, SIDS victims are not 'normal', but rather, have an underlying disorder that puts him/her at risk for sudden death as he/she passes through the critical developmental period and meets a specific exogenous stressor. SIDS may result from multiple causes, with different underlying abnormalities in vulnerable infants, e.g. systemic inborn error of metabolism in one infant, primary brainstem lesion in another. Consequently, the same stressor may not be present in every SIDS case. By corollary, the infant may survive as 'normal' if the stressor is avoided, or if the underlying vulnerability is ameliorated by therapeutic intervention. In this way, the triple-risk model helps explain the apparently asymptomatic behavior of most SIDS victims, and explains why eliminating an external stressor, e.g. prone sleeping position, may reduce the incidence of SIDS. The model also helps explain why the overwhelming majority of infants who sleep prone do not die of SIDS, as they are 'normal' and do not have an underlying vulnerability.

The concept that an external stressor precipitates sudden death is derived from epidemiologic studies indicating that minor respiratory or gastrointestinal illness occurs around the time of death in some SIDS victims, as well as symptoms suggestive of more severe illness in the 2 days before death.[78,79] Potential stressors linked to SIDS other than infection include prone sleeping position, fever, hyperthermia by over-blanketing, and soft bedding.[1,2,6] Of note, exogenous stressors associated with SIDS, such as fever and infection, tend to cause an increased rate of CO_2 production, alter the demand for cardiac output and/or thermoregulation, and/or decrease arousal. The prone sleeping position is associated with the spontaneous face-down sleeping position in infants.[7] The face-down position is associated with rebreathing exhaled gases and increased end-tidal CO_2 in normal infants, particularly those sleeping on soft bedding where pockets of exhaled gas form and trap CO_2.[6] The prone position may also lead to partial or complete upper airway obstruction, by repositioning the mandible and occluding the pharynx, by compressing the nose directly, or by reflex laryngeal closure as part of the 'diving' response. At least 26% of SIDS victims are found in the face-down position,[8] and 71% are found in the prone position.[8]

We now propose that the underlying vulnerability in at least a subset of SIDS victims is an abnormality in the medullary serotonergic network, including the the arcuate nucleus cell populations of the ventral medulla. The critical developmental period concerns maturation of homeostatic control. Although changes in cardioventilatory function and state organization continue throughout life, a relatively stable configuration is achieved by the end of the sixth month, the end of the period during which infants are most at risk for SIDS. We speculate that the external stressor is hypoxia or asphxyia that results from upper airway obstruction and/or asphyxial rebreathing in the face-down (prone) sleeping position. A normal infant's nervous system detects progressive asphyxia or hypoxia, and responds by arousal and a series of protective reflexes and behaviors to ensure airway patency. Due to the underlying abnormality in the medullary serotonergic network, the vulnerable SIDS infant fails to arouse, cry, increase ventilation, and move his/her head in response to the asphyxia, hypercapnia, and/or hypoxia: death results. Other mechanisms may involve improper responses of the medullary serotonergic network to hypotension, arousal, or hyperthermia.[76] If the medullary serotonergic network/arcuate nucleus abnormality is eventually shown to be a defect of timing of medullary serotonergic/arcuate development, then the triple-risk model serves as a conceptual framework that merges the cardioventilatory/arousal hypothesis with the developmental hypothesis in SIDS.

References

1. Fleming PJ, Gilvert R, Azaz Y *et al*. Interaction between bedding and sleeping position in the sudden infant death syndrome: a population based case-control study. *Br Med J* 1990;301:85–9.
2. Ponsonby AL, Dwyer T, Gibbons LE, Cochran JA, Wang YG. Factors potentiating the risk of sudden infant death syndrome associated with the prone position. *N Eng J Med* 1993;329:377–82.
3. Taylor JA, Krieger JW, Reay DT, Davis RL, Harruiff, Cheney LK. Prone sleep position and the sudden infant death syndrome in King County, Washington. *J Pediatr* 1996;128:626–30.
4. Dwyer T, Ponsonby AL, Blizzard L, Newman NM, Cochrane JA. The contribution of changes in the prevalence of prone sleeping position to the decline in sudden infant death syndrome in Tasmania. *JAMA* 1995;273:783–9.
5. Thach BT. Neuromuscular control of upper airway patency. *Clin Perinatol* 1992; 19: 773–88.

6. Kemp JS, Thach BT. Sudden death in infants sleeping on polystryrene-filled cushions. *N Eng J Med* 1991;324:1858–64.
7. Chiodini BA, Thach BT. Impaired ventilation in infants sleeping face-down: potential significance for sudden infant death syndrome. *J Pediatr* 1993;123:686–92.
8. Kemp JS, Kowalski RM, Burch PM, Graham MA, Thach BT. Unintentional suffocation by rebreathing: A death scene and physiologic investigation of a possible cause of sudden infant death. *J Pediatr* 1993;122:874–80.
9. Harper RM, Kinney HC, Fleming PJ, Thach BT. Sleep influences on homeostatic functions: implications for sudden infant death syndrome. *Resp Physiol* 2000;19: 123–32.
10. Hunt CM, McCulloch K, Brouillette RT. Diminished hypoxic ventilatory responses in near-miss sudden infant death syndrome. *J Appl Physiol* 1981;50:1212–17.
11. McCulloch K *et al.* Arousal responses in near-miss sudden infant death syndrome and in normal infants. *J Pediatr* 1982;101:911–17.
12. Shaw CM, Siebert JR, Haas JE, Alvord EC. Megalencephaly in sudden infant death syndrome. *J Child Neurol* 1989;4:39–42.
13. Aranda FU, Teixeira F, Becker LE. Assessment of growth in sudden infant death syndrome. *Neuroepidemiology* 1990;9:95–105.
14. Kinney HC, Brody BA, Finkelstein DM, Vawter GF, Mandell F, Gilles FH. Delayed central nervous system myelination in the sudden infant death syndrome. *J Neuropathol Exp Neurol* 1991;50:29–48.
15. Naeye RL. Brain stem and adrenal abnormalities in the sudden infant death syndrome. *Am J Clin Pathol* 1966;66:526–39.
16. Takashima S, Armstrong D, Becker LE, Bryan C. Cerebral hypoperfusion in the sudden infant death syndrome? Brain stem gliosis and vascular. *Ann Neurol* 1978; 4:257–62.
17. Kinney HC, Burger PC, Harrell FE, Hudson RP. 'Reactive gliosis' in the medulla oblongata of victims of the sudden infant death syndrome. *Pediatrics* 1983;72: 181–7.
18. Bruce Y, Becker LE. Quantitation of medullary astrogliosis in sudden infant death syndrome. *Pediatr Neurosurg* 1991;92:74–9.
19. Summers GC, Parker VC. The brainstem in the sudden infant death syndrome: A postmortem survey. *Am J Forensic Med Pathol* 1981;2:23–30.
20. Yamanouchi H, Takashima S, Becker LE. Correlation of astrogliosis and substance P immunoreactivity in the brainstems of victims of sudden infant death syndrome. *Neuropediatrics* 1993;24:200–3.
21. Storm H, Nylander G, Saugstad OD. The amount of brainstem gliosis in sudden infant death syndrome (SIDS) victims correlates with maternal cigarette smoking during pregnancy. *Acta Paediatr* 1999;88:13–8.
22. Naeye RL, Olsson JM, Combs JW. New brain stem and bone marrow abnormalities in victims of the sudden infant death syndrome. *J Perinatol* 1989;9:180–3.
23. Filiano JJ, Kinney HC. Arcuate nucleus hypoplasia in the sudden infant death syndrome. *J Neuropathol Exp Neurol* 1992;51:394–403.
24. Gilson TP, Balko MG, Blisard KS, Taylor KL. Morphological variations of the external arcuate nucleus in the sudden infant death syndrome. *J Forensic Sci* 1994;39: 1076–80.

25. Schlaefke M, Hukuhara T, See WR. Loss of central chemosensitivity, experimental studies on a clinical problem. *Adv Physiol Soc* 1981;10:609–16.
26. Matturri L, Biondo B, Mercurio P, Rossi L. Severe hypoplasia of medullary arcuate nucleus: quantitative analysis in sudden infant death syndrome. *Acta Neuropathol* 2000;99:371–5.
27. Mallard C, Tolcos M, Leditschke J, Campbell P, Rees S. Reduction in choline acetyl-transferase immunoreactivity but not muscarinic-m2 receptor immunoreactivity in the brainstem of SIDS infants. *J Neuropathol Exp Neurol* 1999;58:255–64.
28. Kubo S, Orihara Y, Gotoda T *et al.* Immunohistochemical studies on neuronal changes in brain stem nucleus of forensic autopsied cases. II. Sudden infant death syndrome. *Nippon Hoigaku Zasshi – Jap J Legal Med* 1998;52:350–4.
29. Kinney HC, Filiano JJ, Sleeper LA, Mandell F, Valdez-Dapena M, White WF. Decreased muscarinic receptor binding in the arcuate nucleus in sudden infant death syndrome. *Science* 1995;269:1446–59.
30. Panigrahy A, Filiano JJ, Sleeper LA *et al.* Decreased kainate receptor binding in the arcuate nucleus of the sudden infant death syndrome. *J Neuropathol Exp Neurol* 1997; 56: 1254–61.
31. Panigrahy A, Filiano JJ, Sleeper LA *et al.* Decreased serotonergic receptor binding in rhombic lip derived regions of the medulla oblongata in the sudden infant death syndrome. *J Neuropathol Exp Neurol* 2000;59:377–84.
32. Quattrochi JJ, McBride PT, Yates AJ. Brainstem immaturity in sudden infant death syndrome: A quantitative rapid Golgi study of dendritic spines in 95 infants. *Brain Res* 1985;325:39–48.
33. Takashima S, Mito T. Neuronal development in the medullary reticular formation in sudden infant death syndrome and premature infants. *Neuropediatrics* 1985;16:76–9.
34. Takashima S, Becker LE. Delayed dendritic development of catecholaminergic neurons in the ventrolateral medulla of children who died of sudden infant death syndrome. *Neuropediatrics* 1991;22:97–9.
35. Takashima S, Becker LE. Developmental abnormalities of medullary 'respiratory centers' in sudden infant death syndrome. *Exp Neurol* 1985;90:580–7.
36. O'Kusky JR, Norman MG. Sudden infant death syndrome: Increased number of synapses in the hypoglossal nucleus. *J Neuropathol Exp Neurol* 1995;54:627–34.
37. O'Kusky JR, Norman MG. Sudden infant death syndrome: Postnatal changes in the numerical density and total number of neurons in the hypoglossal nucleus. *J Neuropathol Exp Neurol* 1992;51:577–84.
38. O'Kusky JR, Norman MG. Sudden infant death syndrome: Increased synaptic density in the central reticular nucleus of the medulla. *J Neuropathol Exp Neurol* 1994; 53:263–71.
39. O'Kusky JR, Kozuki DE, Norman MG. Sudden infant death syndrome: Postnatal changes in the volumes of the pons, medulla, and cervical spinal cord. *J Neuropathol Exp Neurol* 1995;54:570–80.
40. Denoroy L, Kopp N, Gay N, Bertrand E, Pujoi F, Gilly R. Activités des enzymes de synthèse des catecholamines den des régions du bone cérèbral au cours de la mort subité du nourrisson. *CR Acad Sci Paris* 1980;291:217–20.
41. Denoroy L, Gay N, Gilly R, Tayor J, Pasquier B, Kopp N. Catecholamine synthe-sizing enzyme activity in brainstem areas from victims of sudden infant death syn-drome. *Neuropediatrics* 1987;18:187–90.

42. Chigr R, Najimi M, Jordan D *et al.* Absence of adrenergic neurons in medulla oblongata in sudden infant death syndrome. *CR Acad Sci Paris* 1989;309:543–9.

43. Kopp N, Chigr F, Denoroy L, Gilly R, Jordan D. Absence of adrenergic neurons in nucleus tractus solitarius in sudden infant death syndrome. *Neuropediatrics* 1993; 24:25–9.

44. Bergstrom L, Lagercrantz H, Terenius L. Post-mortem analysis of neuropeptides in brains from sudden infant death victims. *Brain Res* 1984;323:279–85.

45. Chigr F, Jordan D, Najimi M *et al.* Quantitative autoradiographic study of somato-statin and neurotensin binding sites in medulla oblongata of SIDS. *Neurochem Int* 1992;20:113–8.

46. Sparks DC, Hunsaker JC. Increased ALZ-50 immunoreactivity in sudden infant death syndrome. *J Child Neurol* 1996;11:101–7.

47. Kopp N, Denoroy L, Eymin C *et al.* Studies of neuroregulators in the brain stem of SIDS. *Biol Neonate* 1994;65:189–93.

48. Waters KA, Meehan B, Huang JQ, Gravel RA, Michaud J, Cote A. Neuronal apop-tosis in sudden infant death syndrome. *Pediatr Res* 1999;45:166–72.

49. Oehmichen M, Linke P, Zilles K, Saternus KS. Reactive astrocytes and macrophages in the brain stem of SIDS victims? Eleven age- and sex-matched SIDS and control cases. *Clin Neuropathol* 1989;8:276–83.

50. Reske-Nielsoen E, Gregersen M, Lund E. Astrocytes in the postnatal nervous sys-tem. *Acta Pathol Microbiol Immunol Scand* 1987;95:347–56.

51. Pearson J, Brandeis L. Normal aspects of morphometry of brainstem astrocytes, carotid bodies, and ganglia in SIDS. In: Tilton JT, Roeder LM, Steinschneider A, (eds). *Sudden Infant Death Syndrome*. Academic Press, New York; 1983; pp.115–22.

52. Takashima S, Mito T, Becker LE. Dendritic development of motor neurons in the cervical anterior horn and hypoglossal nucleus of normal infants and victims of the sudden infant death syndrome. *Neuropediatrics* 1990;2:24–6.

53. Lamont P, Murray G, Halliday G, Hilton J, Pamphlett. Brain stem nuclei in sudden infant death syndrome (SIDS): volumes, neuronal numbers and positions. *Neuro-pathol Appl Neurobiol* 1995;2:262–8.

54. Kuich TE, Franciosi RA. A study of the endogenous opioid system in the sudden infant death syndrome. *Med Hypotheses* 1983;10:365–84.

55. Kinney HC, Filiano JJ, Assman SF *et al.* Tritiated-naloxone binding to brainstem opioid receptors in the sudden infant death syndrome. *J Auto Nerv Sys* 1998;69: 156–63.

56. Nachmanoff DB, Panigrahy A, Filiano JJ *et al.* Brainstem ^{3}H-nicotine receptor binding in the sudden infant death syndrome. *J Neuropathol Exp Neurol* 1998;57: 1018–25.

57. Mansouri J, Panigrahy A, Filiano JJ, Sleeper LA, St John WM, Kinney HC. Alpha2–adrenergic receptor binding in the medulla oblongata in the sudden infant death syndrome. *J Neuropath Exp Neurol* (under revision, 2000).

58. Ambler MN, Neave C, Sturner WQ. Sudden and unexpected death in infancy and childhood: Neuropathologic findings. *Am J Forensic Med Pathol* 1981;2:23–30.

59. Cruz-Sanchez FF, Lucena J, Ascaso C, Tolosa E, Quinto L, Rossi ML. Cerebellar cortex delayed maturation in sudden infant death syndrome. *J Neuropathol Exp Neurol* 1997;56:240–6.

60. Sparks DL, Hunsaker JC. Sudden infant death syndrome: altered aminergic-cholinergic synaptic markers in the hypothalamus. *J Child Neurol* 1991;6:335–9.

61. Kalaria RN, Fiedler C, Hunsaker JC, Sparks DL. Synaptic neurochemistry of human striatum during development: changes in sudden infant death syndrome. *J Neurochem* 1993;60:2098–105.

62. Carey EM, Foster PC. The activity of 2'3'-cyclic nucleotide 3'- phosphohydrolase in the corpus callosum, subcortical white matter, and spinal cord in infants dying of the sudden infant death syndrome. *J Neurochem* 1984;42:924–9.

63. Gadson DR, Emery JL. Fatty change in the brain in perinatal and unexpected death. *Arch Dis Child* 1976;51:42–8.

64. Esiri MM, Urry P, Keeling J. Lipid-containing cells in the brain in sudden infant death syndrome. *Dev Med Child Neurol* 1990;32:319–24.

65. Takashima S, Armstrong D, Becker LE, Huber J. Cerebral white matter lesions in the sudden infant death syndrome. *Pediatrics* 1978;62:155–9.

66. Lucena J, Cruz-Sanchez FF. Ependymal changes in sudden infant death syndrome. *J Neuropathol Exp Neurol* 1996;55:348–56.

67. Lamont P, Sachinwalla T, Pamphlett R. Myelin in SIDS: Assessment of development and damage using MRI. *Pediatrics* 1995;95:409–13.

68. Cann-Moisan C, Girin E, Giroux JD, Le Bras P, Caroff J. Changes in cerebrospinal fluid monoamine metabolites, tryptophan, and gamma-aminobutyric acid during the 1st year of life in normal infants. Comparison with victims of sudden infant death syndrome. *Biol Neonate* 1999;75:152–9.

69. Caroff J, Girin E, Alex D, Cann-Moisan C, Sizun J, Barthelemy L. Neurotransmission and sudden infant death. Study of cerebrospinal fluid. *C R Acad Sci - Ser Iii, Sci Vie* 1992;314:451–4.

70. Sturner WQ, Lunch HJ, Deng MH, Gleason RE, Wurtman RJ. Melatonin concentrations in the sudden infant death syndrome. *Forensic Sci Int* 1990;45:171–180.

71. Trouth CO, Millis RM, Kiwull-Schoene H, Schlaefke ME (eds). *Ventral Brainstem Mechanisms and Control of Respiration and Blood Pressure.* Marcel Dekker, New York, 1995.

72. Filiano JJ, Choi JC, Kinney HC. Candidate cell populations for respiratory chemosensitive fields in the human infant medulla. *J Comp Neurol* 1990;293: 448–65.

73. Zec N, Filiano JJ, Kinney HC. Anatomic relationships of the human arcuate nucleus of the medulla: A DiI-Labeling study. *J Neuropathol Exp Neurol* 1997;56:509–22.

74. Folgering H, Kuyer F, Kille JF. Primary alveolar hypoventilation (Ondine's Curse Syndrome) in an infant without external arcuate nucleus. Case report. *Bull Eur Physiopathol Resp* 1979;15:659–65.

75. Gozal D, Hathout GM, Kirlew KAT *et al.* Localization of putative neural respiratory regions in the human by functional magnetic resonance imaging. *J Appl Physiol* 1994;76:2076–83.

76. Kinney HC, Filiano JJ, White WF. Serotonergic deficits in the medulla oblongata in the sudden infant death syndrome: review of a 15–year study of a single data set. *J Neuropathol Exp Neurol* 2000, (in press).

77. Filiano JJ, Kinney HC. A perspective on neuropathologic findings in victims of the sudden infant death syndrome: the triple-risk model. *Biol Neonate* 1994;65:194–7.

78. Hoffmann RJ, Damus K Hillman L, Krongrad E. Risk factors for SIDS. Results of

the National Institute of Child Health and Human Development SIDS cooperative epidemiological study. *Ann NY Acad Sci* 1988;533:13–30.

79. Taylor BU, Williams SM, Mitchell EA, Ford RP. Symptoms, sweating and reactivity of infants who die of SIDS compared with community controls. New Zealand National Cot Death Study Group. *J Pediatr Child Health* 1996;32:316–22.

CHAPTER 9

Rebreathing of exhaled air

JAMES S. KEMP AND BRADLEY T. THACH

Introduction   138
Early reports postulating rebreathing   140
Later doubts about rebreathing   141
Face-down deaths and SIDS   142
Rebreathing of exhaled air and soft bedding   143
Evidence for lethality of rebreathing   145
Rebreathing and newer epidemiology   150
Conclusions   151
Acknowledgement   152
References   152

Introduction

Twenty to 52% of victims of SIDS have died prone with their face straight down, so that their nose and mouth had been covered by bedding.[1–8] This conclusion is based on consistent findings from at least eight case series and case–control studies performed over the last 60 years (Table 9.1; Fig. 9.1). It thus seems

Table 9.1.   Percentage of face-down deaths among infants dying suddenly and unexpectedly

Percentage	Location and source
43%	New York City (1943)[1]
29%	Cleveland (1956)[2]
20%	London and Cambridge (1965)[3]
27%	Seattle (1972)[4]
52%	New Zealand Cot Death Study (1989)[5]
39%	Hobart, Tasmania (1992)[6]
29%	USA, many cities (1998)[7]
43%	Netherlands (1998)[8]

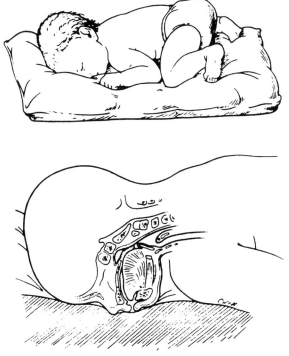

Fig. 9.1 Infants placed prone to sleep on soft items may turn their nose and mouth down into the underlying bedding. Before the Back-to-Sleep interventions, 20–52 per cent of sudden deaths diagnosed as SIDS occurred in this position.[9]

apparent that, although prone infants rarely sleep with nose and mouth down,[10] those dying are often found that way.[3] Parents and others outside of the SIDS field might be surprised to learn, however, that this position of nose and mouth down at death was believed to be insignificant, at least until recently. For example, a manual prepared for parents of victims in 1972 stated:

> Your finding of the baby perhaps face down in its cot or with bedclothes over it may make you think that death was due to suffocation. Many babies normally sleep face down, or get blankets over their faces, with no harmful effects. While it is possible for a child to suffocate accidentally this is, we are quite certain, not 'the cause of death' in children who have died in this particular way.[11]

How did this become the conventional wisdom used for many years by those directly concerned with SIDS? What evidence is there in epidemiologic and physiologic studies for an instrumental role for soft bedding and the face-down position among infants dying prone? What is the evidence that rebreathing of air polluted with exhaled CO_2 and depleted of O_2 is a key mechanism of death among prone infants? Will this mechanism be averted when all infants go to sleep on their back?

These questions will be addressed in this chapter.

Early reports postulating rebreathing and emphasizing face-down position

At the outset it is necessary to provide a definition of terms. 'Face down' in this chapter is meant to imply face straight-down, or nearly so, with nose and mouth covered (Fig. 9.1).[7,9,12] Those reviewing records of death-scene investigations should be aware that, in many jurisdictions, 'face down' is meant to imply both not face up and not supine. An infant who was prone with face to side may still be described in the records as 'face down'. Unless there is specific mention of where the nose and mouth were, or unless their position is clearly implicit from other scene findings, one should not conclude from the records that a 'face-down' infant had its nose and mouth encumbered by bedding. In our work, and in others references cited, face down means nose and mouth down into bedding.

Current interest in face position and rebreathing was foreshadowed by reports done 60 years ago.

ARCHIBALD'S OBSERVATIONS

Herbert Archibald MD, 1942: Asphyxia from pillows, blankets and other items of bedding

Dr Archibald proposed a series of opinions and theories, based on his observations, that we believe to have been correct, for the most part.[13] Archibald postulated that exhaled gases could be lethal if rebreathed from bedding. He surmised 'that a well baby might anesthetize himself by breathing back and forth in to the mattress or pillow, or under the blanket, and then be unable to resist smothering.' Archibald noted that 'in the case of smothering the factors of mattress, pillow, or blankets are constant,' and the infant could be asphyxiated 'from breathing in a confined space.' In fact, we have measured the effective deadspace for items of bedding on which infants have died face down using techniques developed to measure the effective deadspace of anesthesia equipment.[14,15] The imposed deadspace in bedding ranged from 600 ml to >1600 ml. As Archibald predicted, this space was much too large for an infant to entrain only fresh air with every breath, as small infants have tidal volumes <100 ml.

Archibald's statements were based on anecdotal observations. He likely overstated the importance of CO_2 narcosis in the early pathogenesis of deaths where rebreathing has been implicated. Nevertheless, his speculation regarding bedding's more or less 'constant' role appears to have been correct, based on recent findings.

ABRAMSON'S OBSERVATIONS

Harold Abramson MD, 1944: The extent of the problem in New York City

Harold Abramson was a physician who worked in New York City. It is not clear if he was familiar with the theories of Archibald, who was from Oakland, CA, but he was concerned about the same problems. He pointed out that for infants in New York City under 1 year of age, the 'annual deaths from accidental mechanical suffocation have exceeded those from measles, scarlet fever, and diphtheria combined, and have equaled those from whooping cough.' Because of these concerns, he investigated factors that might contribute to unexpected infant deaths.[1]

With the cooperation of the Medical Examiner of the City of New York, Abramson analysed 139 deaths attributed to accidental mechanical suffocation occurring between January, 1939, and December, 1943. The median age at death was between 2 and 3 months. Sixty-eight per cent of the infants were found prone and almost half 'were discovered with nose and mouth in occluding contact with . . . soft pillows, mattresses, or mattress coverings . . .' Abramson recognized the importance of visiting the death scene in understanding these deaths. He speculated that the 'lack of apprehension of this situation may be due in part to the infrequency with which the practicing physician and the hospital are called upon to attend these accidental cases of smothering. The investigation of such deaths falls within the province of the local police department and the office of the medical examiner. Stress is placed (by them) on determining the existence of suspicious violence.'[1]

Abramson went on to recommend supine sleep and avoidance of loose bedding as ways to prevent these deaths. He thus anticipated, over 50 years ago, how the death-scene investigation and studies of soft bedding might contribute to our understanding of many sudden unexpected infant deaths.[16,17]

Later doubts about rebreathing

DISAGREEMENT WITH ABRAMSON AND MUSINGS OF DR WOOLEY

Jacob Werne MD and Irene Garrow MD were two pathologists from New York who disagreed with Abramson's explanation for the deaths of infants found with their nose and mouth down and covered. In 1947, they wrote that claims that accidental suffocation caused many deaths unfairly increased 'the feeling of culpable negligence experienced by the mother.'[18] Furthermore, they reviewed the pathologic specimens from Abramson's cases of accidental suffocation and announced 'findings . . . which were adequate to establish a natural cause of death, therefore excluding suffocation.' Their ultimate diagnoses for the 43 cases included mastoiditis and otitis media (20 cases), unspecified congenital heart disease (seven cases), pneumonia (seven cases), and 'idiopathic cardiac hypertrophy' (three cases). Werne and Garrow believed that they had refuted Abramson's claims, but it appears, in retrospect, that most of their explanations for death were inadequate substitutes for accidental suffocation. Werne and Garrow's long paper also represents an early effort to assuage parental guilt, a sentiment that, unfortunately, may have steered discussion away from safe sleep practices that could have saved lives.

Another paper from the late 1940s by Paul Wooley MD, a pediatrician from Portland, OR, also influenced thinking about mechanisms for face-down deaths.[19] Wooley, like Werne and Garrow, wrote in response to Abramson's findings. Wooley also shared their strong sympathy for grieving families. 'To leave the family with a clear conscience is a duty secondary in importance only to saving the patient, and (after the child's death) the physician should take all measures to be able to do this.' In studies done with a colleague, they 'attempted to induce anoxemia by having the subjects sleep with nose and mouth closely approximated to mattresses and pillows, but here again we were unsuccessful since the smallest was capable of rolling to obtain an airway and the larger were generally out of accord with the position.' Unfortunately, Wooley's paper does not tell how many infants he studied, their ages or weights, or how he was able to document the absence of 'anoxemia'.

If one reviews Wooley's paper, it is clear what motivated him to write it, but the bases for his conclusions are not recorded. Nevertheless, Wooley's paper has been quoted often over the years, and at the dawn of the SIDS era it apparently buttressed conventional wisdom regarding how an infant tolerates soft bedding.[20]

Face-down deaths and SIDS

In her landmark paper entitled 'Sudden and Unexpected Death in Infancy: A Review of the World Literature 1954–1966', Dr Maria Valdes-Dapena made many fundamental observations about infant mortality. She realized that her ideas would lead to new approaches to understanding causation of infant deaths. Dr Valdes-Dapena concluded, emphatically, that 'when criteria are held at their most rigid and no minimal or questionable changes are accepted as causes of death, great numbers of these deaths remain inexplicable.'[20] These words also seem to refute Werne and Garrow's explanations, which, in retrospect, seem to have been based on 'minimal or questionable changes.'

Dr Valdes-Dapena did not cite Abramson or Archibald, but did cite Wooley from the pediatric literature. When considering the 30% of deaths known at that time to be face down,[2] she seemed to conclude that 'I don't know' was the proper response to questions of causation when infants are found face down. She wrote that 'the experiments of Wooley ... have established the fact that a well child – even a newborn – cannot be suffocated by ordinary bedclothing; in the face-down position the infant will adjust his position sufficiently to obtain an airway.'[20] Thus, in the context of this key paper, the work of Wooley, which in retrospect seems biased and lacking in hard data,[21] came to have a critical influence on thinking about face-down deaths. Face-down deaths were believed to be as mysterious as all of SIDS, and the bedding and sleep position as incidental.[11,22]

Because of the importance of Dr Valdes-Dapena's paper, the influence over the last 30 years of Dr Wooley's musings cannot be overstated. For example, Jess Kraus PhD, in reviewing vital statistics from California,[23] noted that 'with the introduction of a new rubric for SIDS in 1973, most of the deaths previously assigned strangulation or suffocation diagnoses by California coroners were called "SIDS".' Therefore, since 1973, in the absence of postmortem findings distinguishing SIDS from subtle suffocation in soft bedding,[24,25] many deaths which we believe can be explained by rebreathing,[1,13] have been classified as SIDS.

We will now review results, which taken together, have begun to change the conventional wisdom.

Rebreathing of exhaled air and soft bedding

CASE–CONTROL STUDIES AND CASE SERIES

Table 9.1 shows results indicating that 20–52% of infants dying suddenly and unexpectedly are found face down. All studies since the early 1970s have included these deaths among cases diagnosed as SIDS. The fraction from the USA has been consistently near 30%.[1,2,7] The rates of face-down deaths were higher in New Zealand and Tasmania where distinctive items of soft bedding – sheepskins and natural fiber mattresses – increased risk associated with prone sleeping.[5,6]

Five case–control studies linking soft bedding to sudden unexplained infant death

In 1965, Carpenter and Shaddick reported 'an analysis of some sociological data' pertinent to 110 sudden infant deaths and to two matched controls per case.[3] The deaths occurred in England (London and Cambridge). Compared to controls, infants dying were: (1) less likely to have been placed supine for sleep; (2) more likely to have used a pillow or soft mattress; and (3) more likely to have been found with their nose and mouth completely covered by bedding (*P*<0.001). Twenty per cent of victims had their nose and mouth completely covered, and another 18% had their external airway partially covered. One per cent of controls were found with their nose and mouth covered on the designated day used for comparison.

Fleming and colleagues in England have shown that in general, using more bedding increases the OR for sudden death among prone infants.[26] Using duvets, or comforters, in particular, yields a significant OR (1.88), when controlling for other factors in the sleep environment. Recent reports from Fleming's group do not mention nose and mouth position, however.[27,28]

Use of sheepskins by prone infants from the New Zealand Cot Death Study increased their OR for dying to 1.70 (95% CI, 1.08 to 2.67). In that study, 52% of infants were found face down.[5]

Another type of distinctive bedding was of interest in case–control studies from Australia.[29] In the study done in Hobart, Tasmania, soft mattresses filled with natural fibers were identified as 'effect modifiers' that increased risk when infants were placed prone. The natural fibers used as filling for pillows and mattresses included kapok and shavings of bark from the ti tree. The OR for use of natural fiber bedding was not increased (OR=1.3, 95% CI=0.6–2.9) unless infants slept prone. Among infants prone on natural fiber bedding, the OR increased dramatically (OR=10.0, 95% CI=2.5–43.0). A related report from Tasmania showed that '39% (of SIDS cases there) . . . were found face down in the prone position.'[6]

There are no published reports of case–control studies from the USA addressing the interaction among soft bedding, sleep position, and sudden death. However, preliminary results form a large infant mortality study in Chicago show an adjusted OR=20.3 (5% CI=7.5–54.5) for prone sleep on soft bedding. The adjusted OR for prone sleep on firm bedding was significant but much smaller (2.0, 95% CI=1.1–3.5).[30]

Case series linking soft bedding to death with nose and mouth covered

A recent case–comparison study from the USA[7] shows that 59 (29%) of 206 SIDS victims died with their nose and mouth covered by bedding. All but two of the 59 were prone and face-down, based on findings from the death-scene investigations. The case–comparison design of their study allowed Scheers *et al.* to identify factors associated with death with nose and mouth covered. The associated factors were prone sleep, soft bedding, and use of pillows and comforters.

After attempting to summarize the epidemiologic data, it seems appropriate to address an important tangential issue. It has been suggested that the face-down posture is 'agonal'.[11,31] While it is conceivable that the face-down posture is agonal in some cases, the strong and consistent association with soft bedding undermines arguments that this is usually the case. Why, if it is agonal, is the face-down posture more common on soft items, as Scheers *et al.*[7] have shown? Why is the face-down posture so common (>70%) among infants dying prone when they are exposed to that position for the first or second time, as discussed below?[8] In addition to these questions arising from epidemiologic studies, physiologic findings, provide further evidence that death in the face-down position on soft bedding is often instrumental, and not only 'incidental', or 'agonal'.

In summary, several case series and case–control studies strongly implicate a role for soft bedding in prone deaths, particularly when infants are found face down. Mechanisms for this type of prone death are discussed next.

Evidence for lethality of rebreathing

BEDDING ASSOCIATED WITH FACE-DOWN DEATHS

When one breathes into comforters, sheepskins, natural fiber mattresses or pillows, items associated with face-down SIDS, the effect is not stifling. That is, the impression is that the items themselves, and their covers, are of low resistance to airflow. We have used modifications of the model shown in Fig. 9.2, inserting a pressure transducer and flow meter, to show that the measured resistance is low. The resistance to airflow measured on these items, with the model in the face-down position, is less than the total resistance of an infant's respiratory system.[33–35] This may explain why infants coming to lie face down on these soft items did not awaken quickly, because they would not sense a high imposed resistive load that could cause arousal from sleep.[36,37]

REBREATHING OF EXHALED AIR: EVIDENCE FROM MODELS

Fig. 9.3 shows a rabbit breathing through a model of an infant's upper airway. When airway CO_2 is recorded, capnometric tracings are obtained (Fig. 9.4).[34,38] Rebreathing is occurring in simulations such as that in Fig. 9.3 when inspired CO_2% increases above ambient levels (0.04%). The degree of rebreathing shown in Fig. 9.4 caused profound arterial blood gas changes in rabbits (Fig. 9.5),[34] with lethal effects in 3 of 4. Fig. 9.5 shows that the rabbits were both hypercarbic and profoundly hypoxemic. Using readily available recording equipment, rebreathing of exhaled CO_2 is easier to document than is hypoxia in the inspired air. Nevertheless, the arterial blood gas levels leave no doubt that inspired air

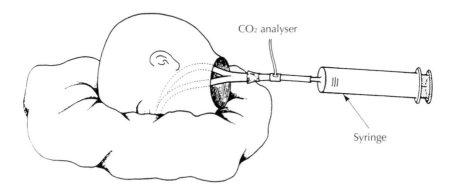

Fig. 9.2   System used to quantify rebreathing consisted of a 100-ml syringe filled with 5 per cent CO_2, tubing connecting syringe to mannequin's head, and bedding studied. Dispersal of CO_2 using 30-ml 'breaths' was recorded by plotting signals from a CO_2 analyser. Half-time for dispersal of CO_2 $(t_{1/2})$ uniquely defines the capacity of the bedding to cause rebreathing.[32]

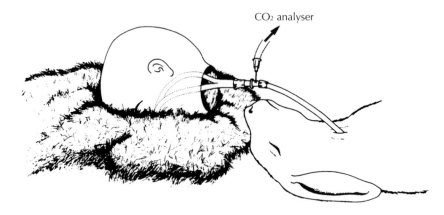

Fig. 9.3   Rabbit breathing through a weighted mannequin's head on a sheepskin. Dotted lines represent tubes from the nares that insert into a Y-connector. A tracheostomy tube with a sideport for CO_2 monitoring has been placed in the sedated rabbit. This preparation was used to show that severe and lethal rebreathing occurred in reconstructions of the scene of sudden infant deaths.[34]

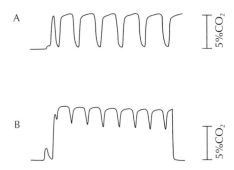

Fig. 9.4 $CO_2\%$ as measured from the endotracheal tube in Fig. 9.3. Exhalation causes an increase or plateau of $CO_2\%$ in the tube. Inspiration causes a decrease of $CO_2\%$ in the tube. (A) Baseline recording with rabbit breathing through the mannequin's head alone. Inspired $CO_2\%$ was 0.21. (B) Recording after 5 minutes of breathing through a mannequin's head while face down on a sheepskin. Note that the lowest inspiratory $CO_2\%$ rose to 4.4%, confirming marked rebreathing.[34]

was markedly depleted of O_2. Thus, it is more correct to describe this scenario as one causing rebreathing of exhaled air, rich in CO_2 and depleted of O_2, rather than to explain the rabbits' demise by hypercarbia alone.

In addition to sheepskins, we have also used rabbits to demonstrate lethal rebreathing on comforters, soft pillows and polystyrene bead-filled cushions.[35,39]

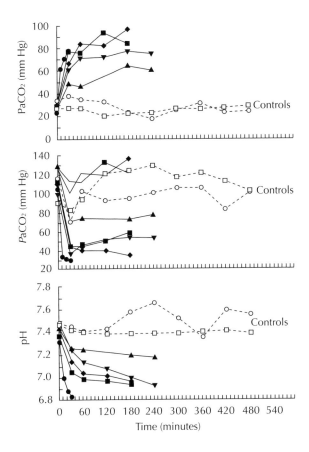

Fig. 9.5 Levels of arterial blood gases for five study rabbits and two controls. Solid lines indicate rabbits breathing into sheepskins; stippled lines, control rabbits that breathed through the mannequin's head alone. Blood gas levels at time 0 were obtained after 30 minutes of breathing through the mannequin's head alone. One rabbit (solid circles) was studied only 30 minutes while rebreathing, as part of a shorter protocol. Three of four rabbits studied for longer than 30 minutes died while breathing into the sheepskin.[34]

Campbell *et al.* used a piglet model to show rapid onset of marked rebreathing on several items of infant bedding in common use in New Zealand. Deaths occurred among piglets rebreathing from sheepskins.[40]

Mechanical models have also been useful in studying bedding associated with face-down SIDS. The mechanical model we developed (Fig. 9.2) was validated by comparison to changes in $PaCO_2$ in rabbits.[32] We filled the syringe with 5% CO_2 and ventilated the mannequin head and bedding ensemble with 30 ml breaths at 15 breaths per minute. Disappearance of CO_2 from this microenvironment followed a single exponential 'decay' curve. The ability of bedding to limit CO_2 dispersal is thus quantifiable via the half-time for CO_2 removal ($t_{1/2}$). Figure 9.6 shows that bedding associated with face-down SIDS, in contrast with firm bedding, has much greater propensity to limit CO_2 dispersal. In all cases, the soft bedding's $t_{1/2}$ exceeds the threshold associated with lethality in rabbit studies. Others have developed sophisticated mechanical models to describe and quantify rebreathing potential[40–44] imposed by bedding, and related their results to abnormalities in animal models.[45]

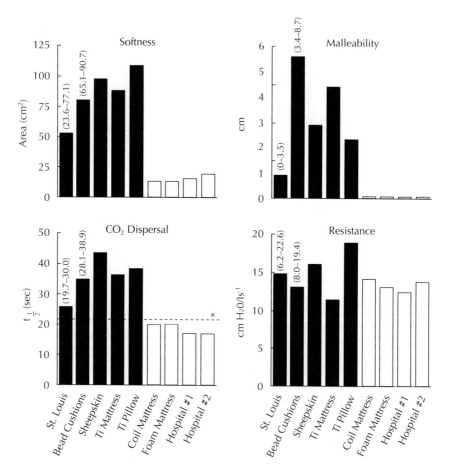

Fig. 9.6   Comparison of physical properties of bedding associated with SIDS to those of presumably safe bedding. Open bars refer to firm mattresses covered with a sheet. Bedding associated with face-down SIDS (solid bars) is softer and has greater propensity to limit CO_2 dispersal than does bedding on which face-down deaths are rare. Line drawn at $t_{1/2}=22.4$ s corresponds to the threshold above which deaths occurred in studies using the rabbit rebreathing model.[15]

Figure 9.6 also shows that bedding causing rebreathing and associated with face-down SIDS is softer than items on which face-down deaths have not been reported. We quantified the softness of the bedding by measuring the area of apposition between the mannequin's face and the underlying bedding.[15] Putting the mannequin head face down on a firm mattress made of foam brings 12.6 cm² into apposition; if it is face down, e.g. on a sheepskin or comforter the areas of apposition are 97.1 cm² and 52.9 cm², respectively.

Figure 9.6 thus shows the important physical properties that distinguish items of bedding on which infants have died face down.

Our mechanical model has also been useful in showing that softness alone may not predict the propensity of an item of bedding to limit CO_2 dispersal. The porosity of an item may also contribute to its ability to cause rebreathing. For example, a soft comforter was shown to cause more rebreathing than an equally soft plastic air mattress.[32] We presume this is because a comforter can trap exhaled air within the interstices of its filling.[46] The additive effects of softness and porosity may explain, in particular, why natural fiber mattresses and bead-filled cushions were associated with many deaths in microenvironments causing rebreathing.[29,39] Those items have permeable covers, and complex, porous interiors.

STUDIES IN INFANTS DEMONSTRATING REBREATHING

Infants have been shown to rebreathe exhaled air from bedding in at least four studies. We will discuss some of them now. Before beginning, however, we should emphasize that the threat to infants would be even greater if the infant had blunted ventilatory or arousal responses to hypoxia and hypercarbia.[47-49]

Perhaps the most dramatic example of rebreathing by an infant is found in a paper by Waters *et al.* from Montreal.[12] They studied 10 healthy infants sleeping at home in prone sleep scenarios chosen by their parents. Their primary goal was to study the face-down position in a 'natural' sleep environment. Waters *et al.* used an infrared video camera to record position and the face's relationship to bedding, and a Respitrace^R to document breathing movements. Sao_2 and transcutaneous Pco_2 and heart rate were also recorded. The median number of times per night that the infants turned their faces straight down – or nearly so – was between 5 and 6. The prone infant of particular interest was one who pulled a loose mattress pad over her nose and mouth. The pad stayed there for 20 minutes. During this time her $Ptco_2$ rose from 50 to 87 mmHg. The infant survived this encounter, but this vignette seems to confirm the profound abnormalities in gas exchange possible when prone infants cover their nose and mouth with bedding. In a related finding, we described the scene of death of a 2-month-old infant who was found prone with a blanket between his flexed arm and face.[50] Our case reinforces the idea that the microenvironment encountered by the subject of Waters *et al.* could indeed be lethal.

Chiodini and Thach[51] used capnometry to show that prone face-down infants rebreathe in soft bedding. Inspired CO_2% increased to as high as 6.4% (mean 3.2%) among 11 infants sleeping on a sheepskin. There was also a significant increase in end-tidal $CO_2\%$ for the infants as a group, suggesting that gas exchange abnormalities occurred. (The $CO_2\%$ in fresh, ambient air is quite low, approximately 0.04%.)

Malcolm *et al.* also used capnography to study 11 newborn infants.[52] They were studied prone and supine, on sheepskins and sheets, and with their heads covered or uncovered. They showed that inspired $CO_2\%$ rose quickly to as high as 2.8%, particularly when the infants were prone beneath blankets. They emphasized that a steady state with elevated inspired $CO_2\%$ was attained by their subjects, who became hyperpneic while rebreathing.

In Norway, Skadberg and Markestad[53] studied whether infants are able to gain access to fresh air when they begin to rebreathe. They studied both prone and supine infants with their heads covered by duvets (comforters). Inspired $CO_2\%$ increased to as high as 4.5%, with small but consistent rises in $PtCO_2$. Only one infant among 30 was able to uncover his head while prone, as compared with 18 of 30 studied supine.

Finally, Lijowska *et al.* studied response sequences leading to access to fresh air while prone infants were rebreathing from a sheepskin covered by a sheet.[54] Inspired $CO_2\%$ rose to as high as 4.8%. Interestingly, head lifting and turning did not always provide these infants with access to fresh air when the head returned to the horizontal, because the nose and mouth was still covered.

In summary, studies in infants have shown that they will rebreathe exhaled air for variable periods when their nose and mouth are in soft bedding. They will rebreathe whether they are placed face down, or turn face down themselves. In most reports, the infants turned and/or lifted their head to gain access to fresh air. However, this was often after many minutes of rebreathing, and this behavior did not always gain them access to fresh air, even when they fully aroused from sleep. One chilling vignette showed that an infant's $PtCO_2$ can rise to very high levels (87 mmHg) during spontaneous rebreathing in bedding. Studies in infants both suggest and document dangers from rebreathing in bedding.

Rebreathing and newer epidemiology

DEATHS WITH HEAD COVERED AND AMONG INFANTS UNACCUSTOMED TO PRONE SLEEPING

Success in reducing SIDS rates by discouraging prone sleep position has generated interest in other sleep practices that could be modified to further reduce mortality. Thus, sleep practice data have been re-examined from both before and after interventions to increase the supine sleep.

Before 'Back-to-Sleep', 14.3 to 28.0% of victims were found with their heads completely covered by bedclothes.[55] The rate appears to be even higher in some locales, after the intervention.[56] In Norway, for example,[57] 48% of SIDS victims (27 of 56) were found with their head covered by a duvet, but none of 133 reference living infants had heads covered. And in England, after the Back-to-Sleep campaign,[27] a case–control study showed that being found with bedcovers over the head was associated with a multivariate OR for death of 21.58 (95% CI=6.21–74.99).

Physiologic studies are beginning to show the dangers of head-covered sleep, also. Using a mechanical model, Campbell *et al.* were able to predict a very high level of rebreathing for supine head-covered infants beneath blankets and duvets.[55] Skadberg and Markestad and Lijowska *et al.* have shown in both prone and supine infants that head covering leads to inspired CO_2% >4% while rebreathing is occurring.[53,54]

Re-examination of data from the New Zealand Cot Death Study has revealed a huge risk associated with prone sleeping among a subgroup of infants. These infants were unaccustomed to the prone position. The OR for infants who usually slept supine or on their side, but who turned prone, or were placed prone inadvertently was 19.3 (95% CI, 8.2–44.8).[58] Of the infants from New Zealand unaccustomed to the prone position, 71% were found face down. Similar results from a more recent study were obtained by L'Hoir *et al.* in the Netherlands in 1996.[8] Victims found prone but unaccustomed to that position had an OR = 17.89 (95% CI, 5.98–53.48). Twelve of the infants were found face down in the Netherlands study; 11 were unaccustomed to prone sleep.[8]

Other studies may offer an explanation for the high rate of face-down deaths among infants unaccustomed to prone sleep.[59] Preliminary physiologic and behavioral studies in living infants indicate that unaccustomed prone sleepers are much less adept at gaining access to fresh air when rebreathing in the face-down position, compared with habitual prone sleepers.[60]

It thus appears that rebreathing remains an important mechanism for death among infants at very high risk after the Back-to-Sleep campaign. Marked rebreathing occurs among infants whose heads are covered by soft bedding. Finally, the position most favoring rebreathing, face straight-down, is over represented among victims unaccustomed to prone sleeping.

Conclusions

A robust framework for attempting to understand sudden unexpected infant death is the triple-risk model developed by Filiano and Kinney.[61] They propose that vulnerable infants at a vulnerable developmental stage are exposed to stressors that lead to death. The success of the Back-to-Sleep program suggests, among other explanations, the importance of environmental stressors associated with prone sleeping.

The case for rebreathing of exhaled air as a lethal mechanism for sudden unexpected infant deaths is supported by: (1) information from death-scene investigations; (2) case–control studies and case series; (3) physiologic studies in infants, and using animal and mechanical models. Rebreathing offers an explanation, among many possible and complementary explanations, for the strong epidemiologic interaction between prone sleeping and soft, porous bedding. It is a mechanism that can be averted by placing infants supine for sleep, provided they do not turn prone, or get their head covered.

Acknowledgement

The research of the authors is supported by the national SIDS Alliance (USA) and the NICHD (HD-10993).

References

1. Abramson H. Accidental mechanical suffocation in infants. *J Pediatr* 1944;25: 404–13.
2. Adelson L, Kinney ER. Sudden and unexpected death in infancy and childhood. *Pediatrics* 1956;17:663–97.
3. Carpenter RG, Shaddick CW. Role of infection, suffocation, and bottle feeding in cot death: an analysis of some factors in the histories of 110 cases and their controls. *Br J Prev Soc Med* 1965;19:1–7.
4. Bergman AB, Ray CG, Pomeroy MA, Wahl PW, Beckwith JB. Studies of the sudden infant death syndrome in King County, Washington III. Epidemiology. *Pediatrics* 1972;49:860–70.
5. Taylor BJ. A review of epidemiological studies of sudden infant death syndrome in southern New Zealand. *J Paediatr Child Health* 1991;27:344–8.
6. Ponsonby A-L, Dwyer T, Gibbons LE, Cochrane JA, Jones ME, McCall MJ. Thermal environment and sudden infant death syndrome: case–control study. *Br Med J* 1992;304:277–82.
7. Scheers NJ, Dayton CM, Kemp JS. Sudden infant death with external airways covered: case comparison study of 206 deaths in the United States. *Arch Pediatr Adolesc Med* 1998;152:540–7.
8. L'Hoir MP, Engelberts AC, Van Well GTJ *et al.* Risk and preventive factors for cot death in the Netherlands, a low-incidence country. *Eur J Pediatr* 1998;157:681–8.
9. Gilbert-Barness E, Barness LA. Cause of death: SIDS or something else? *Contemp Pediatr* 1992;9:13–29.
10. Hassal IB, Vandenberg M. Infant sleep position: a New Zealand survey. *NZ Med J* 1985;98:97–9.
11. Emery JL. Information for parents of a child who died unexpectedly in infancy. In: Camps FE, Carpenter RG (eds). *Sudden and Unexpected Deaths in Infancy*. John Wright and Sons, Bristol, 1972.
12. Waters KA, Gonzalez A, Jean C, Morielli A, Brouillette RT. Face-straight-down and face-near-straight-down in healthy, prone-sleeping infants. *J Pediatr* 1996;128: 616–25.
13. Archibald HC. Sudden unexplained death in childhood – can it be prevented? *Arch Pediatr* 1942;59:57–61.
14. Nunn JF. *Applied Respiratory Physiology*. 3rd edn. Butterworths, Stoneham, MA, 1987,166pp.
15. Kemp JS, Nelson VE, Thach BT. Physical properties of bedding that may increase risk of sudden infant death syndrome in prone-sleeping infants. *Pediatr Res* 1994;36: 7–11.
16. Willinger M, James LS, Catz C. Defining the sudden infant death syndrome. *Pediatr Pathol* 1991;11:677–84.

17. Kattwinkel J, Brooks J, Keenan ME, Malloy M, Willinger M. Positioning and SIDS: update. *Pediatrics* 1996;98:1216–18.

18. Werne J, Garrow I. Sudden deaths in infants allegedly due to mechanical suffocation. *Am J Pub Health* 1947;37:675–87.

19. Wooley PV. Mechanical suffocation during infancy: a comment on its relation to the total problem of sudden death. *J Pediatr* 1945;26:572–5.

20. Valdes-Dapena MA. Sudden and unexpected death in infancy: a review of the world literature 1954–1966. *Pediatrics* 1967;39:123–38.

21. Thach BT. Sudden infant death syndrome: old causes rediscovered? *N Engl J Med* 1986;315:126–8.

22. Guntheroth WG, Spiers PS. Are bedding and rebreathing suffocation a cause of SIDS? *Pediatr Pulmonol* 1996;22:335–41.

23. Kraus JF. Effectiveness of measures to prevent unintentional deaths of infants and children from suffocation and strangulation. *Public Health Rep* 1985;100:231–40.

24. Gordon I, Shapiro HA. *Forensic medicine: a guide to principles.* 2nd edn. Churchill Livingstone, Edinburgh, 1982, 31 pp.

25. Polson CJ, Gee DJ. *The essentials of forensic medicine*, 3rd edn. Pergamon Press, Oxford, 1985, 583 pp.

26. Fleming PJ, Gilbert R, Azaz Y, Berry PJ, Rudd PT, Stewart A, Hall. Interaction between bedding and sleep position in the sudden infant death syndrome: a population based case–control study. *Br Med J* 1990;301:85–9.

27. Fleming PJ, Blair PS, Bacon C *et al.* Environment of infants during sleep and risk of the sudden infant death syndrome: results of the 1993–5 case–control study for confidential inquiry into stillbirths and deaths in infancy. *Br Med J* 1996;313:191–5.

28. Ponsonby A-L, Dwyer T, Couper D, Cochrane J. Association between use of a quilt and sudden infant death syndrome: case–control study. *Br Med J* 1998;316:195–6.

29. Ponsonby A-L, Dwyer T, Gibbons LE, Cochrane JA, Wang Y-G. Factors potentiating the risk of sudden infant death syndrome associated with the prone position. *N Engl J Med* 1993;329:377–82.

30. Hauck FR. Findings from the Chicago Infant Mortality Study. *Presented at the SIDS Alliance National Conference*, Atlanta, Georgia, 1999.

31. Guntheroth WP, Spiers PS. Sleeping prone and the risk of sudden infant death. *JAMA* 1992;267:2359–62.

32. Kemp JS, Thach BT. Quantifying the potential of infant bedding to limit CO_2 dispersal and factors affecting rebreathing in bedding. *J Appl Physiol* 1995;78:740–5.

33. Crossfill ML, Widdicombe JG. Physical characteristics of the chest and lungs and the work of breathing in different mammalian species. *J Physiol* 1961;158:1–14.

34. Kemp JS, Thach BT. A sleep position-dependent mechanism for infant death on sheepskins. *AJDC* 1993;147:642–6.

35. Kemp JS, Kowalski RM, Burch PM, Graham MA, Thach BT. Unintentional suffocation by rebreathing: a death scene and physiological investigation of a possible cause of sudden infant death. *J Pediatr* 1993;122:874–80.

36. Tan S, Duara S, Neto GS, Afework M, Gerhardt T, Bancalari E. The effects of respiratory training with inspiratory flow resistive loads in premature infants. *Pediatr Res* 1992;3:613–18.

37. Fewell JE, Williams BJ, Szabo JS, Taylor BJ. Influence of repeated upper airway

obstruction on the arousal and cardiopulmonary response to upper airway obstruction in lambs. *Pediatr Res* 1988;23:191–5.

38. Swedlow DB. Capnometry and capnography: the anesthesia disaster and early warning system. *Semin Anesth* 1986;5:194–205.

39. Kemp JS, Thach BT. Sudden death in infants sleeping on polystyrene-filled cushions. *N Engl J Med* 1991; 423:1858–64.

40. Campbell AJ, Taylor BJ, Bolton DPG. Comparison of two methods of determining asphyxial potential of infant bedding. *J Pediatr* 1997;130:245–9.

41. Ryan EL. Distribution of expired air in carry cots: a possible explanation for some sudden infant deaths. *Austr Phys Eng Sci Med* 1991;14:112–18.

42. Bolton DPG, Cross KW, McKettrick AC. Are babies in carry cots at risk from CO_2 accumulation? *Br Med J* 1972; iiii: 80–1.

43. Bolton DPG, Taylor BJ, Campbell AJ, Galland BC, Cresswell CA. A potential danger for prone sleeping babies: rebreathing of expired gases when face down into soft bedding. *Arch Dis Child* 1993;69:187–90.

44. Carleton JN, Donoghue AM, Porter WK. Mechanical model testing of rebreathing potential in infant bedding materials. *Arch Dis Child* 1998;78:323–8.

45. Kemp JS, Livne M, White DK, Arfken CL. Softness and potential to cause rebreathing: differences in bedding used by infants at high risk and low risk for sudden infant death syndrome. *J Pediatr* 1998;132:234–9.

46. Batchelor GK. *An introduction to fluid mechanics.* Cambridge University Press, Cambridge, 1967, 233 pp.

47. McCulloch K, Brouillette RT, Guzzetta AJ, Hunt CE. Arousal responses in near-miss sudden infant death syndrome and in normal infants. *J Pediatr* 1982;101: 911–7.

48. Davidson-Ward SL, Bautista DB, Woo MS *et al.* Responses to hypoxia and hypercapnia in infants of substance-abusing mothers. *J Pediatr* 1992;121:704–9.

49. Mograss MA, Ducharme FM, Brouillette RT. Movement/arousals: description, classification, and relationship to sleep apnea in children. *Am J Respir Crit Care Med* 1994;150:1690–6.

50. Kemp JS. Sudden infant death syndrome: the role of bedding revisited. *J Pediatr* 1996;129:946–7.

51. Chiodini BA, Thach BT. Impaired ventilation in infants sleeping facedown: potential significance for sudden infant death syndrome. *J Pediatr* 1993;123:686–92.

52. Malcolm G, Cohen G, Henderson-Smart D. Carbon dioxide concentrations in the environment of sleeping infants. *J Paediatr Child Health* 1994;30:45–9.

53. Skadberg BT, Markestad T. Consequences of getting head covered during sleep in infancy. *Pediatrics* 1997;100;E6.

54. Lijowska AS, Reed NW, Mertins-Chiodini BA, Thach BT. Sequential arousal and airway-defensive behavior of infants in asphyxial sleep environments. *J Appl Physiol* 1997;83:219–28.

55. Campbell AJ, Bolton DPG, Williams SM, Taylor BJ. A potential danger of bedclothes covering the face. *Acta Pediatr* 1996;85:281–4.

56. Brooke H, Gibson A, Tappin D, Brown H. Case–control study of sudden infant death syndrome in Scotland, 1992–5. *Br Med J* 1997;314:1516–20.

57. Markestad T, Skadberg B, Hordvik E, Morild I, Irgens LM. Sleeping position and sudden infant death syndrome: effect of the intervention programme to avoid prone sleeping. *Acta Paediatr* 1995;84:375–8.

58. Mitchell EA, Thach BT, Thompson JMD, Williams S. Changing infants' sleep position increases risk of sudden death. *Arch Pediatr Adolesc Med* 1999;153:1136–41.

59. Burns B, Lipsitt LP. Behavioral factors in crib death: toward an understanding of the Sudden Infant Death Syndrome. *J Appl Dev Psychol* 1991;12:159–84.

60. Paluszynska DA, Harris KA, Thach BT. Ability of prone sleeping infants to escape from asphyxiating microenvironments by changing head position: influence of age and sleep position experience. (Abstract) *Presented at the SIDS Alliance National Conference*, Atlanta, Georgia, 1999.

61. Filiano JJ, Kinney HC. Perspective on neuropathologic findings in victims of the sudden infant death syndrome: the triple-risk model. *Colloquium on Control of Breathing during Development and Apnea in the Newborn and in SIDS*. Universite de Nancy I, September, 1992.

CHAPTER 10

Airway inflammation and peripheral chemoreceptors

ERNEST CUTZ AND ADELE JACKSON

Introduction   156
Respiratory pathogens and inflammatory changes in SIDS infants   157
Pulmonary neuroepithelial bodies as airway chemoreceptors   166
Model linking airway inflammation with chemoreceptor dysfunction   171
Summary, conclusions and the future   174
Addendum: protocol for investigation of lung pathology in SIDS   176
Acknowledgements   176
References   176

Introduction

The observation of airway inflammation in lungs of infants who died of SIDS was first reported in 1953 by Werne and Garrow.[1] This classical study identified up to 33% of infants who died suddenly and unexpectedly had a recent history of upper respiratory tract infection (URI), and their lungs showed changes of airway and/or pulmonary inflammation. Tracheobronchitis with or without associated bronchiolitis has been repeatedly observed by a number of investigators examining the lung tissue of SIDS victims.[2-4] The finding of airway inflammation and/or interstitial pneumonitis-like pattern in SIDS infants was thought to represent lesions related to viral etiology.[5] Previous epidemiologic studies identified in up to 45% of SIDS infants evidence of mild infection preceding death, making this one of the most consistent findings in SIDS.[6] In addition, occurrence of URI has been linked to higher incidence of SIDS during the winter months when these infections are more common.[7] Over the years, the significance of both airway inflammation and viral pathogens isolated in SIDS cases has been questioned.[8] In fact, the SIDS literature is divided on this question with some authors suggesting that these changes may be possible epiphenomen and not related to the pathophysiology of SIDS.[9] In contrast, others view these findings as potentially significant triggering factors leading to SIDS.[5,10] These findings, however, cannot be ignored since SIDS cases with airway inflammation continue to represent a significant subgroup.[4]

The first section of this chapter reviews recent literature on this topic as well as our experience on the incidence, histopathology and immunopathology of airway changes in SIDS. In addition, methods for the recovery and tissue diagnosis of pathogens in the lung are briefly discussed.

The second section focuses on airway chemoreceptors represented by neuroepithelial bodies (NEB), located within the airway epithelium, and hence possible direct or indirect targets of the airway inflammation. Since NEB may represent first-line defense in hypoxia signaling, recent findings of cellular and molecular mechanisms of oxygen sensing are reviewed.

The third section presents an integrated hypothesis linking minor respiratory infection, airway inflammation and its potential effects on NEB airway sensors. Since NEB innervation is derived from the vagus nerve and their function appears to be developmentally regulated, these sensors made vulnerable via airway inflammation may represent the 'missing link' in a triple-risk model of SIDS.[11] In fact, minor respiratory infection causing airway inflammation and thus affecting the function of airway sensor (NEB) could represent the actual triggering factor leading to SIDS. Ongoing and future studies exploring these hypotheses are also discussed.

Respiratory pathogens and inflammatory changes in SIDS infants

It is presumed that the inflammatory changes observed in the airways and/or lungs of infants dying of SIDS are a result of an infection, most commonly of viral origin. The spectrum of histopathologic changes observed in the respiratory tract of SIDS infants has been recently reviewed and classified by Bajanowski and Brinkmann.[10] The classification scheme proposed by these authors includes four grades, with grade zero reflecting minimal, early stages of viral infection. The presence of interstitial and peribronchial inflammatory cell infiltrate constitutes grades two and three. This classification is partially based on a previously described pattern of viral pneumonitis in infants and children with documented respiratory syncytial virus (RSV), parainfluenza and influenza virus infections.[12] The presence of tracheitis and/or bronchiolitis was included as part of 'classic' or typical histopathologic findings in SIDS reported in AFIP Histopathology Atlas for SIDS.[13] These lesions, characterized by acute and chronic inflammatory cell infiltrate of the mucosa and/or submucosa associated with epithelial changes (i.e. loss of cilia), were not considered to represent an adequate cause of death, although these cases were classified as SIDS. The incidence of clinical history of mild URI within 24 hours of death was reported in 29% of cases amongst SIDS infants in the NICHD study.[6] The incidence of URI increased to 44% when the last 2 weeks of life were included.

At our institution, review of 178 consecutive cases of SIDS during a 5-year period (1987–1992) identified 69 (or 39%) of cases of SIDS with inflammatory changes in the lung (tracheobronchitis, bronchiolitis) and/or increased numbers of alveolar macrophages (Fig. 10.1). In the majority of our cases (<80%) there was a clinical history of URI prior to death.[4]

HISTOPATHOLOGY AND IMMUNOPATHOLOGY

To provide baseline data on airway inflammation, we performed detailed analysis of lungs from 21 cases of SIDS and nine age-matched control infants dying of other causes. The main criteria for selection was preservation of airway epithelium, excluding cases with long postmortem interval. For assessment of histopathology combined with immunohistology, a minimum of five blocks of each lung were examined. First we analysed routine hematoxylin and eosin (H&E) sections of trachea and lung (including the lung hilus) for the presence of inflammation and its distribution. Amongst 21 cases of SIDS, nine cases showed evidence of 'minor' airway inflammation whereas in the other 11 cases no inflammation was apparent in routine sections. None of the nine control cases showed evidence of airway inflammation. In positive SIDS cases, the inflammatory cell infiltrate consisting mostly of lymphocytes with few plasma cells and occasional eosinophils was distributed within the submucosa of different size airways, sometimes infiltrating the epithelium (Fig. 10.2). Between 10 to 60% of airways showed inflammatory changes. In some cases, small clusters of

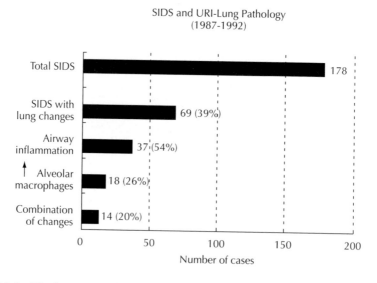

SIDS and URI-Lung Pathology
(1987-1992)

Fig. 10.1 The frequency of inflammatory changes in the lungs and airways in a cohort of 178 infants who died of SIDS during a 5-year period (1987–1992) in Metropolitan Toronto area.

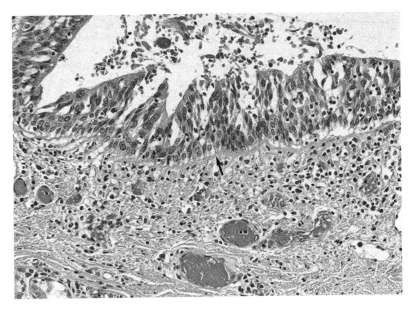

Fig. 10.2   Early inflammatory changes in bronchial epithelium of a 7-month-old infant who died of apparent SIDS. The airway epithelium shows loss of cilia and mild intraepithelial inflammatory cell infiltrate. Similar inflammatory cell infiltrate is present in the lamina propria. Epithelial basement membrane (arrow). (H & E stain, × 400.)

polymorphs were noted within the airway lumen. The epithelium of inflamed airways usually showed loss of cilia with flattening and early regenerative changes.

To quantitate the number and distribution of inflammatory cells we have used a pan-leukocyte marker (CD45) and counted positive cells (Fig. 10.3) localized within airway epithelium, submucosa and alveolar septae using immunohisto-chemical and morphometric methods similar to those reported by Haley *et al.*[14] For the sake of simplicity we only used a single, general marker of inflammatory-type cells. In future studies it will be possible to identify specific inflammatory cell subsets and to define immunophenotypes as shown for specific viral[15] or hypersensitivity-type[14,15] responses.

In our preliminary study we have found up to 10-fold increase in the number of inflammatory cells (CD45-positive) in various pulmonary tissue compart-ments including the airway epithelium, submucosa and to a lesser extent alveo-lar septae (Table 10.1). There was no significant difference between non-SIDS control infants and SIDS infants without apparent inflammatory changes in routine lung sections. Since SIDS is considered a multifactorial disorder, this finding confirms subsets of SIDS cases with and without airway inflammation. Hence, inflammation in the airway is likely to be a relevant risk factor only in some cases of SIDS. These findings are also in agreement with those reported by Howat *et al.*[16] who examined 48 consecutive cases of SIDS and 30 controls

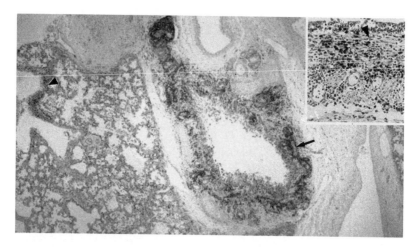

Fig. 10.3 Low magnification view of a hilar bronchus and adjacent lung parenchyma from a lung of a 2½-month-old infant who died of SIDS. The section was immunostained for CD45, a pan-leukocyte marker. Cells positive for CD45 (dark areas) are concentrated around bronchial wall (arrow). A smaller airway within the lung parenchyma shows focal CD45 positivity (arrowhead). (Immunoperoxidase method for CD45, ×100.)

Insert: Higher magnification of a bronchial wall in a section immunostained for CD45. Numerous CD45-positive cells are localized in submucosa with fewer cells in the epithelium (arrowhead). (Immunoperoxidase method for CD45, ×250.)

dying of other non-pulmonary causes. This study reported up to threefold increase in the number of eosinophils, T and B lymphocytes in lungs of SIDS infants suggesting an abnormal pulmonary inflammatory response in SIDS. Although no specific viral or other pathogens were identified in this study, the presence of increased numbers of inflammatory cells was postulated to alter (via locally produced cytokines) the normal pulmonary responses and in a susceptible infant lead to SIDS.

Table 10.1 Quantitative assessment of inflammation in lungs of SIDS and controls

	(A) SIDS with inflammation	(B) SIDS without inflammation	Control
Number of cases	10	11	9
Inflammatory cells (CD45)/unit surface area in:			
Airway epithelium	6.5±0.9*	0.5±0.1	1.0±0.2
Submucosa	30.5±5.4**	5.2±0.9	8.9±1.4
Alveolar septae	12.0±1.4***	9.4±1.0	9.3±1.4

* $P<0.001$ vs both SIDS-B and control;
**$P<0.001$ vs SIDS-B;
*** $P<0.01$ vs control.

IDENTIFICATION OF RESPIRATORY PATHOGENS

Previous studies using viral cultures identified several viral respiratory pathogens in a small proportion of SIDS infants.[5,8] The most frequently reported viruses recovered from samples of lungs of SIDS infants are respiratory syncytial virus (RSV), influenza, parainfluenza, and adenoviruses.[5,8] The low yields of positive viral cultures have been interpreted as being due to the samples taken late in the course of the illness and/or due to postmortem changes.[8] The use of new molecular techniques for detection of viral pathogens have increased the positive yields.[17] The choice of appropriate culture and detection methods in the diagnosis of viral respiratory infections in infants and children has been recently discussed.[18] The advances in immunohistochemistry combined with availability of specific antibodies against a variety of viral antigens has facilitated direct identification and localization of viral antigens in lung and other tissues. In a prospective study (since 1994) we have used a panel of antibodies against RSV, adenovirus and cytomegalovirus (CMV) on lung sections from all infants dying of SIDS or sudden unexpected death (SUD). So far, we have identified 10 cases of SIDS with positive immunostaining for RSV and one case positive for CMV. Amongst cases positive for RSV two types of patterns were identified. The most common acute form was characterized by marked peribronchial inflammatory cell infiltrate affecting different size airways (Fig. 10.4). The airway epithelial cells were devoid of cilia, their apical surface had a spheroid shape and some cells were seen detaching from the epithelium into the airway lumen (Fig. 10.5a). These features are consistent with viral effects. Immunostaining for RSV showed positive reactivity in the apical cytoplasm of airway epithelial cells

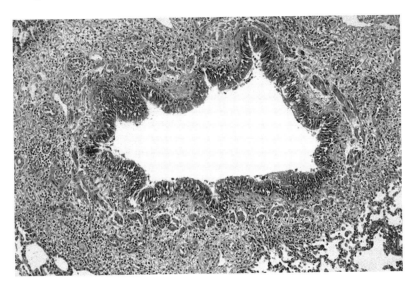

Fig. 10.4   Marked peribronchial inflammatory cell infiltrate in a lung of a 3-month-old infant dying of SIDS with BAL positive for RSV. (H&E stain, ×250.)

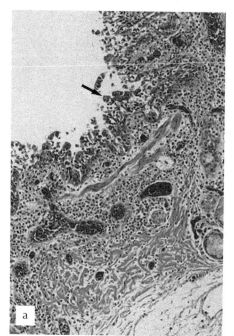 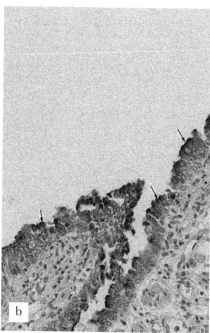

Fig. 10.5 (a) Close-up of bronchial wall from the same case as in Fig. 10.4 showing extensive epithelial changes with detachment of surface epithelial cells (arrow) and dense mononuclear cell infiltrate in subepithelium area. (H&E stain, x250.) (b) Immunostaining with anti-RSV antibody on the same section as in (a). Positive reactivity for RSV protein is localized in apical cytoplasm of airway epithelial cells (arrows). (Immunoperoxidase method for RSV, ×400.)

(Fig. 10.5b). Significantly, in all cases the areas of RSV-positive immunoreactive epithelial cells showed prominent inflammatory cell infiltrate of the epithelium and submucosa indicating active, acute infection.

The second, less common pattern was the presence of positive-RSV-immunoreactivity within the cytoplasm of alveolar macrophages (Fig. 10.6). In the latter cases, the airways were either normal or showed mild chronic inflammation but without RSV-positive epithelial staining. This may indicate a recovery stage or a chronic process with clearing of the virus from the epithelium, and residual viral protein retained in the alveolar macrophages. This pattern is also consistent with recent experimental studies in a guinea pig model of RSV infection demonstrating persistence of RSV protein and genomic RNA in the lung for up to 60 days after acute infection.[19,20] In these animals, immunohistochemistry for RSV viral protein was identified in alveolar macrophages without airway epithelial cell staining and viral cultures were negative. Recent studies on the identification of respiratory viral pathogens in SIDS, using molecular techniques such as non-isotopic *in situ* hybridization (ISH) have reported increased

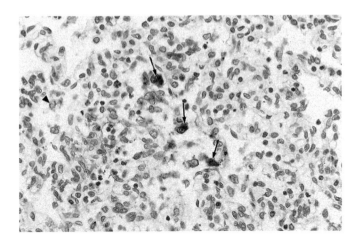

Fig. 10.6 Immunostaining for RSV on lung section from another 3-month-old infant who died of SIDS. Immunoreactivity for RSV is localized in the cytoplasm of a few alveolar macrophages (arrows). Note other alveolar macrophages in adjacent alveoli (arrowhead) are negative, ruling-out non-specific endogenous peroxidase reactivity. (Immunoperoxidase method for RSV, ×500.)

sensitivity of detection. The study of An *et al.*[17] using ISH technique found eight cases of adenovirus type five, two cases of RSV and one parainfluenza type two in a cohort of 45 cases of SIDS. This represented 24% of SIDS with positive findings in contrast to three per cent of non-SIDS controls ($n = 30$). In another recent study of 99 SIDS cases and 58 matched controls, using ISH for RSV, 27% of SIDS were positive compared with 18% of controls.[21] The latter two studies, however, did not correlate findings of viral genome with airway inflammation to differentiate between acute, active infection (clinically significant) with persistence of viral genome without inflammation (i.e. an innocent bystander). Ideally, a combination of methodologies for virus detection (i.e. detection of viral protein, ISH, culture) in conjunction with assessment of airway inflammatory changes could provide more meaningful data relevant to the pathophysiology of SIDS (*see* Addendum for Protocol at end of chapter).

BRONCHO-ALVEOLAR LAVAGE (BAL) IN DIAGNOSIS OF RESPIRATORY PATHOGENS

In the clinical setting, the role of BAL in the diagnosis of respiratory pathogens, interstitial lung disease and other disorders is well established.[22] To determine the potential usefulness of this technique for the detection of viral and microbial pathogens in cases of SIDS and other sudden death we have carried out a prospective study (since 1995) using BAL from autopsy lung samples. In the initial study, we have analysed BAL from consecutive cases of SIDS ($n = 14$) and SUD ($n = 6$) under 8 months of age. The samples of BAL were obtained by instilling 30 ml of saline solution into the main stem bronchus of left lung and withdrawal of the fluid into a syringe. BAL samples were processed for routine cytology (Fig. 10.7a) and residual pellets fixed in formalin, embedded in paraffin for immunohistochemical and other studies (Fig. 10.7b). Aliquots of each BAL sample together with small fragments of lung tissue and a tracheal ring were submitted for routine virological cultures. Although postmortem bacterial and particulate contamination may cause a problem in BAL samples from autopsies, we have found that the overall preservation of cells was excellent in the majority of samples (Fig. 10.7a,b). Routine cytologic examination with special fungal stains identified two SIDS cases positive for *Pneumocystis carini* (P. c.) (Fig. 10.8). The lung tissue from both cases showed areas with prominent hyperplasia of peribronchial and septal lymphoid tissues (Fig. 10.9). These features are

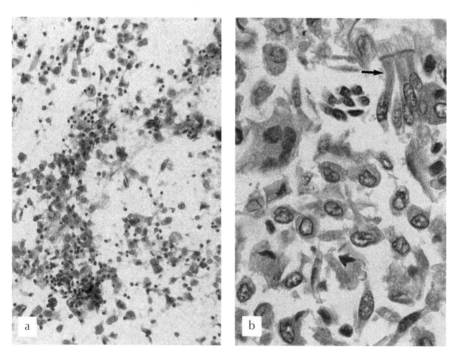

Fig. 10.7   (a) Cytologic preparation of BAL sample from a 3½-month-old infant who died of SIDS and whose lung sections showed airway inflammation. This cell preparation contains a mixture of alveolar macrophages, epithelial cells and inflammatory cells (small dark nuclei). (PAP stain, ×250.) (b) High magnification view of a BAL sample fixed in formalin and processed as a cell pellet. There is excellent cytologic preservation of ciliated epithelial cells (arrow). Most other cells in this field are alveolar macrophages. (H&E stain, ×1000.)

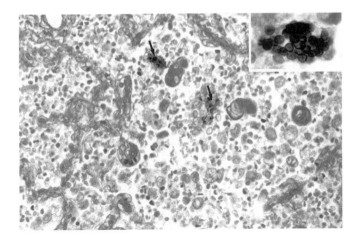

Fig. 10.8 Section of lung from a 2-month-old infant who died of apparent SIDS and in whom BAL revealed *Pneumocystis carini* (P. c.) organisms. Few clusters of P. c. organisms (arrows) are seen within an alveolus also containing red cells and macrophages. (Grocott silver methanamine method, ×400.)

Insert: Cluster of typical P. c. organisms in a BAL cytology sample. (Grocott silver methanamine method, ×1000.)

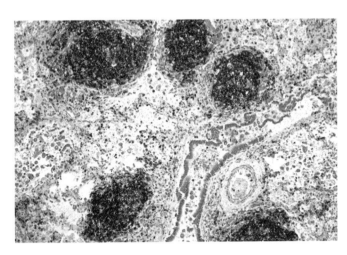

Fig. 10.9 Peribronchial and interstitial lymphoid hyperplasia in another area of lung from the case as in Fig. 10.8 with early P. c. pneumonitis. The section was immunostained for CD45 to highlight the lymphoid areas (dark staining). Testing for HIV and congenital immune deficiency was negative. (Immunoperoxidase method for CD45, ×250.)

compatible with early P. c. pneumonitis (testing for HIV and inherited immuno-deficiencies was negative). Therefore, SIDS cases with bronchial lymphoid hyperplasia may represent a subgroup of P. c. or other pulmonary infections rather than a non-specific, normal response as recently suggested.[23] It should be stressed that without BAL examination these cases would be missed due to the low number of organisms present.

Virology studies on our BAL samples gave positive yields comparable to clinical samples with 10 cases positive for RSV by immunofluorescence or culture, three cases of parainfluenza type two or three, and two cases of CMV. Thus far, no cases of adenovirus have been identified amongst our SIDS cohorts examined recently. It should be noted, however, that viral isolation methods, seasonality and geographical variability may account for differences in viral pathogen isolation identified in different centers.

We recommend the use of BAL since we found this to be a useful adjunct in the investigation of respiratory infections in SIDS. Furthermore, routine use of BAL in these cases may increase detection of pathogens.

Pulmonary neuroepithelial bodies as airway chemoreceptors

GENERAL STRUCTURAL AND FUNCTIONAL FEATURES OF NEB IN MAMMALIAN LUNGS

Intrapulmonary pulmonary neuroepithelial bodies (NEBs) form distinct intra-epithelial corpuscles or clusters of amine- and neuropeptide-containing cells associated with nerve endings usually entering at the basal pole of the cells. NEB cells produce a number of neurotransmitters/neuromodulators including amine (serotonin) and peptides (bombesin, calcitonin, calcitonin gene-related peptide, enkephalin), and others (for review *see* Cutz[24]). NEBs are widely distributed throughout the mucosa of intrapulmonary airways and are often situated at branch points where gas flow rates are higher, allowing for rapid sensing of changes in lung gases.[25–27] Using scanning electron microscopy, the apical surfaces of NEB cells, at least in rabbit fetuses and neonates, form distinct microvilli fully exposed to the airway lumen.[28] There is growing evidence that NEBs function as hypoxia-sensitive airway chemoreceptors,[26,29] and together with other peripheral chemoreceptors (e.g. the carotid body, CB), are involved in the autonomic control of breathing. The prominence of NEBs during the perinatal period suggests that they may be particularly important in the transition from fetal to neonatal life.

The function of NEBs as intrapulmonary sensors is an attractive theory, since there would be a mechanism for direct and immediate local response to hypoxia detected within the respiratory tract in advance of a decrease in blood Po_2 monitored by the CB. In a neonatal rabbit model, NEBs were shown to react to airway hypoxia by a heightened release of serotonin.[26] Subsequent cross-circulation studies confirmed that this secretory response was due to airway hypoxia rather than hypoxemia.[30] In addition, this secretory response appears to be locally mediated since unilateral hypoxia (with the other lung ventilated with hyperoxic gas) caused a significant decrease in 5-HT content in the hypoxic lung despite no change in blood gas values.[31] Various vagotomy procedures have demonstrated that sensory innervation of rabbit NEB is derived from the vagus nerve with nerve cell bodies residing in the nodose ganglion.[32,33] These initial studies helped to solidify the view that NEB cells were connected to the CNS and thus NEBs were seen as part of a respiratory sensory or feedback circuit.

Stimulus-evoked secretion of transmitters from NEBs target two areas: the intracorpuscular nerve endings and basal cell membrane. Transmitters secreted at the basal cell membrane can be taken up by blood capillaries and affect local changes in pulmonary blood flow and airway tone (e.g. vasoconstriction or vasodilation). Some of these same transmitters (e.g. bombesin) also regulate growth and maturation in early lung development.[34,35]

CELLULAR AND MOLECULAR MECHANISMS OF O_2 SENSING IN NEB CELLS

At the cellular level, NEBs share many features with conventional chemoreceptors (e.g. CB), including the presence of amine and peptide mediators, sensory innervation and chemosensitivity to O_2. Similar to CB glomus cells, NEB cells express a membrane-bound O_2-sensing mechanism comprised of an O_2-sensor protein complex (NADPH oxidase) linked to an O_2-sensitive K^+ channel[29] (for review *see* Cutz and Jackson[36]). NADPH oxidase, first identified in professional phagocytes, is composed of several protein subunits that once assembled catalyze the one-electron reduction of molecular oxygen to superoxide (O_2^-), using electrons supplied by NADPH.[37] The oxidase components include two membrane proteins (gp91[phox] and p22[phox]) that together form a b-type cytochrome, two cytosolic peptides (p47[phox] and p67[phox]) and a cytosolic small GTPase (Rac 2). Most of the NADPH oxidase components were shown to be expressed in NEB cells of fetal rabbit lung as well as in glomus cells of rat and human carotid body.[29,38,39] Unlike the oxidase in professional phagocytes, NADPH oxidase in NEBs appears to be active even under basal conditions.[40]

Currently, the preferred mechanism of O_2 chemotransduction in NEB cells is based on the 'membrane' model proposed for CB glomus cells.[41–43] In this model, a primary event in response to a decrease in Po_2 is the closure of O_2-sensitive K^+ channels.[41,43] The actual O_2 sensor is thought to be a heme-linked NADPH oxidase which is closely associated with an O_2-sensitive K^+ channel.[40,43–45] During hypoxia, due to decreased substrate (O_2) availability, NADPH oxidase fails to maintain superoxide (and hence H_2O_2) production and as a result cannot keep redox couples preferentially in the oxidized state. Modulation of the redox status of a cysteine residue in the K^+ channel protein [46] is thought to alter the protein conformation of this H_2O_2-sensitive K^+ channel, leading to channel closure. The resulting membrane depolarization leads to activation of voltage-sensitive Ca^{2+} channels, followed by an influx of extracellular Ca^{2+} triggering secretion of neurotransmitter(s) onto terminals of sensory nerve fibers in contact with NEB cells which, in turn, relay afferent impulses to the brainstem

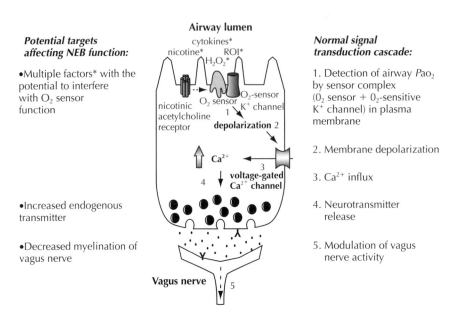

Potential targets affecting NEB function:

•Multiple factors* with the potential to interfere with O_2 sensor function

•Increased endogenous transmitter

•Decreased myelination of vagus nerve

Normal signal transduction cascade:

1. Detection of airway Pao_2 by sensor complex (O_2 sensor + O_2-sensitive K^+ channel) in plasma membrane

2. Membrane depolarization

3. Ca^{2+} influx

4. Neurotransmitter release

5. Modulation of vagus nerve activity

Fig. 10.10 Schema of normal signal transduction cascade in NEBs and sites of potential targets for NEB dysfunction in SIDS. Under normal conditions (right hand panel) during exposure to hypoxia the decreased availability of O_2 substrate causes a reduction in the level of byproducts of O_2 reduction by NADPH oxidase (i.e. O_2^- and H_2O_2). This, in turn, alters the redox potential of the cells, causing a change in the protein conformation of the O_2-sensitive K^+ channel. The resulting closure of these channels prevents the outward flux of K^+ ions, leading to membrane depolarization and/or increase action potential frequency, calcium influx and neurotransmitter secretion. The binding of neurotransmitter to sensory afferent terminals of the vagus nerve (for NEBs) and carotid sinus nerve (for carotid body) causes a relay of information to the respiratory center in the brainstem. Since NEB cell surfaces are exposed to the airway lumen, they make direct contact with the external environment containing a multitude of biological and chemical agents (left hand panel), including nicotine (i.e. smoking mother). In addition, airway infection and inflammation may directly expose NEB cells to inflammatory cytokines, hydrogen peroxide (H_2O_2) and other reactive oxygen intermediates (ROI). All of these 'exogenous or environmental stressors' could directly or indirectly 'blunt' the oxygen-sensing capabilities of NEBs cells by interfering with their O_2 signaling cascade. In addition, findings in SIDS cases of decreased myelination of vagus nerve,[65] increased levels of endogenous transmitters in the carotid body[67] and hyperplasia of NEB cells [48,49] indicate that there are long-term modifications to chemoreceptors which may have increased the vulnerability of these infants to SIDS.

(Fig. 10.10). The role of an oxidase in the regulation of O_2-sensitive K^+ channel has been strengthened by recent studies demonstrating modulation of these channels by the by-products of oxidase, e.g. H_2O_2. Indeed, external application of H_2O_2 on NEB cells, either in culture or in fresh lung slice preparations, under normoxia showed increased outward K^+ current.[40,47] Furthermore, diphenylene iodonium (DPI), an inhibitor of NADPH oxidase, reduced the O_2-sensitive K^+ current in NEBs.[29,47] These findings may be particularly relevant to SIDS, since reactive oxygen intermediates (ROI) are significant by-products of airway inflammation.

PULMONARY NEB IN SIDS

Hyperplasia of pulmonary neuroendocrine cell (PNEC) system including NEB has been reported in two independent studies. Gillan *et al.*[48] used modification of Grimelius silver impregnation method to demonstrate argyrophilic cells in lungs of 25 victims of SIDS and compared them with 20 control infants. This study found up to twofold increase in the percentage of positive airways and numbers of PNEC/NEBs in lungs of SIDS victims versus lungs of control infants dying of other causes. An additional feature of SIDS lungs was increased number and size of NEBs located at bronchio-alveolar junctions. The majority of SIDS cases (21 out of 25) showed values greater than any of the control cases. SIDS cases with values comparable to controls were considered a possible subset with alternate mechanisms leading to death. We studied PNEC/NEB in lungs of SIDS and controls using a combination of immunohistochemistry and radioimmunoassay for detection of bombesin-like peptide.[49] In our control infants, the frequency of PNEC/NEB was high at birth and during the first month, but declined during the first year of life. In contrast, in SIDS infants, the frequency of PNEC and the size of NEBs (Fig. 10.11), as well as the mean concentration of bombesin-like peptide detected in lung extracts, were significantly increased compared to those of age-matched controls.[49] These findings suggest hyperplasia or persistence of the PNEC system in the airways of SIDS infants, which may be a reactive or an adaptive phenomenon to a variety of physical or chemical agents, but a precise mechanism is unknown.

PATHOBIOLOGY OF NEB IN SIDS

In experimental animals, chronic hypoxia in particular has been shown to be a potent stimulus for hyperplasia of PNEC and NEB. Adult Sprague Dawley rats (but not Wistar rats) exposed to chronic normobaric hypoxia (10% O_2) for 3 weeks showed a significant increase in the number of PNEC and enlargement of NEBs to more than double that of control rats.[50] These animals also showed changes associated with prolonged, severe hypoxia, including increased hematocrit, enlarged carotid body, and right ventricular hypertrophy. An increased number of NEBs have also been reported in young rabbits kept in hypobaric chambers,[51] as well as in those raised at high altitude.[52] Hence, chronic hypoxia

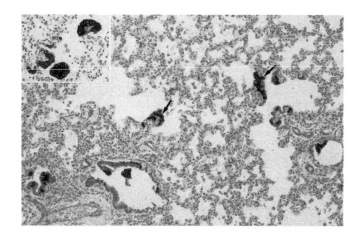

Fig. 10.11 Hyperplasia of NEB in lung of a 3-month-old infant who died of SIDS. The section was immunostained for bombesin, a marker of NEB cells. Clusters of positive NEBs (arrows) composed of 10–20 cells are located in small terminal bronchioles and bronchio-alveolar junction. In contrast, NEB in lungs of age-matched control infants are composed of three to five cells (*see* Ref 49). (Immunoperoxidase method for bombesin, ×400.) Insert: Higher magnification of hyperplastic NEB located at bronchio-alveolar junction ×400).

may reduce the maturation-dependent decrease in NEB cell number and or stimulate the differentiation of NEBs from precursor cells.

An additional factor for PNEC/NEB hyperplasia may relate to maternal smoking, a well-defined risk factor for SIDS.[53] Recent findings suggest that SIDS infants whose mothers smoked during pregnancy and postnatally develop significant structural changes in their airways, i.e. a greater inner airway wall thickness in the larger airways, compared with SIDS infants of non-smoking mothers. This increased thickness may contribute to exaggerated airway narrowing and may help explain abnormalities observed in neonatal lung function in infants of smoking mothers.[53] In addition, we have shown recently that in infants who died of SIDS and who were born to smoking mothers, PNEC frequency was increased significantly compared with that in SIDS infants born to non-smoking mothers.[54] Therefore, it appears that maternal smoking potentiates PNEC/NEB hyperplasia in SIDS lungs possibly via cholinergic/nicotinic receptors expressed on the plasma membrane of these cells.

Numerous experimental studies have shown that cigarette smoke and nicotine are potent stimuli for PNEC hyperplasia. For example, repeated subcutaneous injections of nicotine in pregnant rabbits induced hyperplasia of NEBs in the offspring.[55] In a hamster model, chronic exposure to cigarette smoke resulted in elevation of calcitonin and bombesin concentration in lung extracts correlating with increased numbers of immunoreactive PNEC in lung sections.[56] Similarly, Nylen *et al.*[57] demonstrated that nicotine stimulates replication of hamster PNEC *in vitro*. As stated above, nicotine exposure *in utero* also increased the size and number of NEBs and conversely decreased solitary PNEC in fetal rhesus monkey lung.[58] The latter finding suggests that nicotine may stimulate mitogenesis in already differentiated PNECs leading to formation of NEBs rather than differentiation of new PNEC.[58] All of these studies suggest that NEB cells are directly sensitive to nicotine via nicotinic receptors expressed on their plasma membrane. This belief has now been confirmed by Sekhon *et al.'s*[58] demonstration of α7 nAChRs on fetal monkey NEB cells. In fact, the proliferative effect of nicotine may be mediated by α7 receptors, since Quik *et al.*[59] have shown that α-BGT, a specific antagonist of α7 receptors, blocks the nicotine-induced proliferation in a PNEC-related tumor cell line. Hence, nicotine acting through nicotinic receptors (possibly α7 receptors) may cause a developmental proliferation of PNEC/NEB, which, in turn, may release a variety of growth factors that effect lung development.

Model linking airway inflammation with chemoreceptor dysfunction

It is now recognized that SIDS is a multifactorial disorder rather than a disease entity with a single etiology and uniform pathophysiology. A number of clinicopathological studies on SIDS have identified subgroups of SIDS cases exhibiting different features.[1-4] This variability can also explain apparent discrepancies amongst different studies on SIDS pathology, neurobiology, biochemistry, etc. Therefore, the following discussion is directly relevant to a subgroup of SIDS cases (≤30%) with identified history of mild URI, viral infection and airway inflammation.

At present, there is no universally accepted explanation for the role of the above findings in the pathophysiology of SIDS. In fact, no direct link between respiratory tract infection and SIDS has been established. A main argument against such a direct role is that respiratory tract infections are very common in young infants, yet the incidence of SIDS is relatively low. Additional arguments, advanced mostly by forensic authorities, consider it inconceivable that a mild respiratory infection with minor pathology can be a contributing factor to cause death. Previous studies addressing the role of respiratory tract infection accompanied by 'trivial' airway and/or pulmonary inflammation and SIDS have advanced a number of hypotheses, including: (a) SIDS infants exhibit an abnormal inflammatory reaction, caused by a viral or bacterial infection, with release of toxic eosinophil-derived cytokines which, in turn, initiate abnormal airway responses and/or induce pulmonary edema.[16] (b) Alternatively, an increased release of interleukin-1 by inflammatory cells was postulated to depress ventilation via its effects on brainstem neurons.[60] A similar mechanism proposed by Howatson implicates alpha-interferon (produced by cells in response to a viral infection) affecting the function of brainstem neurons involved in the control of breathing.[61] (c) Blackwell *et al.*[62] have proposed that mild URI could be a route of entry for super infection by toxin-producing bacteria. (d) Lindgren[63] postulated the involvement of laryngeal chemoreceptors based on the well documented association between RSV infection and infantile apnea. He speculated that RSV infection may affect the sensitivity of these chemoreceptors resulting in attenuated inputs to proximal centers of respiratory control.[64] Our hypothesis introduces dysfunction of peripheral chemoreceptors as a key element for interaction between mild URI, airway inflammation and SIDS. This proposal does not negate above noted hypotheses and is in agreement with the so-called triple-risk model for SIDS linking underlying biological vulnerability, critical developmental period, and exogenous stressors or triggering factors.[11]

We postulate that dysfunction of peripheral chemoreceptors (i.e. NEB in the airways and/or CBs) together with previously documented abnormalities in the brainstem and vagus nerve[65,66] may represent the basis for biological vulnerability in infants dying of SIDS. In fact, defects in some or all of these components of the autonomic control of breathing can be documented in the same SIDS cases (unpublished observation). Our earlier studies implicated CB dysfunction based on findings of increased dopamine and norepinephrine content of CBs of infants who died of SIDS.[67] Although the mechanism for CB dysfunction is not known, possible involvement of nicotine (i.e. maternal smoking) has been suggested.[68] In a rat pup model, Holgert et al.[68] have shown recently that nicotine attenuates the respiratory drive generated by the CBs. The proposed mechanism for inhibition of the hypoxic drive involves nicotine-induced release and increased synthesis of dopamine acting via dopamine type two receptors expressed on CB glomus cells. In addition, Jackson and Nurse[69] have exposed dissociated rat carotid body cultures to chronic nicotine to study the mechanisms by which nicotine can interfere with the protective chemoreflex response to hypoxia. Chronic nicotine dramatically elevated basal dopamine levels *in vitro* and this response was attenuated by acute or chronic treatment with mecamylamine, a nicotinic acetylcholine receptor antagonist. Using a potent blocker of the dopamine transporter (i.e. nomifensine), it was demonstrated that nicotine caused the accumulation of extracellular dopamine, at least in part, by inactivating or down-regulating dopamine transporters on glomus cells.

Hyperplasia of PNEC/NEB has been documented in the majority of SIDS infants.[48,49] As discussed earlier, this hyperplastic response could relate to chronic hypoxia or developmental delay, and in some cases may be further potentiated by maternal smoking.[54] The postulated dysfunction of hyperplastic NEBs is based on analogy with findings in CBs of animals exposed to chronic hypoxia where CB hyperplasia and increased neurotransmitter content is accompanied by blunted CB response to hypoxia.[70,71] It should be noted, however, that in contrast to the well documented role of CB in the control of breathing, evidence for involvement of NEB in respiratory control is at present indirect. Supporting evidence includes striking morphologic and biochemical similarities between NEB cells and CB glomus cells, including their O_2-sensing mechanism (for review see Cutz and Jackson[36]). In addition, the innervation of NEB is derived from the vagus nerve[32,33] and there is evidence for modulation of hypoxic breathing by vagal afferents in a chemodenervated rabbit model.[72]

Functionally, NEBs as airway chemoreceptors may complement rather than duplicate CB activity, particularly during the perinatal period when NEBs are most prominent and CBs are relatively inactive. Hence, the dysfunction of NEBs during a critical developmental period, when CBs are resetting their sensitivity towards adult values,[73,74] may make the infant particularly vulnerable to SIDS. Such vulnerability may remain latent until the system is challenged (i.e. exposure to hypoxia induced by sleeping position or mild respiratory infection).

There are several plausible scenarios for potential cellular and molecular mechanisms leading to altered NEB function during respiratory infection and resulting airway inflammation (Fig. 10.10). Although NEB cells are part of the airway epithelium and as such could be a direct target of a viral infection, this mechanism alone could not account for fatal outcome, since inflammatory changes in the airways of SIDS infants tend to be focal. A more likely scenario involves the effects of inflammatory cells and various by-products of inflammation, including generation of H_2O_2 by alveolar macrophages (Fig. 10.10). We have already demonstrated the effects of exogenous H_2O_2 on O_2-sensitive K^+ channels in NEB cultures or *in situ* using fresh lung slices.[29,47] In these experiments H_2O_2 was shown to increase the open probability of H_2O_2-sensitive K^+ channels under normoxia. The sustained opening of these K^+ channels would be expected to prevent repolarization of NEB cell membrane, effectively abolishing signal generation. In the intact animal or an infant the consequence would be failure to signal hypoxia or a generation of an erroneous signal.

The direct effects of cytokines on NEB function have not as yet been investigated. However, the effects are likely to be significant and widespread as there is a vast array of cytokines known to be generated during airway inflammation.[75] Cytokines are low molecular weight glycoproteins released by inflammatory and other cells to self-activate or activate adjacent cells. For example, interleukin-1 subtypes are derived from macrophages and monocytes and increase markedly during respiratory infections. Interleukin-2 subtypes are generated by lymphocytes and are particularly up-regulated during viral infection. In addition, tumor necrosis factor (TNF) released from neutrophils and lymphocytes is abundant during URI. In theory, cytokines generated during URI could affect signal transduction of NEB cells either through its effects on O_2-sensing protein (NADPH oxidase) and/or O_2-sensitive K^+ channels. It is also likely that these humoral substances could affect NEB cells over a large area, not limited to specific inflammatory foci.

There is also recent evidence that the O_2-sensing mechanism, similar to the one expressed on NEB cells, is operational on solitary PNEC distributed within the epithelium of trachea and bronchi. Skogvall *et al.*[76] have shown recently that O_2-sensing PNEC are involved in modulation of contractile responses of airway smooth muscle in isolated guinea pig trachea preparations. This data provide further support for previous studies showing that removal of airway epithelium increases the contractile responses evoked by acetylcholine, histamine or 5-HT.[77] This suggests that airway epithelium generates an inhibitory signal to dampen the effects of contractile stimuli on bronchial smooth muscle and to augment the effectiveness of inhibitory stimuli.[78] Therefore, PNEC and NEB as part of airway epithelium could play a significant role in this process. The above mechanism could also explain the basis for increased airway responsiveness observed in patients with airway inflammation. In the setting of SIDS infants with airway inflammation and/or epithelium damage, the resultant bronchoconstriction could lead to hypoxia and thus trigger the chain of events leading to SIDS (Fig. 10.12).

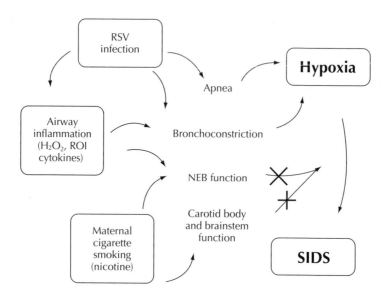

Fig. 10.12 Schema outlining possible interactions between URI, airway inflammation and chemoreceptor dysfunction leading to SIDS. The organoid arrangement of NEBs, their sensory innervation and direct exposure to the airway lumen make them ideally suited as sensors for airway oxygen. These features, however, make NEB cells vulnerable to a variety of 'exogenous stressors', namely nicotine, respiratory infection and by-products of airway inflammation and/or epithelium damage. Therefore, dysfunction of NEB, which may normally serve as a bridge linking the external environment (i.e. airway lumen) to the nervous system (e.g. respiratory control center in brainstem), may interfere with the signaling of airway hypoxia and trigger a cascade of events leading to SIDS. Similarly, dysfunction of the carotid body and brainstem neurons, as a result of the effects of nicotine on O_2–sensing and nervous system development, respectively, may lead to a failure to respond appropriately to hypoxia and result in SIDS. Among the numerous pathways and circumstances by which an infant can become hypoxic, RSV infection and airway inflammation may trigger apnea and bronchoconstriction, respectively.

Summary, conclusions and the future

The association between mild URI, airway inflammation and SIDS has been a subject of speculation since the first report of these findings. At present there is no definitive evidence for a direct link between specific respiratory viral infection and SIDS. However, in this context, RSV appears to be the most significant pathogen due to its epidemiologic characteristics as well as its selective targeting of the airway epithelium and known association with apnea in both infants[79] and animals.[64] Studies using animal models of RSV infection can be useful in defining further the precise pathophysiologic mechanisms. Recent advances in molecular techniques should facilitate the identification of additional viral pathogens important in SIDS. Improvements in virus detection at the tissue level combined with detailed immunophenotyping of airway inflammatory cells should define more closely the cause and effect of these airway lesions. These data will also be helpful in better understanding the airway responses invoked by local mediator release (i.e. bronchoconstriction).

Our hypothesis predicts that in normal infants who develop mild URI, the effects of local inflammation on airway sensors (with all other components of respiratory control mechanism intact) is not sufficient to induce system failure and in fact may invoke compensatory responses leading to recovery. In contrast, a vulnerable infant with single or multiple abnormalities involving some or all of the components of respiratory control mechanism (i.e. NEB and/or CB chemoreceptors, vagal neural pathways, brainstem neurons) will fail to respond appropriately to the hypoxia challenge (Fig. 10.12). The precise mechanism or etiology of these defects or abnormalities are not known. The proposed hypotheses include adverse intrauterine environment, such as maternal smoking, sub-optimal prenatal care, or intrinsic abnormalities affecting fetal neural development.[65] The testing of SIDS hypotheses is difficult as multiple factors seem to play a role and potential interactions are likely to be complex. Although it may not be possible to develop a complete SIDS animal model, recent advances in cellular and molecular biology offer new avenues for investigation, not available previously. For example, it is now possible to test individual components of our hypothesis, by examining directly the effects of by-products of airway inflammation on O_2 sensing by NEB cells using the patch clamp technique. Furthermore, a mouse knock-out model with deficiency of NADPH oxidase is available.[80] In a recent study using this model, we have shown that NEB cells in oxidase-deficient mice fail to respond to hypoxia by closure or inactivation of O_2-sensitive K^+ channel as occurs in wild type mice.[81] We have also shown that viable NEB cells can be recovered from lungs of SIDS infants[82] allowing direct examination of these cells by electrophysiologic or molecular (single cell PCR) techniques. Therefore, there are now unprecedented opportunities to prove or disprove the 'armchair SIDS theories' by direct hypothesis testing.

Irrespective of the progress in SIDS research to better understand its biology, the ultimate test of these hypotheses may involve simple interventional studies as has been the case with change in the sleeping position. In particular, avoidance of smoking during pregnancy, improved prenatal care, prompt recognition and treatment of respiratory infections including the use of new antiviral drugs and/or effective vaccinations may remove the known triggering factors and further reduce the incidence of SIDS.

Addendum: Proposed Protocol for Investigation of Lung Pathology in SIDS

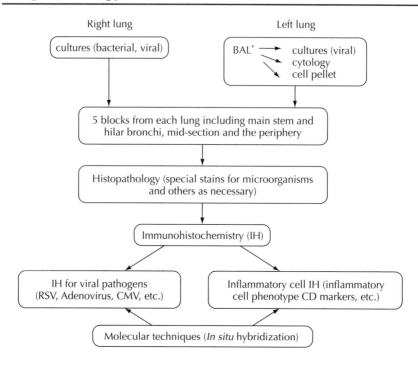

*BAL may be suitable for *in vitro* studies, since it is possible to recover viable cells from SIDS autopsy lungs (Forsyth *et al.*, 1988[83]).

Acknowledgements

The authors thank Dr D.G. Perrin for numerous contributions to this project. Dr A. Jackson is a recipient of a Sydney Segal Research Fellowship from The Canadian Foundation for the Study of Infant Deaths. This study was supported in part by grants from the Medical Research Council of Canada (MT-12742) Ontario Thoracic Society and Nicole Fealdman fund for SIDS research.

References

1. Werne J, Garrow I. Sudden apparently unexplained death during infancy: Pathologic findings in infants found dead. *Arch Pathol* 1953;29:633–75.
2. Krous HF. The pathology of sudden infant death syndrome: An overview. In: Culbertson YL, Krous HF, Bendel RD (eds). *Sudden Infant Death Syndrome*:

Medical Aspects and Psychological Management. The John Hopkins University Press, Baltimore, 1989, pp.18–47.

3. Berry PJ. Pathological findings in SIDS. *J Clin Path* 1992;45 (Suppl.):11–16.
4. Czegledy-Nagy EN, Cutz E, Becker LE. Sudden death in infants under one year of age. *Pediatr Pathol* 1993;13:671–84.
5. Williams AL, Uren EC, Bretherton L. Respiratory viruses and sudden infant death. *Br Med J* 1984;288:1491–3.
6. Hoffman HJ, Damus K, Hillman L, Krongrad E. Risk factors for SIDS: results of the National Institute of Child Health and Human Development SIDS Cooperative Epidemiological Study. *Ann NY Acad Sci* 1988;533:13–30.
7. Carpenter RG, Gardner A. Environmental findings and sudden infant death syndrome. *Lung* 1990;168 (Suppl.):358–67.
8. Fleming KA. Viral respiratory infection and SIDS. *J Clin Pathol* 1992;45 (Suppl.): 29–32.
9. Byard RW, Krous HF. Minor inflammatory lesions and sudden infant death: cause, coincidence, or epiphenomenon? *Pediatr Pathol Lab Med* 1995;15:649–54.
10. Bajanowski T, Brinkmann B. Pulmonary viral infection in SIDS. In: Rognum TO (ed.) *Sudden Infant Death Syndrome. New Trends in the Nineties*. Scandinavian University Press, Oslo, 1995, pp.199–202.
11. Filiano JJ, Kinney HC. A perspective on neuropathologic findings in victims of the sudden infant death syndrome: The triple-risk model. *Biol Neo* 1994;65:194–7.
12. Aherne W, Bird T, Court SDM, Gardner PS, McQuillin J. Pathological changes in virus infections of the lower respiratory tract in children. *J Clin Pathol* 1970;23:7–18.
13. Valdes-Dapena M, McFeeley PA, Hoffman HJ. *Histopathology Atlas for the Sudden Infant Death Syndrome*. Armed Forces Institute of Pathology, Washington DC, 1993.
14. Haley KJ, Sunday ME, Wiggs BR *et al*. Inflammatory cell distribution within and along asthmatic airways. *Am J Respir Crit Care Med* 1998;158:565–72.
15. Fraenkel DJ, Bardin GP, Sanderson G, Lampe F, Johnston SL, Holgate ST. Lower airways inflammation during rhinovirus colds in normal and asthmatic subjects. *Am J Respir Crit Care Med* 1995;15:879–86.
16. Howat WJ, Moore IE, Judd M, Roche WR. Pulmonary immunopathology of sudden infant death syndrome. *Lancet* 1994;343:1390–2.
17. An SF, Gould S, Keeling JW, Fleming KA. Role of respiratory viral infection in SIDS: Detection of viral nucleic acid by *in situ* hybridization. *J Pathol* 1993;171: 271–8.
18. Zuppan CW, Robinson CC, Langston C. Viral pneumonia in infants and children. In: Askin FB, Langston C, Rosenberg HS, Bernstein J (eds). *Pulmonary disease. Perspect Pediatr Pathol*. Karger, Basel, 1995;18:111–13.
19. Hegele RG, Robinson PJ, Gonzalez S, Hogg JC. Production of acute bronchiolitis in guinea-pigs by human respiratory syncytial virus. *Eur Respir J* 1993;6:1324–31.
20. Hegele RG, Hayashi S, Bramley AM, Hogg JC. Persistance of respiratory syncytial virus genome and protein after acute bronchiolitis in guinea pigs. *Chest* 1994;105: 1848–54.
21. Cubie HA, Duncan LA, Marshall LA, Smith NM. Detection of respiratory syncytial virus nucleic acid in archival postmortem tissue from infants. *Pediatr Pathol Lab Med* 1997;17:927–38.
22. Buchino JJ, Ballard ET. Pulmonary cytology in children. In: Askin FB, Langston C,

Rosenberg HS, Bernstein J (eds). *Pulmonary Disease. Perspect Pediatr Pathol.* Karger, Basel, 1995;18:154–82.

23. Tschernig T, Kleemann WJ, Pabst R. Bronchus-associated lymphoid tissue (BALT) in the lungs of children who had died from sudden infant death syndrome and other causes. *Thorax* 1995;50:658–60.

24. Cutz E. Studies on neuroepithelial bodies under experimental and disease conditions. In: Cutz E (ed.) *Cellular and Molecular Biology of Airway Chemoreceptors.* Texas, Landes Bioscience, 1997, pp.109–29.

25. Lauweryns JM, Cokelaere M. Hypoxia-sensitive neuro-epithelial bodies. Intrapulmonary secretory neuroreceptors modulated by the CNS. *Zeits Zellfors Mikroskop Anat* 1973;145:521–40.

26. Lauweryns JM, Cokelaere M, Deleersnyder M, Liebens M. Intrapulmonary neuroepithelial bodies in newborn rabbits. Influence of hypoxia, hypercapnia, nicotine, reserpine, L-dopa and 5–HT. *Cell Tissue Res* 1977;182:425–40.

27. Cutz E, Gillan JE, Perrin DG. Pulmonary neuroendocrine system: an overview of cell biology and pathology with emphasis on pediatric lung disease. In: Askin F.B, Langston C, Rosenberg HS, Bernstein J (eds). *Pulmonary Disease. Perspect Pediatr Pathol.* Karger, Basel, 1995;18:32–70.

28. Cutz E, Chan W, Sonstegard K. Identification of neuroepithelial bodies in rabbit fetal lungs by scanning electron microscopy. *Anat Rec* 1978;192:459–66.

29. Youngson C, Nurse C, Yeger H, Cutz E. Oxygen sensing in airway chemoreceptors. *Nature* 1993;365,153–6.

30. Lauweryns JM, Cokelaere M, Lerut T, Theunynck P. Cross-circulation studies on the influence of hypoxia and hypoxemia on neuro-epithelial bodies in young rabbit. *Cell Tissue Res* 1978;193: 373–86.

31. Lauweryns JM, de Bock V, Guelinckx P, Decramer M. Effects of unilateral hypoxia on neuroepithelial bodies in rabbit lungs. *J Appl Physiol* 1983;55;1665–8.

32. Lauweryns JM, Van Lommel AT, Dom RJ. Innervation of rabbit intrapulmonary neuroepithelial bodies. Quantitative and qualitative ultrastructural study after vagotomy. *J Neurol Sci* 1985;67:81–92.

33. Lauweryns JM, Van Lommel A. Effects of various vagotomy procedures on the reaction to hypoxia of rabbit neuroepithelial bodies. *Exp Lung Res* 1986;11:319–39.

34. Lebacq-Verheyden AM, Trepel J, Susville EA, Battey JF. Bombesin and gastrin releasing peptide: neuropeptides, secretagogues and growth factors. In: Sporn M, Roberts A (eds). *Handbook of Experimental Pharmacology.* Heildelberg, Germany, Springer-Verlag, 1990;95 (part 2):71–124.

35. Sunday ME, Hua J, Dai HB, Nusrat A, Torday JS. Bombesin increases fetal lung growth and maturation *in utero* and in organ culture. *Am J Respir Cell Mol Biol* 1990;3:199–205.

36. Cutz E, Jackson A. Neuroepithelial bodies as airway oxygen sensors. *Respir Physiol* 1999;115:201–14.

37. Cross AR, Jones OTG. Enzymatic mechanisms of superoxide production. (Review.) *Biochim Biophys Acta* 1991;1057:281–98.

38. Youngson C, Nurse C, Yeger H *et al.* Immunocytochemical localization of O_2-sensing protein (NADPH oxidase) in chemoreceptor cells. *Microsc Res Tech* 1997;37: 101–6.

39. Kummer W, Acker H. Immunohistochemical demonstration of four subunits of

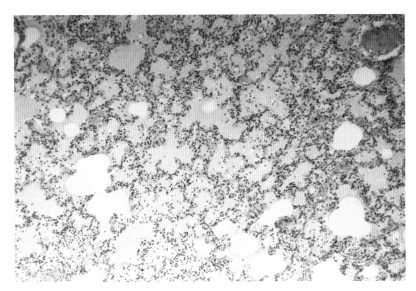

Plate 2.13
Lung section from a SIDS case. Note edema and a slight
thickening of the alveolar septae.

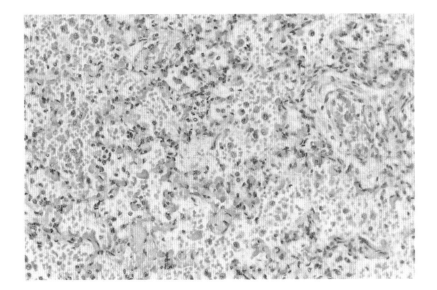

Plate 2.15

Lung section from a SIDS case. Note intra-alveolar hemorrhage and
macrophages.

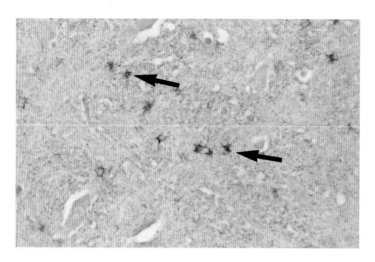

Plate 8.1
Reactive astrocytes (arrows) in the medullary reticular formation (nucleus centralis) of a SIDS victim are highlighted by immunostaining for an astrocytic marker, glial fibrillary acidic protein (GFAP). ×10, GFAP immunostain.

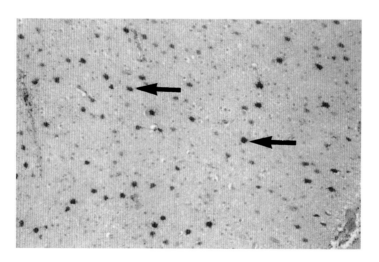

Plate 8.4
Reactive astrocytes (arrows) in the cerebral white matter of a SIDS victim are highlighted by immunostaining for GFAP. ×10, GFAP immunostain.

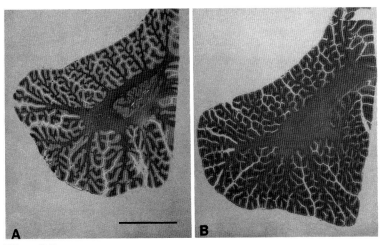

Plate 8.5
Myelin-stained sections of the white matter of the lateral cerebellar hemisphere between an infant dying of congenital heart disease (A) and SIDS victim (B) at 16 postconceptional months. Myelin degree is 0 in the SIDS victim, compared with degree 3 ('mature') in the control. Myelin was graded in each against an internal standard of degree 3 (inferior cerebellar peduncle). Hematoxylin and eosin/Luxol fast blue. Bar: 1 cm. Reprinted with permission from the *Journal of Neuropathology and Experimental Neurology.*

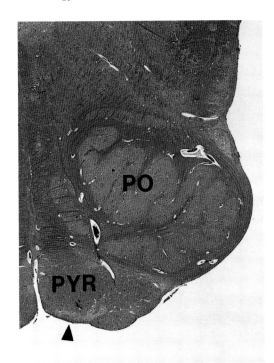

Plate 8.7
The arcuate nucleus (arrow) is located on the ventral surface of the medulla in a human infant. Hematoxylin and eosin/Luxol fast blue. Abbreviations: PO, principal inferior olive; PYR, pyramid.

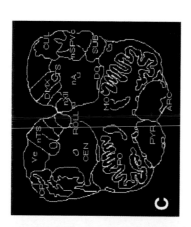

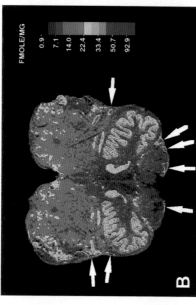

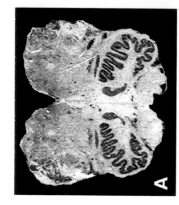

Plate 8.8

(A) Autoradiogram of representative level of the human infant medulla for 3H-kainate binding to kainate receptors. The arcuate nucleus is located along the ventral surface, superficial to the pyramid. (B) Color-coded image of specific activity (fmol/mg tissue) in the same section. The white arrows point to the arcuate nucleus. (C) Anatomic boundaries of nuclei. Abbreviations: ARC, arcuate nucleus; CEN, n. centralis; CUL, n. cuneatus lateralis; DMX, dorsal motor nucleus of the vagus; DO, dorsal accessory olive; ICP, inferior cerebellar peduncle; MO, medial accessory olive; nXII, hypoglossal nucleus; nSPVc, nucleus of the spinal trigeminal nerve, pars caudalis; nTS, nucleus of the solitary tract; PO, principal inferior olive; PYR, pyramid; ROLL, nucleus of Roller; SUB, nucleus subtrigeminalis; VE, vestibular nucleus. Reprinted with permission of *Neuroscience*.

neutrophil NAD(P)H oxidase in type I cells of carotid body. *J Appl Physiol* 1995;78:1904–9.

40. Wang D, Youngson C, Wong V *et al.* NADPH-oxidase and a hydrogen peroxide-sensitive K^+ channel may function as an oxygen sensor complex in airway chemoreceptors and small cell lung carcinoma cell line. *Proc Natl Acad Sci USA* 1996;93: 13182–7.

41. Lopez-Barneo J, Lopez-Lopez JR, Urena J, Gonzalez C. Chemotransduction in the carotid body: K^+ current modulated by Po_2 in type I chemoreceptor cells. *Science* 1988;24:580–2.

42. Gonzalez C, Almarez L, Obeso A, Rigual R. Potassium channel types in arterial chemoreceptors and their selective modulation by oxygen. *TINS* 1992;15:146–53.

43. Lopez-Barneo J. Oxygen-sensing by ion channels and the regulation of cellular functions. *Trends Neurosci* 1996;19:435–40.

44. Acker H, Bolling B, Delpiano MA, Dufau E, Gorlach A, Holtermann G. The meaning of H_2O_2 generation in carotid body cells for Po_2 chemoreception. *J Aut Nerv Syst* 1992;4:41–52.

45. Acker H, Xue D. Mechanisms of O_2 sensing in the carotid body in comparison with other O_2–sensing cells. *News Physiol Sci* 1995;10:211–16.

46. Ruppersberg JP, Stocker M, Pongs O, Heinemann SH, Frank R, Koenen M. Regulation of fast inactivation of cloned mammalian IK(A) channels by cysteine oxidation. *Nature* 1991;352:711–14.

47. Fu XW, Nurse CA, Wang YT, Cutz E. Selective modulation of membrane currents by hypoxia in intact airway chemoreceptors from neonatal rabbit. *J Physiol (Lond)* 1999;514:139–50.

48. Gillan JE, Curran C, O'Reilly E, Cahalane SF, Unwin AR. Abnormal patterns of pulmonary neuroendocrine cells in victims of sudden infant death syndrome. *Pediatrics* 1989;84:828–34.

49. Perrin DG, McDonald TJ, Cutz E. Hyperplasia of bombesin-immunoreactive pulmonary neuroendocrine cells and neuroepithelial bodies in sudden infant death syndrome. *Pediatr Pathol* 1991;11:431–47.

50. Pack RJ, Barker S, Howe A. The effects of hypoxia on the number of amine-containing cells in the lung of the adult rat. *Eur J Respir Dis* 1986;68:121–30.

51. Keith IM, Will JA. Hypoxia and the neonatal rabbit lung: neuroendocrine cell numbers, 5-HT fluorescence intensity, and relationship to arterial thickness. *Thorax* 1981;36:767–73.

52. Taylor W. Pulmonary argyrophil cells at high altitude. *J Pathol* 1977;122:137–44.

53. Elliot J, Vullermin P, Robinson P. Maternal cigarette smoking is associated with increased inner airway wall thickness in children who die from sudden infant death syndrome. *Am J Respir Crit Care Med* 1998;158:802–6.

54. Cutz E, Perrin DG, Hackman R, Czegledy-Nagy EN. Maternal smoking and pulmonary neuroendocrine cells in sudden infant death syndrome. *Pediatrics* 1996;98: 668–72.

55. Chen MF, Diotallevi MJ, Kimizuka G, King M, Wang NS. Nicotine-induced neuroepithelial cell changes in young rabbits: a preliminary communication. *Pediatr Pulmonol* 1985;1:303–8.

56. Tabassian AR, Nylen ES, Linnoila RI, Snider RH, Cassidy MM, Becker KL.

Stimulation of pulmonary neuroendocrine cells and their associated peptides by repeated exposure to cigarette smoke. *Am Rev Respir Dis* 1989;140:436–40.

57. Nylen ES, Becker KL, Snider RH, Tabassian AR, Cassidy MM, Linnoila RI. Cholinergic-nicotine control of growth and secretion of cultured pulmonary neuroendocrine cells. *Anat Rec* 1993;236:129–35.

58. Sekhon HS, Jia Y, Raab R, Kuryatov A, Pankow JF, Whitsett JA, Lindstrom J, Spindel ER. Prenatal nicotine increases pulmonary $\alpha7$ nicotinic receptor expression and alters fetal lung development in monkeys. *J Clin Invest* 1999;103:637–47.

59. Quik M, Chan J, Patrick J. alpha-Bungarotoxin blocks the nicotinic receptor mediated increase in cell number in a neuroendocrine cell line. *Brain Res* 1994;655:161–7.

60. Guntheroth WG. Interleukin-1 as intermediary causing sleep apnea and SIDS during respiratory infections. *Med Hypotheses* 1989;28:121–3.

61. Howatson AG. Viral infection and (interferon in SIDS. *J Clin Pathol* 1992;45 (Suppl.):25–8.

62. Blackwell CC, Weir DM, Busuttil A *et al.* Infection, inflammation, and the developmental stage of infants: A new hypothesis for the aetiology of SIDS. In: Rognum TO (ed.) *Sudden Infant Death Syndrome. New Trends in the Nineties.* Scandinavian University Press, Oslo, 1995, pp.189–98.

63. Lindgren C. Respiratory syncytial virus and the sudden infant death syndrome. *Acta Paediatr* 1993;389 (Suppl.):67–9.

64. Lindgren C, Jing L, Graham B, Grögaard J, Sundell H. Respiratory syncytial virus infection reinforces reflex apnea in young lambs. *Pediatr Res* 1992;31:381–5.

65. Becker LE. Neural maturational delay as a link in the chain of events leading to SIDS. *Can J Neurol Sci* 1990;17:361–71.

66. Kinney HC, Filiano JJ, Harper RM. The neuropathology of sudden infant death syndrome: A review. *J Neuropathol Exp Neurol* 1992;51:115–16.

67. Perrin DG, Cutz E, Becker LE, Bryan AC, Madapallimatum A, Sole MJ. Sudden infant death syndrome: increased carotid body dopamine and noradrenaline contents. *Lancet* 1984;2:535–7.

68. Holgert H, Hokfelt T, Hertzberg T, Lagercrantz H. Functional and developmental studies of the peripheral arterial chemoreceptors in rat: effects of nicotine and possible relation to sudden infant death syndrome. *Proc Natl Acad Sci USA* 1995;92: 7575–9.

69. Jackson A, Nurse CA. Role of acetylcholine receptors and dopamine transporter in regulation of extracellular dopamine in rat carotid body cultures grown in chronic hypoxia or nicotine. *J Neurochem* 1998;70:653–62.

70. Dhillon DP, Barer GR, Walsh M. The enlarged carotid body of the chronically hypoxic and chronic hypoxic and hypercapnic rat: a morphometric analysis. Q*uart J Exp Physiol* 1984;69:301–17.

71. McGregor KH, Gil J, Lahiri S. A morphometric study of carotid body in chronically hypoxic rats. *J App Physiol* 1988;57:1430–8.

72. Kalhoff H, Kiwull-Schöne H, Kiwull P. Pulmonary vagal afferents involved in the hypoxic breathing without arterial chemoreceptors. In: Eyzaguirre C, Fidone SJ, Fitzgerald, RS (eds). *Arterial Chemoreception.* Springer Verlag, New York, NY, 1990;350–6.

73. Eden GJ, Hanson MA. Maturation of the respiratory response to acute hypoxia in the newborn rat. *J Physiol (Lond)* 1987;392,1–9.

74. Hertzberg T, Hellstrom S, Lagercrantz H, Pequignot JM. Development of the arterial chemoreflex and turnover of carotid body catecholamines in the newborn rat. *J Physiol (Lond)* 1990;425:211–25.

75. Howarth PM, Bradding P, Quint D, Redington AE, Holgate ST. Cytokines and airway inflammation. In: Chignard M, Pretolani M, Renesto P, Vargaftig BB (eds). cells and cytokines in lung inflammation. *Ann NY Acad Sci* 1994;725:69–82.

76. Skogvall S, Korsgren M, Grampp W. Evidence that neuroepithelial endocrine cells control the spontaneous tone in guinea pig tracheal preparations. *J Appl Physiol* 1999;86:789–98.

77. Spina D. Epithelium-dependent regulation of airways smooth muscle tone. In: Raeburn ND, Giembycz MA (eds). *Airways smooth muscle, development and regulation of contractility*. Basel, Birkhauser, 1994, pp.2–32.

78. Morrison KJ, Gao Y, Vanhoutte PM. Epithelial modulation of airway smooth muscle. *Am J Physiol* 1990;258:L254–62.

79. Church N, Arias N, Hall C, Brooks J. Respiratory syncytial virus-related apnea in infants (demographics and outcome). *Am J Dis Child* 1984;138:247–50.

80. Pollock JD, Williams DA, Gifford MA *et al*. Mouse model of x-linked chronic granulomatous disease, an inherited defect in phagocyte superoxide production. *Nature Genet* 1995;9:202–9.

81. Fu XW, Wang D, Nurse CA, Dinauer MC, Cutz E. NADPH oxidase in an O_2 sensor in airway chemoreceptors: Evidence from K^+ current modulation in wild-type and oxidase-deficient mice. *Proc Natl Acad Sci USA* 2000;97:4374–9.

82. Yeger H, Speirs V, Youngson C, Cutz E. Pulmonary neuroendocrine cells in cultures of human infant airway mucosa from postmortem tissues. *Am J Resp Cell Mol Biol* 1996;15:232–6.

83. Forsyth KD, Bradley J, Weeks SC, Smith MD, Skinner J, Zola H. Immunocytologic characterization using monoclonal antibodies of lung lavage cell phenotype in infants who have died from sudden infant death syndrome. *Pediatr Res* 1988;23:187–90.

CHAPTER 11

A microbiological perspective

CAROLINE C. BLACKWELL, DONALD M. WEIR AND
ANTHONY BUSUTTIL

Introduction   182
Risk factors for SIDS   183
Bacteria or viruses?   184
Risk factors for SIDS and bacterial colonization   187
Risk factors and potentially pathogenic bacteria in healthy infants   190
Prone position and induction of staphylococcal toxins   191
Synergy between microorganisms and cigarette smoke   192
Evidence for inflammatory/immune responses in SIDS infants   192
How can risk factors affect inflammatory responses?   193
SIDS and genetic, environmental and developmental factors   197
Next stage in SIDS research   198
Caveat   199
Acknowledgements   200
References   200

Introduction

The epidemiology of SIDS suggests a microbiological etiology as the risk factors are associated with increased susceptibility infection in infants, particularly respiratory tract infections. Early attempts to identify viruses and bacteria in SIDS infants were not particularly helpful, mainly because investigators were searching for a single cause of these deaths. With the exception of infant botulism in a small number of SIDS cases, major bacterial pathogens were not identified in these infants.[1,2] Microbiological findings in autopsy reports have often been dismissed as irrelevant, normal flora or postmortem contamination[3]; however, some members of the normal bacterial flora are capable of producing toxins that can act as superantigens. Pyrogenic toxins of *Staphylococcus aureus* were identified in over half of SIDS cases[4] and *Escherichia coli* isolated from extra-intestinal sites in SIDS infants.[5] The criticisms that detection of endotoxin and Gram-negative bacteria in SIDS cases is due to overgrowth from the gut have been addressed in recent articles.[6,7]

This chapter will examine five areas in relation to the role of infection and inflammation in SIDS: (1) the evidence that infectious agents are involved in some SIDS deaths; (2) risk factors in relation to bacterial colonization and induction of temperature-dependent toxins; (3) risk factors in relation to induction and control of inflammatory responses; (4) the night-time prevalence of these deaths in relation to development of circadian rhythm in infants and the role of cortisol in relation to control of inflammatory responses; 5) the increased incidence of SIDS and serious respiratory infections in some ethnic groups.

Risk factors for SIDS

Many developmental and environmental factors significantly associated with SIDS parallel those associated with susceptibility of infants and young children to infectious agents, particularly bacterial infections of the respiratory tract.[8,9]

The majority of SIDS cases occur between 2–4 months, a time when maternal antibodies to bacteria and viruses are declining and the infant's immune system is immature. Maternal smoking is a major risk factor for SIDS.[10] Investigation of smoking and susceptibility to infection in children found the strongest association was usually with the mother's smoking.[11] SIDS infants often had mild respiratory infections the week prior to death.[12,13] Viral infections are predisposing factors for bacterial colonization by organisms such as staphylococci.[14] In populations in which breastfeeding is not strongly associated with socioeconomic status, breastfed infants were found to be at decreased risk of SIDS compared with formula-fed infants.[15] Breastfeeding reduces the risk of both respiratory and gastrointestinal infections,[16,17] both of which have been implicated in SIDS. Infants who were not immunized against diphtheria, pertussis and tetanus (DPT) or those immunized late were at increased risk of SIDS.[18–20] The prone sleeping position identified as a major risk factor for SIDS[21] could contribute to susceptibility to SIDS by reducing clearance of bacteria from the upper respiratory tract[22] and by contributing to induction of temperature-dependent toxins of *S. aureus*.[23] In industrialized countries, SIDS disproportionately affects families from lower socioeconomic groups,[24] and some ethnic groups have a higher incidence of SIDS than others.[25] Infectious diseases are more common among poorer families, and infants of some ethnic groups (e.g. Australian Aborigines) are colonized earlier and more densely by potentially pathogenic bacteria.[26] There are, however, exceptions to this pattern and proposals for multidisciplinary studies to examine these differences are included at the end of this chapter.

Bacteria or viruses?

SEASONAL INCIDENCE OF SIDS

The winter peak of SIDS observed in many countries parallels increased levels of respiratory diseases, particularly infections spread from older children to infants during periods when schools are in session.[27] Because evidence of invasive bacterial infection would, by definition, be an explainable death and not SIDS, investigations on the role of infection have concentrated on viruses or bacteria that colonize mucosal surfaces, but produce powerful toxins that can cross the membranes and cause damage to the host.

VIRUSES

No single agent has been clearly identified as causing SIDS, but many different viruses affecting both respiratory and gastrointestinal tracts have been identified in 20–30% of these infants (Table 11.1).[28,29] It was suggested that early surveys underestimated the incidence of virus infection because of difficulties in cultivation of viruses or identification of viral antigens; however, recent studies with more

Table 11.1 Evidence for virus infection in SIDS cases

	Associated with SIDS	Not associated with SIDS
Upper respiratory symptoms	Williams (1980)[128]	Gupta *et al.* (1996)[129]
	Williams *et al.* (1996)[130]	Hoffman *et al.* (1988)[131]
	Czegledy-Nagy *et al.* (1993)[132]	
Population mixing	Bentham (1994)[133]	
Influenza virus	Nelson *et al.* (1975)[134]	
	Ford *et al.* (1990)[135]	
	Zink *et al.* (1987)[136]	
RSV	An *et al.* (1993)[30]	Cubie *et al.* (1997)[31]
Rhinovirus	Las Heras & Swanson (1983)[137]	
Adenovirus	An *et al.* (1993)[30]	
	Bajanowski *et al.* (1996)[138]	
	Shimizu *et al.* (1995)[139]	
	Bettiol *et al.* (1994)[140]	
Cytomegalovirus	Bajanowski *et al.* (1996)[138]	
Echovirus		Shimizu *et al.* (1995)[139]
Virus isolation	Carpenter & Gardner (1990)[141]	Gilbert *et al.* (1990)[13]
	Uren *et al.* (1980)[142]	Ford *et al.* (1990)[135]
		Zink *et al.* (1987)[136]
Enterovirus	Shimizu *et al.* (1995)[139]	
	Grangeot-Keros *et al.* (1996)[143]	
Rota virus	Bettiol *et al.* (1994)[140]	
	Yolken & Murphy (1982)[144]	

sophisticated molecular techniques have not found significant associations between any specific virus infection and SIDS.[29–31]

TOXIGENIC BACTERIA

The common bacterial toxin hypothesis[32,33] suggested toxins produced by the normal bacterial flora are absorbed from the respiratory tract. This mathematical model predicted the bacteria responsible would be commonly encountered by infants during the first few weeks/months of life. Toxigenic bacteria or their toxins have been identified in SIDS infants in several different countries (Table 11.2). Many produce toxins that act as superantigens, substances that can non-specifically stimulate powerful inflammatory responses such as those responsible for toxic shock syndrome or septic shock.

ENDOTOXIN

Gram-negative bacteria are not normally isolated from the upper respiratory tract (URT); consequently, their detection in SIDS infants has been dismissed as

Table 11.2 Toxigenic bacteria implicated in SIDS

Species	Toxin	Superantigen	Reference
Staphylococcus aureus	Enterotoxins, TSST-1	Yes	Newbould *et al.* (1989)[47] Malam *et al.* (1992)[48] Zorgani *et al.* (1999)[4]
Bordetella pertussis	Pertussis toxin/ endotoxin	No/yes	Nicholl & Gardner (1988)[50] Lindgren *et al.* (1997)[51]
Hemophilus influenzae	Endotoxin	Yes	Telford *et al.* (1989)[34] Oppenheim *et al.* (1994)[37]
Clostridium perfringens	Enterotoxin A	Yes	Murrell *et al.* (1987)[144] Lindsay *et al.* (1993)[40]
Clostridium botulinum	Botulinum toxin	No	Arnon *et al.* (1978); (1981)[1,39] Sonnabend *et al.* (1985)[2]
Streptococcus pyogenes	Pyrogenic toxins A&B	Yes	Telford *et al.* (1993)[34]
Escherichia coli	Enterotoxins, verotoxins	?	Bettleheim *et al.* (1989;1990;1995)[41–43] Goldwater *et al.* (1990)[146] Pearce & Bettleheim (1997)[44]
	Endotoxin	Yes	Oppenheim *et al.* (1994)[37]
Streptococcus mitis	?	Yes	Matsushita *et al.* (1997)[147]
Helicobacter pylori	Vacuolating toxin	?	Pattison *et al.* (1998)[54,55]
	Endotoxin	Yes	

postmortem contamination or overgrowth. The evidence, however, contradicts these assumptions. Studies on URT flora of SIDS infants indicate that samples taken soon after death are more likely to yield these species than those taken later.[3,34] The bacterial flora observed in SIDS infants, including Gram-negative species, can be reproduced in older children (12–18 months of age) who have upper respiratory tract infection (URTI) and who sleep in the prone position.[35,36]

There is serologic evidence that some SIDS infants 3 months or younger have been exposed to bacterial endotoxin.[37] Endotoxin is a powerful superantigen, but there has been little convincing evidence of increased levels in SIDS infants.[6,38] Raised levels of endotoxin could reflect endotoxemia before death, entrance of endotoxin into the blood as an agonal event or postmortem contamination due to overgrowth of gut flora. An experimental model developed to address these problems found significantly higher levels of endotoxin in rats injected with the lipopolysaccharide (LPS) than in rats injected with saline. Experiments to assess effects of temperature and time after death on detection of endotoxin found storage of the animals at 8°C for up to 102 hours after death had no effect on levels of endotoxin detected in kidney, liver or spleen.[7] Blood endotoxin levels were higher in SIDS infants in whom there was evidence of mild or moderate inflammation compared with those in whom evidence of inflammation was absent or minimal.[6]

TOXINS OF ENTERIC BACTERIA

Toxigenic bacteria and/or their toxins have been identified in SIDS infants in Australia and the United States. Infant botulism due to toxins of *Clostridium botulinum* was identified in some of the earliest studies on sudden infant deaths,[1,2,39] and *Cl. perfringens* and its toxins have been implicated in other studies.[40] Toxigenic *E. coli* isolates have been found in samples from SIDS infants.[41–44]

PYROGENIC TOXINS OF STAPHYLOCOCCUS AUREUS

Pyrogenic toxins of *S. aureus* are potent superantigens that can kill previously healthy adults or older children.[45–47] Staphylococcal enterotoxin C (SEC) and the toxic shock syndrome toxin (TSST), were identified by immunohistochemical methods in tissues of SIDS infants, SEC in 36% of the infants examined and TSST in 19%.[48–49] Both ELISA and flow cytometry have been employed in more recent studies to identify TSST-1, SEC_1, staphylococcal enterotoxins A (SEA) or B (SEB) in tissues of over half the SIDS cases tested: 9/16 (56%) of Scottish infants; 7/13 (55%) French infants; 16/30 (53%) Australian SIDS infants but only 3/19 (16%) non-SIDS cases from the Australian series ($\chi^2 = 5.42$, $P < 0.02$).[4] Toxin-positive specimens were found in approximately three times as many SIDS infants as controls, similar to the proportions observed with the immunohistochemical method used to detect the toxins.[4,48,49]

PERTUSSIS TOXIN

Although *Bordetella pertussis* produces several toxins, evidence for involvement in SIDS is circumstantial. Epidemiologic studies indicated that some cases of SIDS might be due to asymptomatic whooping cough.[50] Infants do not exhibit the characteristic whoop observed in older children. There was a temporal association between SIDS and epidemics of whooping cough in Norway.[51] Laboratory studies found that some of the risk factors for SIDS enhanced binding of *B. pertussis* to epithelial cells.[52]

   B. pertussis is difficult to culture, even from patients with symptomatic whooping cough, and there are no reports of its isolation from SIDS infants. Molecular methods were used to identify *B. pertussis* DNA in infant autopsies. Unfortunately, the molecular studies were not carried out with complementary studies to culture the organism from the same children; however, 9/51 (18%) children who died suddenly had evidence of *B. pertussis* DNA.[53]

HELICOBACTOR PYLORI

At present the evidence for *H. pylori* is based on detection of the DNA from this organism by PCR and microscopy.[54,55] It has been suggested that aspiration of urease produced by these bacteria might lead to lethal levels of ammonia in the blood. While the organism has been identified in SIDS infants, there is no hard evidence as to how they might be triggering the series of events leading to death.

Risk factors for SIDS and bacterial colonization

Density of colonization is a key factor in development of bacterial diseases, both diseases resulting from invasion of tissues as in meningitis or diseases due to production of toxins as in cholera.[56] Epidemiologic surveys and complementary experimental studies indicate that risk factors associated with SIDS can enhance frequency and/or density of colonization by some of the bacteria implicated in SIDS.

DEVELOPMENTAL STAGE

In all surveys of SIDS, the most consistent risk factor is the characteristic age distribution observed for these deaths. During the 2–4 month age range in which most SIDS deaths now occur, 80–90% of infants express the Lewis[a] antigen on their red blood cells. The antigens are also present on epithelial cells as they are adsorbed from secretions. The proportion of infants expressing Lewis[a] decreases with age. By 18–24 months, the antigen is usually found on red cells of 20–25% of children, a proportion similar to that observed in adults.[57] We found Lewis[a] in respiratory secretions of 71% of SIDS infants.[58,59]

Lewis[a] antigen is used as a receptor on epithelial cells by three bacterial species implicated in SIDS: *S. aureus*[52,59–61]; *B. pertussis*[62]; *Cl. perfringens.*[63] Lewis[a] is also one of the receptors on monocytes for pertussis toxin.[64] Binding of some staphylococcal enterotoxins to monocytes can be partially inhibited by pretreating the toxin with anti-Lewis[a].[65,66]

Susceptibility to bacterial disease associated with expression of a host cell antigen during a particular developmental stage is not a new concept. Susceptibility of calves to enterotoxigenic strains of *E. coli* expressing the K99 adhesin parallels expression of a carbohydrate antigen which disappears with age. An analogue of the receptor fed to the calves prevented colonization by the toxigenic strains and disease due to the toxin.[67]

VIRUS INFECTION

Virus infection enhances bacterial colonization in humans[14]; increased staphylococcal disease among influenza patients was observed as early as 1919. In a model system, infection of the human epithelial cell line HEp-2 significantly enhanced binding of *S. aureus* and *B. pertussis* compared with uninfected HEp-2 cells. Both serotype A and serotype B of RSV showed this pattern.[59,62,68] Similar results were observed for some Gram-negative species identified in SIDS infants or those species known to cause respiratory tract infections, *Haemophilus influenzae*, *Neisseria* spp., and *Moraxella catarrhalis.*[68,69] This increased binding of bacteria is due partly to up-regulation of host cell antigens that can act as receptors for some bacteria (Lewis[x], CD14 and CD18).[68,70] Enhanced binding of *S. aureus, B. pertussis* and other Gram-positive species was also observed with HEp-2 cells infected with influenza A.[71]

EXPOSURE TO CIGARETTE SMOKE

Smokers are more frequently colonized by some bacterial pathogens than non-smokers, e.g. staphylococci[14] or *Neisseria meningitidis.*[72] Flow cytometry assays for bacterial binding demonstrated cells from smokers bind significantly more *S. aureus, B. pertussis*, and several Gram-negative bacteria.[62,73] The mechanism of enhancement was not the same as that observed with virus infection. The cells of smokers did not express enhanced levels of antigens on cell surfaces to which the bacteria bind, e.g. Lewis antigens, CD14, CD18, fibronectin or fibrinogen.[73]

Treatment of buccal epithelial cells from non-smokers with a water-soluble cigarette smoke extract (CSE) was shown to enhance bacterial binding. The enhancement was observed with dilutions of the CSE up to 1 in 300. This indicates coating of mucosal surfaces by passive exposure to cigarette smoke might result in adsorption of substances that non-specifically enhance attachment of a variety of bacterial species.[73]

BREASTFEEDING AND FORMULA FEEDING

There have been conflicting reports on the effects of breast feeding in relation to SIDS.[15,74,75] With respect to the hypothesis that toxigenic bacteria are involved in some cases of SIDS, breastfed infants are better protected against both enteric and respiratory tract infections. Human milk contains antibodies specific for viruses, bacteria and their toxins. Both whole and defatted milk was demonstrated to aggregate *S. aureus* and *Cl. perfringens*.[61,63] It also contains non-immunoglobulin fractions that help protect against infection during the first year of life, mainly due to the anti-adhesive activities of oligosaccharides found in milk.[76,78] Oligosaccharides containing sialic acid inhibit binding of influenza A virus and S-fimbriated enteropathogenic *E. coli* to their target cells[79]. Lewis[a] and Lewis[b] antigens are present in human milk and also in infant formula preparations. Human milk contains much higher levels of these antigens than the formula preparations or cow's milk. Synthetic forms of these two antigens inhibited binding of *S. aureus, B. pertussis and Cl. perfringens* to epithelial cells. In experiments with staphylococci, inhibitory activity was not correlated with the levels of either Lewis antigen in human milk or formula preparations but with IgA antibodies in human milk specific for the staphylococcal adhesin obtained by affinity purification with Lewis[a].[60,63]

Unlike infant formula preparations, human milk also contains IgA that binds to staphylococcal toxins and the enterotoxin A of *Cl. perfringens.*[80]

SLEEP POSITION

Recent studies investigated the effect of sleeping position on nasopharyngeal flora in infants aged 0–18 months. All the infants in the study slept in the supine position for the first 5 months. Between 7–11 months of age, although they were put down to sleep in the supine position, the infants turned themselves over to the prone position. Over 50% slept prone and by 11 months 72% regularly slept prone.[35,81] For both adults and infants in the prone position, the normal clearance of bacteria by the secretions appears to be impaired.[22,35] Among infants aged 12–18 months who slept prone and who had an upper respiratory tract infection (URTI), there was increased isolation of staphylococci, streptococci, *H. influenzae* and other Gram-negative bacilli ($P < 0.05$) compared with infants who slept in the supine position. URTI and prone sleeping position appeared to reproduce the bacterial flora often found in the nasopharynx of SIDS infants.[35,36,81]

SOCIOECONOMIC BACKGROUND AND ETHNIC GROUP

In Britain lower social deprivation is reported to be a significant factor contributing to the risk of SIDS.[9,24] Although many Asian families in Britain could be classified as socially deprived, the incidence of SIDS among Indian, Pakistani and Bangladeshi families is lower than in the white population.

Deaths among these infants due to respiratory infections are also lower than in white families.[82] In Hong Kong many families live in suboptimal circumstances, but there is also a very low incidence of SIDS.[83]

'Ethnic origin has an important influence on the incidence of SIDS'.[25] The very high incidence of SIDS among the Maori in New Zealand led to investigations that identified important risk factors associated with these deaths. Several indigenous populations have high incidences of SIDS, e.g. American Indians, Alaskan natives and Australian Aborigines.[84,85] The criticism that the higher incidence of SIDS among Aboriginal infants was due to differences in diagnosis was addressed by re-examination of all Aboriginal cases of SIDS and sudden unexpected death in infancy between 1980 and 1988. These findings were compared with a corresponding random sample of non-Aboriginal infant deaths. There was no evidence of differences in diagnosis of SIDS in the two populations.[86]

Among Native Americans, Eskimos and Australian Aborigines, the incidence of serious respiratory tract and ear infections is also higher.[26,87] Aboriginal and Eskimos infants have been found to be colonized earlier and more heavily by respiratory pathogens.[26,87]

Risk factors and potentially pathogenic bacteria in healthy infants

Do risk factors affect isolation of potentially pathogenic bacteria from healthy infants? The normal upper respiratory tract flora of infants has been examined in three independent studies.[35,88,89] In each, *S. aureus* was the predominant isolate during the 0–3 month age range during which the majority of SIDS now occurs.[90] In Scottish infants, *S. aureus* was isolated from 56% of 253 healthy infants in this age range. Among 37 SIDS cases that occurred during the period of the study, *S. aureus* was isolated from 86.4% of these infants 3 months of age or younger ($P < 0.02$).[89]

THE EFFECTS OF CIGARETTE SMOKE AND METHOD OF FEEDING

These two factors are difficult to separate in the UK. Smoking is more common among socially deprived women than among more affluent groups.[91] In one study, exposure of infants to cigarette smoke ($P < 0.001$) and formula feeding ($P < 0.001$) were significantly more prevalent in the less affluent area studied.[89] Women in higher social classes were more likely to breastfeed and to breastfeed for longer periods.[75] Breastfeeding had no effect on isolation of any species.[81]

Cotinine, a metabolite of nicotine, can be used to assess exposure to cigarette smoke in blood, urine or saliva. The number of cigarettes smoked in the household per day correlated with levels of cotinine in saliva specimens obtained from the infants ($r = 0.71$, $P < 0.001$). If the father or other members of the household smoked, there were higher levels of cotinine in the infant's saliva compared with households in which no one smoked. The strongest association was, however, with maternal smoking.[89,92] Infants ($n = 72$) 3 months of age or younger who were exposed to tobacco smoke were significantly more likely to harbour *S. aureus*.[81]

THE EFFECT OF GENDER AND OLDER SIBLINGS

Male infants are at greater risk of SIDS and some respiratory infections. Male infants had significantly heavier growth of *S. aureus* (P <0.05) compared with females.[35] Other siblings in the home did not affect isolation of *S. aureus* from infants <3 months of age but were associated with increased isolation of *S. aureus*, *Strep. pneumoniae*, *H. influenzae* and *M. catarrhalis* in infants 3–7 months of age. This could reflect increased close contact between siblings and older infants.

VIRUS INFECTION

Increased levels of viral respiratory tract infections are thought to contribute to the winter peak of SIDS observed in some countries. This pattern is also found for bacterial pneumonia and otitis media.[93,94] Previous studies suggested there are two categories of SIDS infants based on age, those less than 3 months and those older than 3 months, and that virus infection might be a more important factor in the older group.[28] Upper respiratory tract infection during the first 3 months of life increased isolation of *S. aureus* ($P = 0.05$), *Strep. mitis* (P <0.01) and other α or non-hemolytic streptococci but not Gram-negative species. In the 3–7 month age range, virus infection was not associated with increased isolation of *S. aureus* from infants but with increased isolation of α or non-hemolytic streptococci (P <0.02). While Gram-negative species were isolated more often from infants with viral infection, the only significant association was with *M. catarrhalis* (P <0.05).[35,81]

PRONE SLEEPING POSITION

For ethical reasons, prone sleeping could not be assessed in infants <12 months of age. In older infants (12–18 months) with respiratory tract infections who slept prone, isolation of *S. aureus*, streptococci, *H. influenzae* and other Gram-negative bacilli was increased compared with those who slept supine ($P < 0.05$). The numbers of bacteria and the variety of species isolated from the infant decreased during the day when the child was upright. The bacterial species isolated from the prone sleepers was very similar to that found in SIDS infants.[35,81]

Prone position and induction of staphylococcal toxins

The three epidemiologic studies of live infants cited above indicated *S. aureus* is the species that best fits the mathematical model proposed by Morris *et al.*[32] It closely predicted the age distribution of SIDS if these deaths were due to a single common toxin which 50% of the population met in any 50-day period.

Although over half of normal infants are colonized by these bacteria during the period in which SIDS is most prevalent and many isolates were genetically capable of producing the toxins, SIDS is a rare event. The pyrogenic toxins of *S. aureus* and *Strep. pyogenes* are produced only between 37–40°C.[46] In healthy children and adults, the temperature of the nasopharynx is usually below 37°C; however, virus infection and the resulting inflammatory reactions might increase local as well as systemic temperatures. We suggested the prone sleeping position might increase the nasopharyngeal temperature by accumulation of secretions or by blocking a nostril by bedding, creating a 'microenvironment' in which the permissive temperature for toxin induction is reached.[95–98] Fever might enhance production of the toxins as they are produced in greater quantities at the higher temperatures.[46] We found the temperatures in the noses of young children are significantly higher than those of adults,[99] and the temperature in the nose is significantly higher in the prone position. In some children in whom there was no evidence of respiratory tract infection, the temperature in the prone, but not the upright position, reached 37°C or higher.[23,100]

Synergy between microorganisms and products of cigarette smoke

Although a number of toxigenic species of bacteria have been isolated from SIDS infants, Koch's postulates are not fulfilled. The same species is not isolated from each case and the syndrome cannot be produced reliably in an animal model.

Because no single microorganism has been implicated in all cases of SIDS, the possibility of additive or synergistic effects between microorganisms or components of cigarette smoke have been examined.[22,40,58,95–98,101–103] We proposed the following hypothesis: some SIDS deaths are due to pathophysiologic responses elicited by a combination of infectious agents and/or exposure to cigarette smoke during a postnatal developmental stage in which infants' endocrine responses are less able to 'damp down' the effects of inflammatory mediators.[96,97] Epidemiologic and experimental evidence for this hypothesis is explored in the following sections.

Evidence for inflammatory/immune responses in SIDS infants

Signs of mild infection and associated inflammatory responses in SIDS infants have been identified at autopsy of SIDS infants.[104,105] SIDS victims had evidence of increased immune stimulation in the upper airways and intestinal tract compared with infants who died of other causes such as violent deaths. Several pro-inflammatory cytokines have been detected in body fluids or tissues of SIDS victims: interleukin-6 (IL-6); interleukin-1β (IL-1β); and tumor necrosis factor α (TNF-α). Mild inflammatory reactions, increased levels of some acute phase proteins, raised immunoglobulin levels in the respiratory tract or gut and changes indicating T-cell activation have been identified in SIDS infants (Table 11.3).

How can risk factors affect inflammatory responses?

With reference to the hypothesis that inflammatory responses similar to those involved in toxic or septic shock could be responsible for some SIDS deaths, we examined the risk factors for SIDS in relation to epidemiologic and experimental studies.

VIRUS INFECTION

Animal models indicate virus infections enhance lethality of bacterial toxins. Influenza virus infection greatly enhanced the lethal effects of staphylococcal α and γ toxins, endotoxin and diphtheria toxin in the infant ferret model.[106] INF-γ produced in response to virus infection enhanced the activities of bacterial components that can act as superantigens. Asymptomatic infection with lymphocytic choriomeningitis virus (LCMV) primed mice for induction of rapid, fatal shock with sublethal concentrations of staphylococcal enterotoxin B (SEB).

Table 11.3 Evidence for inflammatory or immune responses in SIDS

Respiratory tract	Peribronchial inflammatory infiltrates	Howat et al. (1994)[148] Baxendine & Moore (1995)[149]
	Increased IgM cells in trachea	Stoltenberg et al. (1995)[150]
	Mast cell degranulation	Holgate et al. (1994)[151]
Digestive tract	Increased IgA cells in duodenum	Stoltenberg et al. (1995)[150]
Nervous system	Interferon alpha in brain	Howatson (1992)[152]
	Increased levels of IL-6 in spinal fluid	Vege et al. (1996)[153]
Blood	Decreased IgG to core endotoxin	Oppenheim et al. (1994)[37]
	Increased IgM to core endotoxin	Oppenheim et al. (1994)[37]
	Increased levels of mast cell tryptase	Holgate et al. (1994)[151]
	Increased levels of mannan binding lectin	Kilpatrick et al. (1998)[154]
	Cross-linked fibrin degradation products	Goldwater et al. (1990)[146]
	Low proportion of sera with IgG to toxins	Siarakas et al. (1999)[114]

INF-γ produced by viral infection activated macrophages and subsequent exposure to the toxin induced TNF-α and nitric oxide radicals. The mice were protected from the effects of the toxin by TNF receptor-Fc fusion protein or nitric oxide synthase inhibitor.[107] INF-γ has been suggested to enhance cell permeability to the enterotoxins of *Cl. perfringens*.[102] In a mouse model, SEB stimulated the same levels of nitric oxide production as endotoxin from endothelial cells primed by INF-γ. The ability to produce nitric oxide depended on priming by INF-γ. Although mRNA for the nitric oxide synthase was induced by SEB, production of detectable quantities of nitric oxide required both INF-γ and SEB.[108] Influenza infection increased release of TNF-α and interleukin-1β but not interleukin-6 from human peripheral blood leukocytes exposed to endotoxin.[109]

CIGARETTE SMOKE

Synergy between nicotine and bacterial toxins was demonstrated in the chick embryo model.[103] Our preliminary studies demonstrated that a water-soluble extract of cigarette smoke can induce inflammatory mediators from human leukocytes and that it enhances the production of these mediators from virus infected cells.[110,111]

INFANT FEEDING

Maternal antibodies received before birth are the major protection of infants against bacteria and viruses. IgG specific for toxins would be an important defense for neutralization of the toxins implicated in SIDS. An enzyme-linked immunosorbent assay (ELISA) was used to detect IgG antibodies to staphylococcal toxins in sera from 116 women in late pregnancy. There was a significant decline in levels of IgG that bound SEC and TSST, two toxins identified in many SIDS infants. Antibodies to two other staphylococcal enterotoxins A and B rose slightly but significantly.[112,113]

As IgG antibodies decrease, the infant would become more vulnerable to the bacterial toxins. Because the toxins implicated in SIDS are produced on mucosal surfaces, antibodies or oligosaccharides in human milk might be important defenses to reduce the density of colonization or the activities of the toxins before they could cross the mucosal barriers and cause systemic responses. Infant formula lacks these antibodies. Human milk reduced the ability of TSST to elicit nitric oxide from monocytes of eight different donors.[60] IgA antibodies to TSST, SEC and the enterotoxin A of *Cl. perfringens* were identified in human milk.

IMMUNIZATION

Unimmunized infants or infants immunized late are at increased risk of SIDS[18-20]; however, there have been few studies to try to explain these important observations. From October 1990, immunization for DPT was initiated at 2 months rather than 3 months of age for all British infants. If some deaths were due to asymptomatic pertussis or other toxigenic bacteria, we predicted that earlier immunization would result in a reduction in the proportion of SIDS deaths over 2 months of age as a consequence of earlier production by infants of protective antibodies. In south-east Scotland, the proportion of SIDS infants 2 months of age or younger has risen from 16% in 1988 to 44% in 1992[96,97] and more recently to 56% in 1994 (*P* <0.001). Analysis of SIDS deaths for England and Wales during the same period found the greatest decrease in SIDS deaths was observed in the 4–6 month age range[36,81] which might reflect the production of higher levels or more effective antibodies following the booster responses to the vaccines at 3 and 4 months.[113]

Although there is no strong evidence for endotoxemia in SIDS infants,[35] there were significantly lower levels of IgG to endotoxin core among SIDS infants less than 3 months of age compared with other infant groups.[34] A recent study in Australia found the percentage of SIDS infants with IgG to a variety of bacterial toxins was significantly lower than those for age-matched live infants.[114]

In sera of infants sent for virologic analysis, we found a significant correlation between levels of IgG antibodies bound to the DPT vaccine with levels of IgG antibodies bound to pertussis toxin, TSST-1 and SEC_1 but not to SEA or SEB. As predicted, the levels of IgG antibodies to the toxins decreased with age. The mean level of IgG antibodies detected for each of the toxins among infants greater than 2 months of age was lower than those in samples from infants less than 2 months of age. The decline in level of antibodies was significantly less for DPT and PT for infants immunized at 2 months compared with those immunized at 3 months.[112,113] If these toxins are involved in some cases of SIDS, the earlier immunization schedule initiated in October 1990 might have contributed to the decline in cot deaths.

Although the earlier immunization schedule might prevent a small number of deaths due to *B. pertussis*, we suggest the main effect of the earlier immunization is induction of antibodies cross-reactive with adhesins or toxins of other species. These could be antibodies to endotoxin induced by vaccines that contain whole cells of *B. pertussis*. In an ELISA system for detection of cross-reactive antibodies, normal rabbit serum did not bind to DPT or the staphylococcal toxins, but IgG from a rabbit immunized with the current DPT vaccine bound to the vaccine components and to each of the pyrogenic staphylococcal toxins tested, SEB, SEA, SEC_1 and TSST-1. The rabbit anti-DPT serum, but not normal rabbit serum, partially neutralized the ability of staphylococcal toxins to induce nitric oxide from human monocytes.[66,113] Sera from the majority of SIDS infants tested contained lethal activity in the chick embryo assay. The lethal effects of the serum could be neutralized with a commercial preparation of IgG or pooled sera from healthy adults.[115] This suggests passive immunization might be one means of protecting infants with low levels of maternal antibodies to toxins implicated in SIDS.

DEVELOPMENTAL STAGE AND SLEEP

The majority of SIDS deaths occur during the 2–4 month age range and most occur between midnight and 8 a.m. How are these factors related to inflammatory responses?

Almost all components of the inflammatory responses are suppressed by cortisol and other glucocorticoids. In infants, the adrenal gland decreases in weight during the first 2 months after birth. This is associated with a decrease in the plasma cortisol levels.[116] Adults are less able to control inflammatory responses such as TNF elicited by endotoxin during the early hours of the morning.[117] After midnight when a significant number of SIDS deaths occur, there is minimal secretion of cortisol, and the gland is less responsive than it is during the day.

Individuals with obstructive sleep apnea syndrome (OSAS) have deranged sleep patterns and sleep more during the day than at night. Blood specimens taken from these patients and normal controls at different times during the day and night were compared for their responses to endotoxin. TNF-α, interleukin-1 (IL-1), interleukin-6 (IL-6) and interferon-γ (INF-γ) responses were measured in the samples. For normal individuals, the peak of induction of these mediators occurred during late evening or early morning. For patients with OSAS, the peak occurred during the afternoon or evening. Production of high levels of inflammatory mediators corresponded to times of minimal cortisol production.[118]

During the 2–4 month age range, infants are more reliant on their inflammatory responses to deal with infection because of decreasing levels of specific passive immunity against bacteria and viruses. These inflammatory responses are also involved in septic shock. The increasingly severe stages leading from sepsis to septic shock do not reflect increasing severity of infection, but increasing severity of the systemic response to infection.[119] Strong inflammatory responses might be quite common among infants; however, if the events occur when the ability to control these responses is reduced, the result might be SIDS or a 'near miss' episode.

Infants begin to develop circadian rhythms at about 12 weeks of age. The body temperature of infants falls at night to 36.4°C, similar to that of sleeping adults. This change usually occurs between 7–16 weeks. In some groups such as infants of low birthweight or who experienced problems at delivery, this change can be as late as 22 weeks.[120] It was suggested that the 'immature' state is a risk factor because infants who remain in this stage longer share many of the risk factors with SIDS infants. Other work by this group found that Asian infants stay in the 'immature' stage significantly longer than white infants, but they have a lower incidence of SIDS.[121]

An alternative interpretation is related to other physiologic changes that occur in conjunction with the change in body temperature rhythm. There is a dramatic decrease in night-time, but not daytime, cortisol levels the week following the temperature switch. Before the developmental switch, the morning and night-time values for cortisol range from 0.34 to 22.5 μg dl^{-1} and from 0.22 to 15.2 μg dl^{-1} respectively. After the switch, there is no significant change in the daytime levels of cortisol (0.34–23.9 μg dl^{-1}) but a sharp drop in the night-time levels (0.1–7.25 μg dl^{-1}). In an *in vitro* model, we demonstrated that levels of cortisol present at night-time in infants following the developmental switch (<5 μg dl^{-1}) had little or no effect on control of inflammatory responses (IL-6 and TNF) from human buffy coats stimulated with TSST.[122]

If the drop in night-time cortisol levels occurs early when the baby still has maternal antibodies to neutralize viruses or toxins or after it has developed its own antibodies, the probability of uncontrolled inflammatory responses is reduced. If the drop occurs when the infant has low levels of protective antibodies, it might be more vulnerable to inflammatory responses that we postulate contribute to some of these deaths.

There is indirect evidence that younger infants have reduced inflammatory responses to microorganisms. This comes from a large study carried out in conjunction with the change in British infant immunization schedules in which the initial dose of DPT vaccine was administered at 2 months instead of 3 months. One of the unexpected findings associated with the change in immunization schedule was the significant decrease in adverse reactions (fever or local inflammatory reactions) among infants immunized at the earlier age of 2 months compared with the old schedule beginning at 3 months. This was observed regardless of vaccine type, acellular or whole cell pertussis vaccines.[123] If, as the work on night-time levels of cortisol suggests, younger infants are better able to deal with inflammatory mediators, the new immunization schedule is helping to increase levels of antibodies against toxins during a period in which they are better able to handle inflammatory reactions.

SIDS and genetic, environmental and developmental factors

Epidemiologic studies indicate that in groups in which smoking is less prevalent among women, the incidence of SIDS is lower. Studies on American Indians and Alaskan natives compared populations in which there was a significant difference in the incidence of SIDS. From 1984–1986 the incidence of SIDS was 4.6 per 1000 live births among Indians and Alaskan Natives in the northern region of the United States. Among southwestern Indians, this was 1.4 per 1000 live births. There was no difference between the incidence of SIDS in white populations in the two regions: 2.1 live births in the north and 1.6 per 1000 in the southwest. There were no significant differences in socioeconomic status, maternal age, birth weight or prenatal care between the two Indian populations. Maternal smoking during pregnancy was exceptionally high among northern Indians and Alaskan Natives but low among the southwest Indians.[84]

In Britain smoking is more prevalent among socially deprived groups,[91] and both maternal smoking and poorer socioeconomic conditions were found to be significant risk factors for SIDS.[9,24] Among Asian women of all social classes, smoking is rare,[124] and we have suggested that this might contribute to the lower levels of both SIDS and respiratory deaths in these populations. This could be related to reduced frequency or density of colonization by potential pathogens in both mother and infant or to a lower level of absorption of water-soluble components of cigarette smoke that could enhance inflammatory responses to infection.

There appears to be a significant genetic component associated with induction of both pro-inflammatory and anti-inflammatory cytokines.[125–127] Fatal outcome of meningococcal disease was significantly associated with low TNF-α responses and/or high IL-10 responses of first degree relatives of the patient.[126] There have been few comparative studies on differences in pro- and anti-inflammatory responses carried out in different ethnic groups or in relation to the effects of smoking on inflammatory responses to bacterial toxins.

Next stage in SIDS research

The next stage in SIDS research needs to focus on how the risk factors identified for SIDS contribute to the death of these infants. There are no suitable animal models to examine interactions between the genetic developmental and environmental risk factors for SIDS and the proposed role of infectious agents. Examination of the interactions underlying differences in the incidence of SIDS and serious respiratory infection in some ethnic groups is probably one of the best approaches available. Another model could be detailed examination of infants suffering an acute life-threatening episode (ALTE).

There is evidence that many SIDS deaths are associated with bacterial toxins, those of *S. aureus* in particular. Infants in ethnic groups in which there are high incidences of serious respiratory infections and SIDS have been found to be colonized earlier by potentially pathogenic bacteria.[26,87] Studies of mothers and infants from different ethnic groups are needed to determine if genetic, developmental and environmental risk factors for SIDS affect density of bacterial colonization or inflammatory responses to infectious agents.

DEVELOPMENTAL STAGE

The developmental stage of the infant reflected in the age distribution of SIDS could affect expression of receptors for toxigenic bacteria resulting in enhancement of both frequency and density of colonization. There is no information on age and expression of the Lewis[a] antigen on epithelial cells of infants of different ethnic groups.

The studies on Asian infants in Britain suggest there are significant differences in physiologic development that could play an important role in control of inflammatory responses postulated to contribute to the series of events leading to SIDS. Similar studies are needed for groups in which the incidence of SIDS is increased. Comparative studies of temperature and local reactions of infants from different ethnic groups to immunizations might provide significant insights into control of inflammatory responses during this critical period. Asian infants maintain the 'immature' night-time temperature pattern and higher levels of night-time cortisol for longer periods than white infants. This indicates that in many infants in this group, inflammatory responses to infection might be better controlled during the age range in which the peak incidence of SIDS occurs. Analysis of hormone levels and cytokine levels in infants of different ethnic groups who have been hospitalized for severe respiratory infections might provide evidence to support or refute this hypothesis.

ENVIRONMENTAL FACTORS

Environmental risk factors examined can affect both frequency and density of bacterial colonization. Since the mother is probably the source of the infant's normal flora, the significantly enhanced binding of bacteria to buccal cells of adult smokers might result in exposure of the infant to a greater number of bacteria. Passive coating of the infant's mucosa by components of cigarette smoke might also increase the non-specific 'stickiness' of these cells for bacteria. The effects of maternal smoking on density of colonization of mothers and infants of different ethnic group needs to be assessed in countries in which breastfeeding is not associated with socioeconomic status. Cotinine levels in saliva of the infants could be used as a quantitative estimate for exposure to cigarette smoke.

The prone sleeping position enhances the number and variety of bacterial species in nasal secretions of both adults and children with upper respiratory tract infections. The temperature of children in the prone position is significantly increased and in some instances reached 37°C which could result in induction of pyrogenic toxins of both staphylococci and streptococci.[23] The effect of infection and exposure to cigarette smoke (assessed by cotinine levels in saliva or urine) on nasal temperatures needs to be assessed, preferably in the home environment.

Experimental models suggest that components of cigarette smoke induce inflammatory responses in the absence of infectious agents and enhance responses to viral infection.[111] The effects of cigarette smoke on inflammatory responses might be assessed by measuring temperature responses of infants following immunization in relation to maternal smoking and cotinine levels in the infants' secretions. These studies should include families from different ethnic groups.

The quantitative techniques needed for the studies proposed have been developed; however, they require cooperative efforts between research workers in a variety of disciplines. For many years SIDS research has been compartmentalized and focused mainly on epidemiology, descriptive pathology, and developmental physiology. Research workers in these disciplines need to combine their complementary skills to address the studies proposed.

Caveat

The recent increases in SIDS deaths in Britain and examination of historical records on the fluctuations of the rate of SIDS in different communities[5] suggest we must not become complacent and should view the success of the 'reduce the risks' campaigns with caution. We need to examine in detail the mechanisms underlying the dramatic decreases in the incidence of SIDS that occurred following the campaigns initiated in the early 1990s to reduce the risk factors identified in epidemiologic studies.

If bacterial toxins are involved in the series of events leading to SIDS, major efforts need to be made to identify those components and to develop appropriate active or passive immunization protocols to attempt to reduce further the incidence of these infant deaths.

Acknowledgements

This work was supported by grants from the Scottish Cot Death Trust, Babes in Arms and Chest, Heart and Stroke, Scotland. We are grateful to colleagues who have worked with us on the various aspects of the projects – O. Al Madani, O.R. El Ahmer, R.A. Elton, S.D. Essery, A.E. Gordon, V.S. James, J.W. Keeling, D.A.C. MacKenzie, N. Molony, M.M. Ogilvie, M.W. Raza, A.T. Saadi, A.A. Zorgani.

References

1. Arnon SS, Damus K, Chin J. Infant botulism: epidemiology and relation to sudden infant death syndrome. *Epidemiol Rev* 1981;3:45–66.
2. Sonnabend OAR, Sonnabend WFF, Krech U, Molz G, Sigrist T. Continuous microbiological and pathological study of 70 sudden and unexpected infant deaths: toxigenic intestinal *Clostridium botulinum* infection in 9 cases of sudden infant death syndrome. *Lancet* 1985;I:237–41.
3. Rambaud C, Guibert M, Briand E, Grangeot-Keros L, Coulom-L'Hermine A, Dehan M. Microbiology in Sudden Infant Death Syndrome (SIDS) and other childhood deaths. *FEMS Immunol Med Microbiol* 1999;25:59–66.
4. Zorgani AA, Al Madani O, Essery SD *et al.* Detection of pyrogenic toxins of *Staphylococcus aureus* in cases of sudden infant death syndrome (SIDS). *FEMS Immunol Med Microbiol* 1999;25:103–8.
5. Pearce JL, Luke RKJ, Bettleheim KA. SIDS: What questions should we ask? *FEMS Immunol Med Microbiol* 1999;25:7–10.
6. Crawley BA, Morris JA, Drucker DB *et al.* Endotoxin in blood and tissue in the sudden infant death syndrome. *FEMS Immunol Med Microbiol* 1999;25:131–5.
7. Sayers NM, Crawley BA, Humphries K *et al.* Effect of time postmortem on the concentration of endotoxin in rat organs: implications for sudden infant death syndrome (SIDS). *FEMS Immunol Med Microbiol* 1999;25:125–30.
8. Gibson AAM. Current epidemiology of SIDS. *J Clin Pathol* 1992;45 (Suppl.): 7–10.
9. Brooke H, Gibson A, Tappin D, Brown H. Case control study of sudden infant death syndrome in Scotland 1992–1995. *Br Med J* 1997;314:1516–20.
10. Mitchell EA. Smoking: the next major and modifiable risk factor. In: Rognum TO (ed.) *Sudden Infant Death Syndrome, New Trends in the Nineties.* Scandinavian University Press, Oslo, 1995, pp.114–18.

11. Pershagen G. Review of epidemiology in relation to passive smoking. *Arch Toxicol* 1986;9(Suppl.):63–73.
12. Gilbert RE, Rudd PT, Berry PJ *et al*. Combined effect of infection and heavy wrapping on the risk of sudden unexpected infant death. *Arch Dis Child* 1992;67:171–7.
13. Gilbert RE, Fleming PJ, Azaz Y, Rudd PT. Signs of illness in babies preceding sudden unexpected infant death *Br Med J* 1990;300:1237–9.
14. Musher DM Fainstein V. Adherence of *Staphylococcus aureus* to pharyngeal cells from normal carriers and patients with viral infections. In: Jeljaswiecz J (ed.) *Staphylococci and staphylococcal infections*. Gustav Fischer Verlag, New York, 1981, pp.1011–16.
15. Ford RP, Taylor BJ, Mitchell EA *et al*. Breast feeding and the risk of sudden infant death syndrome. *Int J Epidemiol* 1993;22:885–90.
16. Buescher ES. Host defence mechanisms of human milk and their relations to enteric infections and necrotizing enterocolitis. *Clin Perinatol* 1994;21:247–62.
17. Pisacane A, Graziano L, Zona G *et al*. Breast feeding and acute lower respiratory infection. *Acta Paediatr* 1994;83:714–18.
18. Hoffman HS, Hunter JC, Damus K *et al*. Diphtheria–tetanus–pertussis immunization and sudden infant death: results of the National Institute of Child Health and Human Development Co-operative Epidemiological Study of Sudden Infant Death Syndrome Risk Factors. *Pediatrics* 1987;79:598–611.
19. Walker AM, Jick H, Perera DR, Thompson RS, Knauss TA. Diphtheria–tetanus–pertussis immunization and sudden infant death syndrome. *Am J Pub Health* 1987;77:945–51.
20. Jonville-Bera AP, Autret E, Laugier J. Sudden infant death and diphtheria–tetanus–pertussis–poliomyelitis vaccination status. *Fund Clin Pharmacol* 1995;9:263–70.
21. Beal S. Sleeping position and SIDS: Past, present and future. In Rognum TO (ed.) *Sudden Infant Death Syndrome. New Trends in the Nineties*. Scandinavian University Press, Oslo, 1995, pp. 147–51.
22. Bell S, Crawley BA, Oppenheim BA, Drucker DB, Morris JA. Sleeping position and upper airways bacterial flora: relevance to cot death. *J Clin Pathol* 1996;49:170–2.
23. Molony N, Blackwell CC, Busuttil A. The effect of prone posture on nasal temperature in children in relation to induction of staphylococcal toxins implicated in sudden infant death syndrome. *FEMS Immunol Med Microbiol* 1999;25:109–13.
24. Blair PS, Fleming PJ, Bensley D *et al*. Smoking and the sudden infant death syndrome: results from 1993–5 case–control study for confidential inquiry into stillbirths and deaths in infancy. Confidential Enquiry into Stillbirths and Deaths Regional Coordinators and Researchers. *Br Med J* 1996;313:195–8.
25. Nelson EAS. *Sudden Infant Death Syndrome and Childcare Practices*. E.A.S. Nelson, Hong Kong, 1996, pp. 25–8.
26. Leach AJ, Boswell JB, Asche V, Nienhuys TG, Mathews JD. Bacterial colonization of the nasopharynx predicts very early onset and persistence of otitis media in Australian Aboriginal infants. *Pediatr Infect Dis* 1994;13:983–9.
27. Guntheroth WG, Lohman R, Spiers PS. A seasonal association between SIDS deaths and kindergarten absences. *Public Health Rep* 1992;107:319–23.
28. Williams AL, Uren EC, Brotherton L. Respiratory viruses and sudden infant death. *Br Med J* 1984;288:1491–3.

29. Fleming KA. Upper respiratory inflammation and detection of viral nucleic acids. *J Clin Pathol* 1992;45 (Suppl.):77–9.

30. An SF, Gould S, Keeling JW, Fleming KA. The role of viral infection in SIDS: detection of viral nucleic acid by *in situ* hybridization. *J Pathol* 1993;171:271–8.

31. Cubie HA, Duncan LA, Marshall LA, Smith NM. Detection of respiratory syncytial virus nucleic acid in archival post mortem tissue from infants. *Pediatr Pathol Lab Med* 1997;17:927–38.

32. Morris JA, Haran D, Smith A. Hypothesis: common bacterial toxins are a possible cause of the sudden infant death syndrome. *Med Hypotheses* 1987;22: 211–12.

33. Morris JA, The common bacterial toxin hypothesis of sudden infant death syndrome. *Fems Immunol Med Microbiol* 1999;25:11–17.

34. Telford DR, Morris JA, Hughes P *et al.* The nasopharyngeal bacterial flora in sudden infant death syndrome. *J Infect* 1989;18:125–30.

35. Harrison LM, Morris JA, Telford DR, Brown SM, Jones K, The nasopharyngeal flora in infancy: effects of age, gender, season, viral, upper respiratory tract infection and sleeping position. *Fems Immunol Med Microbiol* 1999;25:19–28.

36. Harrison LM, Morris JA, Telford DR, Brown S, Jones K. Sleeping position in infants over six months of age: implications for theories of sudden infant death syndrome (SIDS). *FEMS Immunol Med Microbiol* 1999;25:29–35.

37. Oppenheim BA, Barclay GR, Morris J *et al.* Antibodies to endotoxin core in sudden infant death syndrome. *Arch Dis Child* 1994;70:95–8.

38. Platt MS, Elin RS, Hosseini JM, Smialek JE. Endotoxemia in sudden infant death syndrome. *Am J Forens Med Pathol* 1994;5:261–5.

39. Arnon SS, Midura TF, Damus K, Wood RM, Chin J. Intestinal infection and toxin production by *Clostridium botulinum* as one cause of sudden infant death syndrome. *Lancet* 1978;I:1273–7.

40. Lindsay JA, Mach AM, Wilkinson MA *et al. Clostridium perfringens* type a cytotoxic-enterotoxin(s) as triggers for death in the sudden infant death syndrome: development of a toxico-infection hypothesis. *Curr Microbiol* 1993;27: 51–9.

41. Bettleheim KA, Dwyer BW, Smith DL, Goldwater PN, Bourne AJ. Toxigenic *Escherichia coli* associated with sudden infant death syndrome. *Med J Aust* 1989;15:538.

42. Bettleheim KA, Goldwater PN, Dwyer BW, Bourne AJ, Smith DL. Toxigenic *Escherichia coli* associated with sudden infant death syndrome. *Scand J Infect Dis* 1990;22:467–76.

43. Bettleheim KA, Chang BJ, Elliot SJ, Gunzburg ST, Pearce JL. Virulence factors associated with strains of *Escherichia coli* from cases of sudden infant syndrome (SIDS). *Comp Immunol Microbiol Infect Dis* 1995;18:179–88.

44. Pearce JL, Bettleheim KA. The faecal *Escherichia coli* of SIDS infants are phenotypically different from those of healthy infants. *11th Australian SIDS Conference.* Melbourne, Australia, 1997, No. 124.

45. Schlievert PM. The role of superantigens in human disease. *Curr Opin Infect Dis* 1995;8:170–4.

46. Bohach GA, Fast DJ, Nelson RD, Schlievert PM. Staphylococcal and streptococcal pyrogenic toxins involved in toxic shock syndrome and related illnesses. *Crit Rev Microbiol* 1990;17:251–72.

47. Bentley AJ, Zorgani AA, Blackwell CC, Weir DM, Busuttil A. Sudden unexpected death in a 6 year old child. *Forensic Sci Int* 1997;88:141–6.

48. Malam JE, Carrick GF, Telford DR, Morris JA. Staphylococcal toxins and sudden infant death syndrome. *J Clin Pathol* 1992;45:716–21.

49. Newbould MJ, Malam J, McIllmurray JM, Morris JA, Telford DR, Barson AJ. Immunohistological localisation of staphylococcal toxic shock syndrome toxin (TSST-1) in sudden infant death syndrome. *J Clin Pathol* 1989;42:935–9.

50. Nicholl A, Gardner A. Whooping cough and unrecognized post-perinatal mortality. *Arch Dis Child* 1988;63:41–7.

51. Lindgren C, Milerad J, Lagercrantz H. Sudden infant death and prevalence of whooping cough in the Swedish and Norwegian communities. *Eur J Paediatr* 1997;156:405–9.

52. Saadi AT, Weir DM, Poxton IR *et al*. Isolation of an adhesin from *Staphylococcus aureus* that binds Lewisa blood group antigen and its relevance to sudden infant death syndrome. *FEMS Immunol Med Microbiol* 1994;8:315–20.

53. Heininger U, Stehr K, Schmidt-Schlapfer G *et al*. *Bordetella pertussis* infections and sudden unexpected deaths in children. *Eur J Pediatr* 1996;155:551–3.

54. Pattison CP, Smoot DT, Ashtorab H, Vergara GG, Young TW, Smith GP. Confirmation of *Helicobacter pylori* by PCR in sudden infant death syndrome. *Gastroenterology* 1998;114:G3686.

55. Kerr JR, Al-Khattaf A, Burnie PJ. An association between sudden infant death syndrome (SIDS) and *Heliobacter pylori* infection. *Arch Dis Child* 2000;83: 439–434.

56. Beachey EA. Bacterial adherence: adhesin-receptor interactions mediating attachment of bacteria to mucosal surfaces. *J Infect Dis* 1981;143:325–45.

57. Issit PD. *Applied Blood Group Serology*. 3rd edn. Montgomery, Miami, 1986, pp. 169–91.

58. Blackwell CC, Saadi AT, Raza MW, Stewart J, Weir DM. Susceptibility to infection in relation to sudden infant death syndrome. *J Clin Pathol* 1992;45(Suppl.): 20–4.

59. Saadi AT, Blackwell CC, Raza MW *et al*. Factors enhancing adherence of toxigenic staphylococci to epithelial cells and their possible role in sudden infant death syndrome. *Epidemiol Infect* 1993;110:507–17.

60. Saadi AT, Blackwell CC, Essery SD, Weir DM, Busuttil A. Comparison of human milk and infant formula on inhibition of bacterial binding and neutralisation of toxins. *Fourth SIDS International Meeting*, 1996, p. 166.

61. Saadi AT, Gordon AE, MacKenzie DAC *et al*. The protective effect of breast feeding in relation to sudden infant death syndrome (SIDS): the effect of human milk and infant formula preparations on binding toxigenic *Staphylococcus aureus* to epithelial cells. *FEMS Immunol Med Microbiol* 1999;25:155–165.

62. Saadi AT, Blackwell CC, Essery SD *et al*. Developmental and environmental factors that enhance binding of *Bordetella pertussis* to human epithelial cells in relation to sudden infant death syndrome. *FEMS Immunol Med Microbiol* 1996;16: 51–9.

63. Gordon AE, Saadi AT, MacKenzie DAC *et al*. The protective effect of breast feeding in relation to Sudden Infant Death Syndrome (SIDS): II. The effect of human milk and infant formula preparations on binding of *Clostridium perfringens* to epithelial cells. *FEMS Immunol Med Microbiol* 1999;25:167–173.

64. van t'Wout J, Burnette WN, Mar VL, Rozdzinski E, Wright SD, Tuomanen E. Role of carbohydrate recognition domains of pertussis toxin in adherence of *Bordetella pertussis* to human macrophages. *Infect Immun* 1992;60:3303–8.

65. Essery SD, Saadi AT, Twite SJ, Weir DM Blackwell CC, Busuttil A. Lewis antigen expression on human monocytes and binding of pyrogenic toxins. *Agent Act* 1994;4:108–10.

66. Essery SD. *Studies on the role of the pyrogenic staphylococcal toxins in sudden infant death syndrome*, PhD Thesis, University of Edinburgh, 1997.

67. Mouricourt M, Petit JM, Carias JR, Julien R. Glycoprotein glycans that inhibit adhesion of *Escherichia coli* mediated K99 fimbriae: treatment of experimental colibacillosis. *Infect Immun* 1990;58:98–106.

68. El Ahmer OR, Raza MW, Ogilvie MM, Blackwell CC, Weir DM, Elton RA. The effect of respiratory virus infection on expression of cell surface antigens associated with binding of potentially pathogenic bacteria. In: Ofek I, Kahane I (eds). *Toward anti-Adhesin Therapy of Microbial Diseases.* Plenum, New York, 1996, pp. 95–105.

69. Raza MW, Ogilvie MM, Blackwell CC, Stewart J, Elton RA, Weir DM. Effect of respiratory syncytial virus infection on binding of *Neisseria meningitidis* and type b *Haemophilus influenzae* to human epithelial cell line (HEp-2). *Epidemiol Infect* 1993;110:339–47.

70. Raza MW, Ogilvie MM, Blackwell CC, Saadi AT, Elton RA, Weir DM. Enhanced expression of native receptors for *Neisseria meningitidis* on HEp-2 cells infected with respiratory syncytial virus. *FEMS Immunol Med Microbiol* 1999;23:115–24.

71. El Ahmer OR, Raza MW, Ogilvie MM, Elton RA, Weir DM, Blackwell CC. Binding of bacteria to HEp-2 cells infected with influenza A virus. *FEMS Immunol Med Microbiol* 1999;23:331–41.

72. Blackwell CC, Tzanakaki G, Kremastinou J, Weir DM, Vakalis N, Elton RA, Mentis A. Factors affecting carriage of *Neisseria meningitidis* among Greek military recruits. *Epidemiology and Infection*, 1992;108:441–8.

73. El Ahmer, OR, Essery SD, Saadi AT *et al.* The effect of cigarette smoke on adherence of respiratory pathogens to buccal epithelial cells. *FEMS Immunol Med Microbiol* 1999;23:27–26.

74. Gilbert RE, Wigfield RE, Fleming PJ, Berry PJ, Rudd PT. Bottle feeding and the sudden infant death syndrome. *Br Med J* 1995;310:88–90.

75. Tappin DM. Bottle feeding and the sudden infant death syndrome. Study was not large enough to show effect. *Br Med J* 1995;310:88–90.

76. Andersson B, Porras O, Hanson LA, Lagergard T, Svanborg-Eden C. Inhibitin of attachment of *Streptococcus pneumoniae* and *Haemophilus influenzae* by human milk and receptor oligosaccharides, *J Infect Dis* 1986;153:232–7.

77. Pisacane A, Graziano L, Zona G, Granata G, Dolezalova H, Cafiero M, Coppola A, Scarpallino B, Ummarino M, Mazzarella G. Breast feeding and acute lower respiratory infection. *Acta Pediatrica* 1994;83;714–18.

78. Coppa GV, Gabrielli O, Giorgi P *et al.* Preliminary study of breast feeding and bacterial adhesion to uroepithelial cells. *Lancet* 1990;335:569–71.

79. Kunz C, Rudloff S. Biological function of oligosaccharides in human milk. *Acta Paediatrica* 1993;82:903–12.

80. Gordon AE, Saadi AT, MacKenzie DAC *et al.* The protective effect of breast feeding in relation to sudden infant death syndrome (SIDS): III. Detection of IgA anti-

bodies in human milk that bind to bacterial toxins implicated in SIDS. *FEMS Immunol Med Microbiol* (in press).

81. Harrison L. *The effect of upper respiratory tract infection and sleeping position on the nasopharyngeal bacterial flora in infancy: possible relevance to sudden infant death syndrome.* PhD Thesis, Lancaster University, 1998.

82. Balarajan R, Raleigh VS, Botting B. Sudden infant death syndrome and post neo-natal mortality in immigrants in England and Wales. *Br Med J* 1989;298: 716–20.

83. Davies DP. Cot death in Hong Kong: a rare problem? *Lancet* 1985;ii:1346–9.

84. Bulterys M. High incidence of sudden infant death syndrome among northern Indians and Alaska natives compared with southwestern Indians: possible role of smoking. *J Commun Health* 1990;15:185–94.

85. Alessandri LM, Read AW, Stanley FJ, Burton PR, Dawes VP. Sudden infant death syndrome in aboriginal and non-aboriginal infants. *J Paediatr Child Health* 1994;30:234–41.

86. Alessandri LM, Read AW, Dawes VP, Cooke CT, Margolius KA, Cadden GA. Pathology review of sudden and unexpected death in aboriginal and non-aboriginal infants. *Pediatr Perinatal Epidemiol* 1995;9:406–19.

87. Homoe P, Prag J, Farholt S *et al.* High rate of nasopharyngeal carriage of poten-tial pathogens among children in Greenland: results of a clinical survey of middle ear disease. *J Infect Dis* 1996;23:1081–90.

88. Aniansson G, Alm B, Andersson B *et al.* Nasopharyngeal colonization during the first year of life. *J Infect Dis* 1992;165 (Suppl.):38–42.

89. Blackwell CC, Mackenzie DAC, James VS *et al.* Toxigenic bacteria and sudden infant death syndrome (SIDS): nasopharyngeal flora during the first year of life. *FEMS Immunol Med Microbiol* 1999;25:51–8.

90. Court C. Cot deaths: Britain: Incidence reduced by two thirds in five years. *Br Med J* 1995;310:7–8.

91. Wald N, Kiryluk S, Doll R, Peto, R. *UK Smoking Statistics.* Oxford University Press, Oxford, 1988.

92. Mackenzie DAC, James VS, Elton RA *et al.* Toxigenic bacteria and SIDS: naso-pharyngeal flora in the first year of life. *Fourth SIDS International Conference.* 1996, pp. 166–7.

93. Ruuskannen O, Arola M, Putto-Laurila A *et al.* Acute otitis media and respiratory syncytial virus infections. *Pediatr Infect Dis J* 1989;8:94–9.

94. Bakeletz LO. Viral potentiation of bacterial superinfection of the respiratory tract. *Trends Microbiol* 1995;3:110–14.

95. Blackwell CC, Weir DM, Busuttil A *et al.* The role of infectious agents in sudden infant death syndrome. *FEMS Immunol Med Microbiol* 1994;9:91–100.

96. Blackwell CC, Weir DM, Busuttil A. Infectious agents, the inflammatory responses of infants and sudden infant death syndrome (SIDS). *Mol Med Today* 1995;1:72–8.

97. Blackwell CC, Weir DM, Busuttil A *et al.* Infectious agents and SIDS: a new concept involving interactions between microorganisms the immune system and developmental stage of infants. In Rognum TO (ed.) *Sudden Infant Death Syn-drome, New Trends in the Nineties.* Scandinavian University Press, Oslo, 1995, pp. 189–98.

98. Blackwell CC, Weir DM, Busuttil A. Infectious agents and SIDS: analysis of risk factors and preventive measures. *J SIDS Infant Mort* 1997;2:61–76.

99. Molony N, Kerr AIG, Blackwell CC, Busuttil A. Is the nasopharynx warmer in children than in adults? *J Clin Forens Med* 1996;3:157–60.

100. Molony N, Blackwell CC, Busuttil A. The prone sleeping position, nasal temperature and SIDS. *Fifth SIDS International Conference*. Rouen, France, 1998.

101. Drucker DB, Aluyi HA, Morris JA, Telford DR, Gibbs A. Lethal synergistic action of toxins of bacteria isolated from sudden infant death syndrome. *J Clin Pathol* 1992;45:799–801.

102. Mach AM, Lindsay JA. Activation of *Clostridium perfringens* cytotoxic enterotoxin(s) *in vivo* and *in vitro*: role in triggers for sudden infant death. *Curr Microbiol* 1994;28:261–7.

103. Sayers NM, Drucker DB, Telford DR, Morris JA. Effects of nicotine on bacterial toxins associated with cot death. *Arch Dis Child* 1995;73:549–51.

104. Vege A, Rognum TO. Inflammatory responses in SIDS - past and present views. *FEMS Immunol Med Microbiol* 1999;25:67–78.

105. Forsyth KD. Immune and inflammatory responses in SIDS. *FEMS Immunol Med Microbiol* 1999;25:79–83.

106. Jakeman KJ, Rushton DI, Smith H, Sweet C. Exacerbation of bacterial toxicity to infant ferrets by influenza virus: possible role in sudden infant death syndrome. *J Infect Dis* 1991;163:35–40.

107. Sarawar SR, Blackman MA, Doherty PD. Superantigen shock in mice with inapparent viral infection. *J Infect Dis* 1994;170:1189–94.

108. Leclaire RD, Kell WM, Sadik RA, Dawns MB, Parker GW. Regulation of staphylococcal enterotoxin B-elicited nitric oxide production by endothelial cells. *Infect Immun* 1995;63:539–46.

109. Lundemose JB, Smith H, Sweet C. Cytokine release from human peripheral blood leucocytes incubated with endotoxin with or without prior infection with influenza virus: relevance to the sudden infant death syndrome. *Int J Exp Pathol* 1993;74:291–7.

110. Raza MW, Essery SD, Saadi AT *et al.* Maternal smoking, infection and SIDS. *International Conference on Sudden Infant Death Syndrome*. Dublin, Ireland, 1997, p. 24.

111. Raza MW, Essery SD, Elton RA, Weir DM, Busuttil A, Blackwell CC. Exposure to cigarette smoke, a major risk factor for sudden infant death syndrome: effects of cigarette smoke on inflammatory responses to viral infection and toxic shock syndrome toxin-1. *FEMS Immunol Med Microbiol* 1999;25:145–54.

112. Blackwell CC, Saadi AT, Essery SD, Zorgani AA, Weir DM, Busuttil A. Has the new immunisation schedule contributed to the decline in SIDS in Britain? *Fourth SIDS International Conference*. 1996, p. 54.

113. Essery SD, Raza MW, Saadi AT, Weir DM, Busuttil A, Blackwell CC. The protective effect of immunisation in relation to Sudden Infant Death Syndrome. *FEMS Immunol Med Microbiol* 1999;25:183–92.

114. Siarakas S, Brown AJ, Murrell WG. Immunological evidence for a bacterial toxin aetiology in SIDS. *FEMS Immunol Med Microbiol* 1999;25;37–50.

115. Sayers NM, Drucker DB, Hutchinson IV, Barson AJ. Preliminary investigation of lethally toxic sera of SIDS victims and neutralisation by commercially available immunoglobulins and adult sera. *FEMS Immunol Med Microbiol* 1999;25:193–8.

116. Wittekind CA, Arnold JD, Garth L, Lattrell B, Jones MP. Longitudinal studies of plasma ATCH and cortisol levels in very low birth weight infants in the first 8 weeks of life. *Early Hum Devel* 1993;33:191–200.

117. Pollmacher T, Mullington J, Korth C *et al*. Diurnal variations in the human host response to endotoxin. *J Infect Dis* 1996;174:1040–5.

118. Entzian P, Linnemann K, Schlaak M, Zabel P. Obstructive sleep apnea syndrome and circadian rhythms of hormones and cytokines. *Am J Respir Crit Care Med* 1996;153:1080–6.

119. Bone RC. Gram-negative sepsis: a dilemma of modern medicine. *Clin Microbiol Rev* 1993;6:57–68.

120. Lodemore MR, Peterson SA, Wailoo MP. Factors affecting the development of night-time temperature rhythms. *Arch Dis Child* 1992;67:1259–61.

121. Peterson SA Wailoo MP. Interactions between infant care practices and physiological development in Asian infants. *Early Hum Develop* 1994;38:181–6.

122. Gordon A, Al Madani O, Raza M, Weir D, Busuttil A, Blackwell CC. Cortisol levels and control of inflammatory responses to toxic shock syndrome toxin (TSST-1): The prevalence of night time deaths in Sudden Infant Death Syndrome. *FEMS Immunol Med Microbiol* 1999;25:199–206.

123. Miller E, Ashworth LAE, Redhead K, Thornton C, Waight PA, Coleman T. Effect of schedule on reactogenicity and antibody persistence of acellular and whole-cell pertussis vaccines: value of laboratory tests as predictors of clinical performance. *Vaccine* 1997;15:51–60.

124. Hilder AS. Ethnic differences in the sudden infant death syndrome: what can we learn from immigrants to the UK. *Early Hum Develop* 1994;38:143–9.

125. Westendorp RGJ, Langermanns JAM, de Bel CE *et al*. Release of tumor necrosis factor: an innate host characteristic that may contribute to the outcome of meningococcal disease. *J Infect Dis* 1995;171:1057–60.

126. Westendorp RGJ, Langemans JAM, Huizinga TWJ *et al*. Genetic influence on cytokine production and fatal meningococcal disease. *Lancet* 1997;349:170–3.

127. Read Rc, Camp NJ, di Giovine FS, Borrow R, Kaczmarski EB, Chaudhury AGA, Fox AJ, Duff GW. An interlukin-1 genotype is associated with fatal outcome of meningococcal disease. *J Infect Dis* 2000;182;1557–60.

128. Williams AL. Tracheobronchitis and sudden infant death syndrome. *Pathology* 1980;12,73–6.

129. Gupta R, Helms PJ, Jolliffe IT, Douglas AS. Seasonal variation in sudden infant death syndrome and bronchiolitis– a common mechanism. *Am J Respir Crit Care Med* 1996;154,431–5.

130. Williams SM, Taylor BJ, Mitchell EA. Sudden infant death syndrome: insulation from bedding and clothing and its effect modifiers. The National Cot Death Study Group. *Int J Epidemiol* 1996;25,366–75.

131. Hoffman HJ, Damus K, Hilman L, Krongrad E. Risk factors for SIDS: results of the National Institute of Child Health and Human Development SIDS Cooperative epidemiological study. *Ann NY Acad Sci* 1988;533:13–30.

132. Czegledy-Nagy EN, Cutz E, Becker LE. Sudden infant death syndrome under one year of age. *Pediatr Pathol* 1993;13:671–84.

133. Bentham G. Population mixing and sudden infant death syndrome in England and Wales. *Int J Epidemiol* 1994;23:540–4.

134. Nelson KE, Greenberg MA, Mufson MA, Moses VK. The sudden infant death syndrome and epidemic viral disease. *Am J Epidemiol* 1975;101:423–30.

135. Ford RPK, McCormick HE, Jennings LC. Cot death in Cantebury (NZ); Lack of association with respiratory virus patterns. *Aust NZ J Med* 1990;20:798–801.

136. Zink P, Drescher J, Verhagen W, Filk J, Milbradt H. Serological evidence of recent influenza virus A (H3N2) infections in forensic cases of the sudden infant death syndrome (SIDS). *Arch Virol* 1987;93:223–32.

137. Las Heras J, Swanson VL. Sudden death of an infant with rhinovirus infection complicating bronchial asthma: case report. *Pediatr Pathol* 1983;1:319–23.

138. Bajanwski T, Wiegand P, Pring-Akerblon P, Adrian T, Jorch G, Brinkmann B. Detection and significance of adenoviruses in cases of sudden infant death. *Virchows Arch* 1996;428:113–8.

139. Shimizu C, Rambaud C, Cheron G et al. Molecular identification of viruses in sudden infant death associated with myocarditis and pericariditis. *Pediatr Infect Dis J* 1995;14:584–8.

140. Bettiol SS, Radcliff FJ, Hunt AL, Goldsmid JM. Bacterial flora of Tasmanian SIDS infants with special reference to pathogenic strains of *Escherichia coli*. *Epidemiol Infect* 1994;112:275–84.

141. Carpenter RG, Gardner A. Environment findings and sudden infant death syndrome. *J Infect* 1990;18:125–30.

142. Uren EC, Willaims AL, Jack I, Rees JW. Association of respiratory virus infections with sudden infant death syndrome. *Med J Aust* 1980;1:417–19.

143. Grangeot-Keros L, Broyer M, Briand E et al. Enterovirus in sudden unexpected death in infants. *Pediatr Infect Dis J* 1996;15:123–8.

144. Yolken R, Murphy M. Sudden infant death syndrome associated with rotavirus infection. *J Med Virol* 1982;10:291–6.

145. Murrell WG, Stewart BJ, O'Neill C, Siarakas S, Kariks S. Enterotoxigenic bacteria in the sudden infant death syndrome. *J Med Microbiol* 1993;39:114–27.

146. Goldwater PN, Williams V, Bourne AJ, Byard RW. Sudden infant death syndrome: a possible clue to causation. *Med J Aust* 1990;153:59–60.

147. Matsushita K, Uchiyama T, Igarashi N et al. Possible pathogenic effect of *Streptococcus mitis* superantigen on oral epithelial cells. *Adv Exp Med Biol* 1997;418:685–8.

148. Howat WJ, Moore IE, Judd M, Roche WR. Pulmonary immunopathology of sudden infant death syndrome. *Lancet* 1994;343:1390–2.

149. Baxendine JA, Moore IE. Pulmonary eosinophilia in sudden infant death syndrome. *J Pathol* 1995;177:415–21.

150. Stoltenberg I, Vege A, Opdal SH, Saugstad OD, Rognum TO. Does immunostimulation play a role in SIDS? In: Rognum TO (ed.) *Sudden Infant Death Syndrome. New Trends in the Nineties*. Scandinavian University Press, Oslo, 1995, pp. 179–81.

151. Holgate ST, Walters C, Walls AF et al. The anaphylaxis hypothesis of sudden infant death syndrome (SIDS): mast cell degranulation in cot death revealed by elevated concentrations of tryptase in serum. *Clin Exp All* 1994;24:115–23.

152. Howatson AG. Viral infection and alpha interferon in SIDS. *J Clin Pathol* 1992;45 (Suppl.):25–8.

153. Vege A, Rognum TO, Scott R, Aasen AO, Saugsted OD. SIDS cases have increased levels of interleukin-6 in cerebrospinal fluid. *Acta Paediatr* 1995;84:193–6.

154. Kilpatrick DC, James VS, Blackwell CC, Weir DM, Hallam NF, Busuttil A. Mannan binding lectin and the sudden infant death syndrome. *Forensic Sci Int* 1998;97:135–8.

CHAPTER 12

Differential diagnosis of sudden infant death

ROGER W. BYARD AND HENRY F. KROUS

Introduction   209
Deaths due to accidents   210
Deaths due to inflicted injury   214
Death due to natural diseases   220
Conclusion   222
References   223

Introduction

A wide variety of conditions involving all organ systems may be responsible for the sudden death of an infant who appeared reasonably well prior to death.[1] Infants have a great capacity for not manifesting symptoms and signs even when suffering from quite serious disease. While many unexpected infant deaths may be due to SIDS, the possibility of underlying organic illness, accidents or even homicide must always be considered.

Unfortunately the autopsy findings in SIDS are by definition not diagnostic, and the features of other conditions may be extremely subtle, or even identical to SIDS.[2,3] For this reason there is reliance on the presenting history to guide the autopsy investigation. The veracity of the history may be doubtful, however, in cases of lethal inflicted injury. Given the absence of a history of illness, the possibility of an inaccurate story from caretakers, and the lack of pathognomonic findings at autopsy, establishing an accurate diagnosis in some cases may simply not be possible. The difficulties in separating out individual diagnoses in cases of unexpected infant death has resulted in the suggestion by Emery that the term 'SIDS' has been used as a 'convenient diagnostic dustbin'.[4]

For this reason the investigation of unexpected infant deaths should revolve around a pediatric or forensic pathologist who has a specific interest in SIDS and who is able to liaise with pediatricians, pediatric radiologists, neuropathologists and child abuse physicians. In this way the possibility of uncovering occult diagnoses will be maximized and more credibility will be given to the final conclusion of SIDS, if this is considered most likely.

Estimates of the percentage of cases where death is due to an identifiable cause in infants who present dead in their cots has varied greatly. One report stated that nearly every second case was due to some other entity, however, this has not been supported by other studies which found that the figure was less than one in ten.[5-7] The reasons for this difference are unclear, however, it is possible that the thoroughness with which the clinical history is reviewed or the death scene examined may vary, resulting in significant presenting findings being overlooked prior to autopsy. However, the recent fall in numbers of SIDS deaths has certainly increased the relative percentage of other cases.[8]

Deaths due to accidents

Fatal accidents are quite a common cause of death in the 15 to 24-year-old age group but are uncommon in infancy. The high dependency and relative immobility of infants has resulted in only 3% of fatalities in this age group being caused by accidents.[9] The types of fatal injuries vary between different reports, depending on the community studied. However, generally the most frequent causes of accidental death in infants and young children are drowning, asphyxia, burns, scalds and motor vehicle accidents. Less common causes of fatal accidents in infancy are falls and poisoning.[1,10] Pathologists, because of their continued exposure to such trauma, are in an excellent situation to initiate injury prevention campaigns particularly in this age group.[11]

DROWNING

Infants are most at risk from drowning in the bath, with recent work suggesting that shared bathing with an older sibling may increase this risk (Byard, unpublished observation). Toddlers are more mobile and curious, and are at risk of overbalancing into heavy, industrial buckets filled with water, or falling into swimming pools. Both of these types of accident may be associated with children playing with toys in water and are exacerbated by the relatively high centre of gravity of young children. Unfortunately their poor coordination and muscle strength may not enable them to escape from a potentially dangerous situation.[12,13] The possibility of pre-existing disease initiating the drowning episode in children of all ages should always be considered.[14]

BURNS AND SCALDS

Infants most often die in fires at their home address due to either inhalation of products of combustion, or to burns, or to a combination of both factors.

Infants and young children are particularly vulnerable to the effects of fires due to their relative immobility and inability to move to a safer environment. Although soot in the upper airway and high levels of carbon monoxide indicate that the infant was alive during the fire, interpretation can be complicated, as children tend to have lower carboxyhemoglobin levels than adults in similar circumstances.[15] Cyanide from burning plastic may also be lethal and should be checked for, although blood levels may decline after death. The absence of soot staining of the airways and low levels of carboxyhemoglobin require careful evaluation as the case may represent a homicide.

Scalds from hot water should match the description of the accident, which should be plausible. Re-enactment of the accident should be able to demonstrate the pattern of injury, with the presence of satellite 'splash' scalds suggesting non-inflicted injury.

VEHICLE ACCIDENTS

Motor vehicle deaths usually involve infants who were passengers. The circumstances and cause of death are usually quite obvious from the history and autopsy examination, and injuries tend to be severe with multiple fractures and organ disruption.[16] Numbers of deaths have declined in areas where car capsules have been used to transport infants.

ASPHYXIA

Infants and young children are particularly vulnerable to accidental asphyxia from unsafe cots and sleeping arrangements, with an average age of 10 months and an upper limit of 3 years reported in one recent study.[17] Developmentally delayed children may be at risk at older ages.[18] The two main categories of death are wedging and hanging.

Young children and infants may slide or roll into gaps left between mattresses and cot sides, or between mattresses and the wall, or between cushions and the back of couches. Figures 12.1 and 12.2 illustrate such situations.[19,20] Once within these crevices they are often unable to extricate themselves and tend to move progressively deeper into the gap. This may cause respiratory embarrassment from pressure on the chest or abdomen, or from occlusion of the mouth and nose. The autopsy findings in such cases may be entirely non-specific, and unless a clear and accurate description of the death scene is obtained, an incorrect diagnosis of SIDS may be made.

Hanging occurs when an infant slips and is caught under the neck by loose restraining harnesses, or becomes tangled in curtain cords, or when clothing catches on the side of a cot. The diagnosis may be established at autopsy when a parchmented ligature mark around the neck is found, occasionally with facial petechiae.

Given the relatively non-specific findings at autopsy in infants who have died from wedging, or from other forms of upper airway occlusion, an examination

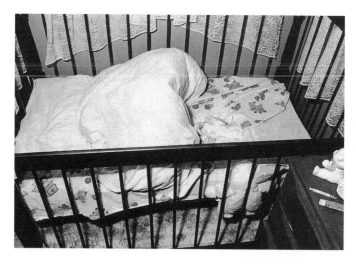

Fig. 12.1 A drop-sided cot were the body of an 8.5-month-old girl was found wedged in the gap between the sliding side and the mattress. A teddy bear has been used in the scene reconstruction.

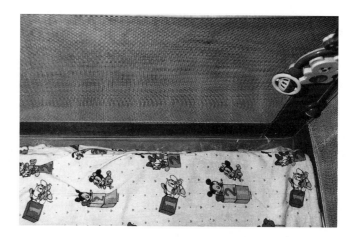

Fig. 12.2 A trough where a 3.5-month-old boy was found wedged between the distensible mesh side of the cot and the mattress.

of the death scene is a vital part of the investigation of such deaths. This has led to the identification of defective cots and dangerous sleeping environments including loose bouncinette harnesses, waterbeds, mesh cots, 'U' shaped pillows, rocking cradles and thin plastic mattress covers.[18,21–24]

The danger of accidental suffocation of an infant sharing a bed with an adult ('overlaying') has been recognized for many hundreds of years. In recent years, however, there has been argument as to whether the benefits of shared sleeping outweigh the risks.[25] Given that the autopsy findings in infants who have died from either upper airway occlusion or SIDS are non-specific,[26] assessment of the likelihood of death from overlaying requires careful scene examination and parental interview. Ultimately it may not be possible to determine accurately the sequence of terminal events. However, a small infant wedged in an adult bed between two intoxicated adults, or being held under the breast of a sleeping mother while feeding, is at risk of accidental asphyxia.[27,28] It has also been reported that an infant sleeping with a mother who smokes has a twofold risk of dying unexpectedly.[29] Accidental suffocation by an adult may not necessarily require that the adult lies fully over the infant, as certain infants are extremely susceptible to even transient upper airway occlusion.[30]

Infants are often enthusiastic about placing objects into their mouths without being aware of possible dangers. Toy parts and food are responsible for most cases of accidental asphyxia due to upper airway occlusion.[31-33]

Large inhaled foreign bodies most often cause immediate symptoms with coughing, vomiting or airway obstruction. This may not always be the case, however, and foreign bodies may cause airway compromise some time after ingestion. This may be due to direct intralumenal obstruction of the trachea/glottis, or obstruction from external pressure when material lodges in the esophagus. Other mechanisms of death include perforation of the heart or great vessels from migrating impacted foreign material. Because of the possible delay between ingestion and airway compromise the presence of an obstructive foreign body may only be recognized after discovery at autopsy.[34,35]

POISONING

Infants and toddlers often ingest a wide variety of objects and substances including caustics, household and garden products and adult medications. Poisonous plants are less commonly swallowed. The autopsy investigation of cases of potential infant poisoning requires a complete inventory of medications and substances in the house, garage and yard that the child may have access to. Visitors to the house should be interviewed about medications, and full toxicological screening should be undertaken for both pharmaceutical products and illegal drugs. Unfortunately not every substance can be screened for and so death scene information may be particularly useful in directing the search.

FALLS

Infants are able to survive falls from considerable heights and usually do not suffer severe injuries from accidental falls around the house. The differences between head injuries sustained in accidental falls compared with those due to inflicted trauma are described later in this chapter.

DEATHS IN HOSPITAL

While surgical intervention in infancy is usually undertaken without problem, there may be an increased risk of death from respiratory or cardiovascular complications. Problems that may arise during surgery that adversely affect an anesthetized infant include airway obstruction, fluid and electrolyte imbalance, cardiac perforation from central catheters,[36] cardiac dysrrhythmias and inadequate ventilation.

If an infant dies while under anesthesia it is imperative that the hospital records are carefully reviewed, including laboratory assessments, that the surgical record is examined, and that the case is discussed with the involved surgeon and anesthetist. It may also be of assistance to consult with physicians from other institutions who did not treat the infant.[37]

HYPO- AND HYPERTHERMIA

Extremes of temperature may put infants at risk of death from hypo- or hyperthermia. For example, infants who are left in rooms with no central heating, or who are exposed to low environmental temperatures following abandonment, may die from hypothermia. Although classic autopsy findings have been described which include pink coloration of the skin, pulmonary edema, acute pancreatitis, acute gastric erosions and perivascular hemorrhages within the brain, the autopsy findings may be minimal.[1] For this reason it is important to obtain full details of the environmental and body temperatures, the humidity and wind-chill factor, the time of exposure to cold and the adequacy of bedding and clothing.

High environmental temperatures or exposure of infants to excessive heating for prolonged periods may result in death from hyperthermia. Infants are particularly at risk as they are not able to remove themselves from hot environments such as cars in the sun,[38] have high metabolic rates and have poorly developed thermoregulatory control. At autopsy infants may appear dehydrated (and so a vitreous electrolyte analysis is required), or have skin slippage and rhabdomyolyis. The autopsy findings may, however, again be quite minimal.[39] Information required from the death scene includes the environmental and body temperatures, the humidity and ventilation, the time of exposure to heat and the amount of clothing worn. Very rarely an underlying organic disease which predisposes to collapse on hot days, such as cystic fibrosis or congenital adrenal hyperplasia, may be detected.[39]

Deaths due to inflicted injury

Inflicted injury may result in death, with infants and young children being particularly susceptible to serious organ and tissue damage because of their inability to adequately defend themselves, or to flee from an adult assailant. Although injuries may be clearly observed at autopsy in cases of assault, inflicted asphyxia may be indistinguishable from SIDS.[40]

The current definition of SIDS clearly specifies the need for a review of the clinical history, as the presence of multiple deaths within the family may suggest homicide. When injuries are detected, the history may be vague regarding the details of the 'accident' and there may have been no attempt to obtain medical help. It is not unusual for injuries detected at postmortem to be blamed on a parent falling with the child en route to the hospital or for an older sibling to be held responsible. A parents explanation for extensive and lethal injuries may be remotely possible, but is usually not plausible.[1]

Given the subtleties of many inflicted injuries in infancy, all cases of unexpected infant death should have a careful scene examination with external examination of the clothed body. If cardiopulmonary resuscitation has taken place it is important to get an idea of the duration and by whom it was performed. The body should then be undressed and all surfaces and orifices of the unwashed body examined under good lighting. This may require transfer back to the mortuary to facilitate a proper examination. Full body radiographs taken by trained personnel are required along with color photographs of all body surfaces, the conjunctivae and inner surfaces of the lips, even if no lesions are observed. The remainder of the autopsy examination should be undertaken according to recognized protocols with involvement of other sub-specialists in cases where bite marks or fractures are found, or where sexual abuse is suspected. The authors would recommend formal neuropathologic examination of the brain and spinal cord in all cases.[40]

HEAD TRAUMA

The most common cause of death in infants with inflicted injury is from cranial trauma involving cerebral concussion, contusion and laceration, skull fractures and intracranial hemorrhage.[41] In addition to complete skeletal surveys, radiologic assessment requires cerebral computerized axial tomography (CT) and magnetic resonance imaging (MRI) if possible.[42]

Fractures of the skull due to accidents in infancy tend to be non-displaced and linear, and do not cross suture lines. This contrasts with skull fractures from inflicted injury which may be similar to those encountered in motor vehicle accidents, in that they tend to be larger, with a complex, comminuted pattern. Inflicted fractures also tend to involve more than one bone and have separation of the edges of more than 3 mm. When depressed fractures occur accidentally they result from falls of greater than four feet, or down stairs, or from an impact with a sharp or moving object. The history should plausibly reflect the injuries sustained and the autopsy findings.[1]

The history that is often given following an inflicted skull fracture is of a fall around the home, however, infants and young children are surprisingly robust when it comes to surviving falls. For example, only two relatively minor skull fractures and two extremity fractures were found in a study of 165 witnessed accidental falls from beds and cots in hospital in children under the age of 16 years.[43] No deaths occurred in falls from three stories or less in another study of 61 children who fell from buildings.[44]

Skull fractures may be accompanied by both intracranial hemorrhage and damage to the brain parenchyma. Hemorrhage may occur in the absence of skull fractures, for example in shearing injuries of the kind seen in whiplash shaking due to tearing of dural bridging veins. There may be associated subarachnoid, retinal and optic nerve hemorrhages as well.[45–47]

Intraparenchymal damage to the brain may occur in the vicinity of the fracture due to direct trauma, or it may be in more distant locations associated with shearing and rotational forces due to violent head movement. Examination of the brains of infants with possible inflicted head injury by a neuropathologist is required, as the nature and degree of injury must be meticulously documented. The 'retraction balls' of diffuse axonal injury[48] can also be more sensitively detected with immunohistochemical staining of brain tissue for amyloid precursor protein. This type of study may enable some estimation of the time course of the fatal injury or may indicate previous trauma.

Shaking-impact syndrome describes a constellation of symptoms and signs associated with intracranial injury without skull fracture or external signs of head trauma.[49,50] It occurs predominantly in infants and results from vigorous shaking. The intracranial injuries consist of marked cerebral edema, subarachnoid and subdural hemorrhage, parenchymal hemorrhage/contusion and retinal hemorrhages.

Infants are thought to be susceptible to this type of injury because of their small size, which enables picking up and shaking, and also because of their unique anatomy and immature physical development; i.e. the infant head is relatively large with poorly developed neck muscles which provide minimal bracing when the infant is shaken. The infant brain is soft and poorly supported due to lack of myelination, and the interior of the skull is relatively smooth with less well developed bony anchoring points than at older ages. These unique characteristics allow considerable movement of the brain within the skull when shaking occurs.

As in many cases of inflicted injury there is often no accurate history of the type of trauma that has been sustained when the infant comes to autopsy. There may, however, be a history of reduced consciousness, apnea, vomiting or convulsions.[51]

Thumb and finger tip bruising of the anterior chest wall may be observed, along with bruising beside the spine where the infant has been held. The anterior fontanelle may be bulging reflecting underlying cerebral swelling.[52,53] In addition to the intracranial features noted above, there may be rib fractures, often situated posteriorly, from chest compression.

SKELETAL TRAUMA

The autopsy evaluation of all cases of unexpected infant death requires a full skeletal survey, with special views, and interpretation by a pediatric radiologist. Not only is radiologic assessment a more accurate way to date fractures, but it will also identify long bone fractures that would not usually be found during a standard autopsy.

Particular features which may be found in cases of inflicted infant trauma include multiple fractures of varying ages (in the absence of bone disease or a plausible history), spiral fractures of the long bones and metaphyseal avulsion fractures.

There is sometimes resistance on the part of hospital staff to assist with radiographs of dead infants if the cause of death has already been established, as unfortunately the significance of other apparently minor injuries may not be understood. Such injuries may be extremely valuable in establishing a pattern of trauma and may enable a chronology of the inflicted injury to be ascertained. These findings may be crucial in the medicolegal evaluation of the death.

SKIN AND SOFT TISSUE TRAUMA

One of the most common findings at autopsy in an abused infant are injuries to the skin in the form of bruises, burns and bites. Although the presence of bruises on the skin of an infant without adequate explanation is a disturbing finding, it may be difficult to distinguish inflicted injury from an accident in individual lesions. The overall pattern may be of far greater significance, particularly if there are bruises of different ages to suggest repeated episodes of trauma. Discerning the pattern of injury in aging bruises may not be possible due to fading and loss of definition of the areas of hemorrhage.

All parts of the body should be examined for bruising including the nasal passages, inside of the mouth and the external ear canals. As bruising may be masked by postmortem lividity or by darkly pigmented skin, extensive skin incisions must be performed in suspected cases of injury. Rarely the cause of death may be subcutaneous hemorrhage.

The site of bruising may assist in determining whether the injuries were inflicted in younger children, with a predilection for the lower back and head.[54] Accidental bruising is found more often on the lower legs, feet and hands, and is more often unilateral.

The pattern of bruising may also be extremely useful in working out the mechanism of injury, as the shape of the object with which the infant has been hit may be discernable. For example, finger marks on the face may occur with slapping or punching, and looped impressions may be left after an infant has been hit with a rope or flex.

Bite marks left by adults are larger than those left by children or animals and are most often found on the cheeks or buttocks. Swabbing of the bite for DNA matching is mandatory and examination by a forensic odontologist may assist in subsequent matching with possible suspects.

ABDOMINAL TRAUMA

Injury to the abdominal organs is the second most common cause of fatalities in inflicted pediatric trauma. Intraperitoneal organs may be trapped between a fist or knee and the vertebral column, resulting in rupture and laceration. The most susceptible organs and tissues are those which are relatively immobile and cross the spinal column such as the liver, pancreas, mesentery, stomach and duodenum. Death results from hemorrhage or sepsis with shock.[1]

POISONING

Deliberate poisoning or drugging of infants is unusual but may occur with homicide, or if there has been a miscalculation in the dose of a drug being used to oversedate a child. Infants may also be given medication by their mothers in an attempt to either create or simulate disease in Munchausen syndrome by proxy.

BURNS

Inflicted burns or scalds account for 10% of cases of non-accidental injury in children.[55-57] Infants may either have hot objects placed next to them, or be held against a hot surface such as a stove. The pattern of the injury may enable identification of the object causing the burn. Cigarettes may be used to inflict injury, causing very characteristic circular burns which may be full thickness. These are most often found on the palms, soles and buttocks.

Infants may be placed into hot water in a bath causing a variety of different but characteristic patterns. A clearly demarcated edge may be seen between scalded and unscalded skin without any satellite splashes indicating that the infant was firmly held in the water and was not able to struggle or splash. Accidental scalds tend to have more irregular edges. A 'doughnut' pattern of scalding may be seen due to perineal sparing if the infant was placed in a sitting position in the water, and 'glove and stocking' burns may be observed if the infant's hands or feet were held underwater.

STARVATION

Malnourished infants demonstrate marked wasting with wrinkling of skin over the thighs and buttocks. The abdomen is scaphoid and the infant may also be dirty and have severe nappy rash. If significant dehydration is present there may be sinking of the fontanelle and eyes with drying of body cavity linings and wrinkling of the liver capsule.

Unfortunately it may be difficult at autopsy to distinguish an infant who is simply malnourished due to an inadequate diet, from an infant who has a rare metabolic disorder, as in the authors' experience starvation appears to cause derangements of certain biochemical tests.

SEXUAL ABUSE

It is important that any injury to the genitalia is fully documented and photographed and that any genital discharge or unexplained bleeding is investigated.

Early involvement of a pediatric forensic physician is a useful exercise as a colposcopic video of lesions may be able to be taken prior to autopsy. Routine oral, pharyngeal, vaginal and anal swabs and smears should be taken if sexual contact is suspected.

MUNCHAUSEN SYNDROME BY PROXY

This refers to a rare condition in which a mother either causes or simulates disease in her child so that there is repetitive medical attention and investigation.[58–60]

Reports of infant death are well recognized in association with this syndrome with several notorious cases involving a number of deaths within the same families due to induced asphyxia. As there are no pathognomonic features at autopsy to enable SIDS to be clearly distinguished from induced suffocation,[3,61] it is often not possible to exclude Munchausen by proxy on purely pathologic grounds. While the occurrence of a second SIDS death in a family is certainly possible, consideration should be given to Munchausen by proxy[62] or to inherited disease.

Although it is possible that an infant who dies of SIDS may have had episodes of difficulty breathing (so-called apparent life-threatening events or ALTEs), this has been questioned following the conviction for homicide of the mother of two infants who were reported in the first paper linking SIDS and ALTEs.[63,64] Covert video camera surveillance of a suspected mother with her infant in hospital has been successfully performed to detect and record episodes.[62,65]

INJURIES FROM CARDIOPULMONARY RESUSCITATION

Infants at autopsy often manifest a wide range of injuries associated with attempts at resuscitation. These consist of impressions from electrocardiograph leads, puncture wounds from intravascular lines, and trauma from endotracheal intubation. Chest trauma in the form of bruising and rib fractures are not seen, presumably due to the greater elasticity of the juvenile rib cage and costal cartilages.[66]

Retinal hemorrhages may be seen in infants' eyes following birth, but then disappear during the first several days of life.[67] Although retinal hemorrhages have been rarely documented after resuscitation,[68] underlying disease of the brain is required to predispose to their occurrence, i.e. studies addressing this issue have not shown an association between retinal hemorrhages and cardiopulmonary resuscitation in the absence of pre-existing brain trauma, seizures, tumors, sepsis, severe dehydration or coagulation defects.[69–73] An experimental study using piglets could not induce retinal hemorrhages through resuscitation.[74] When accompanied by unexplained intracranial hemorrhage and cerebral edema, retinal hemorrhages should suggest shaken impact syndrome. Other injuries are extremely rare and their assessment requires a detailed history of the duration and type of resuscitation.

Death due to natural diseases

Many conditions cause death in infants who were thought to be quite well prior to the fatal episode.[75,76] The following text discusses some of the more common conditions with more detailed analyses and descriptions available elsewhere.[1]

CARDIOVASCULAR CONDITIONS

Both congenital and acquired cardiovascular disease may cause sudden death in infancy. Structural abnormalities of the heart associated with sudden death include tetralogy of Fallot, Ebstein anomaly, Eisenmenger syndrome and transposition of the great vessels. Sudden death may also occur in these conditions after surgical repair, associated with scarring of tissues around conduction tracts or progressive cardiomegaly. Although infants with life-threatening cardiovascular disease are usually symptomatic, this may not always be so. For example, the only indication in some cases may be failure to thrive. Other symptoms and signs may include cyanosis, irritability, episodic breathlessness and difficulty feeding.

Although ventricular septal defect is the most common congenital cardiac anomaly, it is rarely associated with sudden death, and then usually only when there has been left ventricular enlargement.[77,78] Congenital aortic stenosis may also cause sudden death from left ventricular decompensation, but this usually occurs in later childhood. Left ventricular hypoplasia may also be associated with precipitate clinical deterioration and death.

Cardiomyopathies may occur in infancy and can cause sudden death due to involvement of conduction tracts with dysrhythmias, or to outflow obstruction.[79] Endocardial fibroelastosis is rarely primary, and is usually secondary to either a structural defect of the heart with altered hemodynamics, or to an underlying metabolic disorder. It may interfere with myocardial contractility or impede oxygenation of subendocardial myocytes.

Primary cardiac tumors include fibromas and rhabdomyomas, the latter forming part of the spectrum of tuberous sclerosis, a condition characterized by mental retardation, fitting and tumors elsewhere. Although rhabdomyomas may be completely clinically occult, their diagnosis at autopsy is important as tuberous sclerosis is heritable.[33,80]

Congenital or acquired vascular disease may also be an unexpected finding at autopsy that has been responsible for death.[81–83] Abnormally situated coronary arteries may not be perfused adequately, or may be associated with narrowed ostia or reduced caliber. The result of these anomalies may be significant myocardial ischaemia with fatal dysrhythmias.[83–85]

Kawasaki disease, or mucocutaneous lymph node syndrome, is a disease characterized by fever, skin rash, enlarged lymph nodes and coronary artery vasculitis. Unfortunately in infancy the clinical manifestations may be relatively minor and so the diagnosis may not have been made during life. Sudden death may occur from aneurysm rupture or thrombosis, with acute and chronic ischemic damage to the heart. In addition, lethal myocarditis may develop.[86,87]

Other causes of unexpected death due to vascular anomalies and pathology in early life include pulmonary hypertension, pulmonary thromboembolism and total anomalous pulmonary venous drainage, where blood from the lungs drains to the right rather than the left side of the heart.[88–91]

INFECTIOUS DISEASE

One of the most significant historical causes of sudden death in infancy is infection, and this is also still one of the major causes of infant mortality globally. Diseases such as gastroenteritis and malaria continue to account for large numbers of infant and early childhood deaths annually. Death may be due to a side effect of the infection as in fatal dehydration from gastroenteritis, or may occur from septic shock. Fulminant cases of meningitis and septicemia may cause unexpected death, and infants are periodically seen with well established pneumonias and unremarkable histories.

On occasion the location of the infection may be of more significance, with cases of acute upper airway obstruction resulting from *Haemophilis influenzae* acute epiglottitis, and sudden cardiac death occurring from coxsackie B4 viral infection[92] of heart conduction tracts.

RESPIRATORY CONDITIONS

Upper airway obstruction is a rare, but significant cause of unexpected death in infancy cause by inhaled foreign material, or less commonly by an intrinsic lesion of the upper aerodigestive tract. Such intrinsic lesions and conditions include lingual thyroglossal duct cysts, micrognathia, nasopharyngeal tumors and upper airway infections.[93–96] Asthma may be a cause of sudden death in older children.[97]

HEMATOPOEITIC CONDITIONS

Hematologic conditions may result in sudden death in infancy from spontaneous hemorrhage, thrombotic vascular obstruction or sepsis. For example, acquired or congenital conditions such as hemolytic–uremic syndrome, scurvy or hemophilia, may cause sudden death, either due to bleeding within a critical area such as the cranium, or around the upper airway, or to exsanguination.[1,98] Sudden death may also occur in infants and young children who suffer from one of the hemoglobinopathies such as sickle cell disease from sequestration of blood within the spleen.[87]

CENTRAL NERVOUS SYSTEM CONDITIONS

Infants with cerebral malformations and epilepsy are at increased risk of sudden death, often for ill-understood reasons. It is, however, likely that infants with epilepsy may be prone to lethal cardiac dysrhythmias associated with an epileptic discharge. Infants with occult cerebral tumors and vascular malformations are also at risk of premature death.[99] Malformations of posterior fossa structures, such as the cerebellum in Arnold–Chiari syndrome, may predispose to unexpected death associated with pressure on sensitive brainstem structures. Developmentally retarded infants are also at increased risk of gastric aspiration.

GASTROINTESTINAL AND GENITOURINARY CONDITIONS

Although infants may die from a variety of gastrointestinal problems, infectious gastroenteritis would be by far the most common lethal condition found at autopsy. Despite obvious dehydration in some cases, parents may have mistaken extremely watery feces for urine, and thus assumed that hydration was adequate. Rarer gastrointestinal causes of sudden infant and early childhood death include volvulus, intussusception and late presenting congenital diaphragmatic hernia.[100] The antemortem diagnosis of certain of these conditions may be difficult; for example, asymptomatic intussusceptions have been reported in up to 20% of pediatric cases.[101] Genitourinary causes of sudden infant death are very rare and have mostly involved Wilms' tumor embolism or intratumoral hemorrhage.[102]

MISCELLANEOUS CONDITIONS

Rarely endocrine, metabolic, or connective tissue disorders may cause sudden infant death, including Marfan and Ehlers–Danlos syndromes.[87,103] Given the heritable nature of a number of these conditions, genetic counseling and investigation of the family of the deceased infant is required.

Conclusion

Determination of the cause of death in infancy may be difficult as the preceding symptoms and signs may be subtle and the autopsy findings non-specific. In addition the range of rare conditions which may cause unexpected infant death is beyond that normally encountered in adult autopsy practice. For this reason standard autopsy protocols (*see* Appendix I) are useful in providing a template for the autopsy, as well as guidelines for the types of examinations that need to be carried out.[104,105] Despite liaison with pediatricians, extensive laboratory testing, and complete autopsy examinations, however, it must be recognized that the cause of death in a certain proportion of infant deaths is destined to remain 'undetermined'.

References

1. Byard RW, Cohle SD. *Sudden Death in Infancy, Childhood and Adolescence*. Cambridge University Press, Cambridge, 1994.
2. Byard RW. Sudden infant death syndrome: historical background, possible mechanisms and diagnostic problems. *J Law Med* 1994;2:18–26.
3. Byard RW. Sudden infant death syndrome – a 'diagnosis' in search of a disease. *J Clin Forens Med* 1995;2:121–8.
4. Emery JL. Is sudden infant death syndrome a diagnosis? Or is it just a diagnostic dustbin? *Br Med J* 1989;299:1240.
5. Byard RW, Carmichael EM, Beal SM. How useful is postmortem examination in sudden infant death syndrome? *Pediatr Pathol* 1994;14:817–22.
6. Fleming PJ, Berry PJ, Gilbert R *et al*. Categories of preventable unexpected infant deaths. *Arch Dis Child* (letter) 1991;66:171–2.
7. Gilbert-Barness E, Barness LA. Cause of death: SIDS or something else? *Contemp Pediatr* 1992;9:13–29.
8. Mitchell E, Krous HF, Donald T, Byard RW. Changing trends in the diagnosis of sudden infant death. *Am J Forens Med Pathol* 2000;21:311–14.
9. Byard RW. Accidental death and the role of the pathologist. *Perspect Pediatr Pathol* 2000;3:405–18.
10. Corey TS, McLoud LC, Nichols GR, Buchino JJ. Infant deaths due to unintentional injury. An 11 year autopsy review. *Am J Dis Child* 1992;146;968–71.
11. Byard RW. Preventative pathology. *Inj Prevent* 1999;5:292–3.
12. Jumbelic MI, Chambliss M. Accidental toddler drowning in 5 gallon buckets. *JAMA* 1990;263:1952–3.
13. Byard RW, Lipset J. Drowning deaths in toddlers and pre-ambulatory children in South Australia. *Am J Forensic Med Pathol* 1999;20:328–32.
14. Smith NM, Byard RW, Bourne AJ. Death during immersion in water in childhood. *Am J Forens Med Pathol* 1991;12:219–21.
15. Byard RW, Lipset J, Gilbert J. Fire deaths in children in South Australia from 1989 to 1998. *J Paediatr Child Health* 2000;36:176–8.
16. Byard RW, Green H, James RA, Gilbert JD. Pathological features of childhood pedestrian fatalities. *Am J Forensic Med Pathol* 2000;21:101–6.
17. Byard RW, Beal SM, Bourne AJ. Potentially dangerous infant sleeping environments. *Arch Dis Child* 1994;71:497–500.
18. Amanuel B, Byard RW. Accidental asphyxia in severely disabled children. *J Paediatr Child Health* 2000;36;66–8.
19. Byard RW. Hazardous infant and early childhood sleeping environments and death scene examination. *J Clin Forensic Med* 1996;3:115–22.
20. Beal SM, Byard RW. Sudden infant death syndrome in South Australia 1968–1997. Part 3: Is bed sharing safer in infants? *J Paediatr Child Health* 2000;36:552–4.
21. Byard RW, Beal SM. 'V' shaped pillows and unsafe infant sleeping. *J Paediatr Child Health* 1997;33:171–3.
22. Byard RW, Bourne AJ, Beal SM. Mesh-sided cots: yet another potentially dangerous infant sleeping environment. *Forensic Sci Int* 1996;83:105–9.
23. Moore L, Bourne AJ, Beal S, Collett M, Byard RW. Unexpected infant death in association with suspended rocking cradles. *Am J Forensic Med Pathol* 1995;16:177–80.

24. Byard RW, Beal SM, Simpson A, Carter RF, Khong TY. Accidental infant deaths and stroller prams. *Med J Aust* 1996;165:140–1.

25. Byard RW. Is cosleeping in infancy a desirable or dangerous practice? *J Paediatr Child Health* 1994;30:198–9.

26. Byard RW, Stewart WA, Beal SM. Pathological findings in SIDS infants who have died in the supine position compared to the prone. *J SIDS Infant Mort* 1996;1:43–8.

27. Byard RW, Hilton J. Overlaying, accidental suffocation and sudden infant death. *J SIDS Infant Mort* 1997;2:161–5.

28. Byard RW. Is breast feeding in bed always a safe practice? *J Paediatr Child Health* 1998;34:418–19.

29. Scragg R, Mitchell EA, Taylor BJ *et al.* Bedsharing, smoking, and alcohol in the sudden infant death syndrome. *Br Med J* 1993;307:1312–18.

30. Byard RW, Burnell RH. Apparent life threatening events and infant holding practices. *Arch Dis Child* 1995;73:502–4.

31. Byard RW, Gallard V, Johnson A *et al.* Safe feeding practices for infants and young childen. *J Paediatr Child Health* 1996;32:327–9.

32. Byard RW. Unexpected death due to acute airway obstruction in child care centers. *Pediatrics* 1994;94:113–14.

33. Byard RW. Significant coincidental findings at autopsy in accidental childhood death. *Med Sci Law* 1997;37:259–62.

34. Byard RW, Moore L, Bourne AJ. Sudden and unexpected death – a late effect of occult intraesophageal foreign body. *Pediatr Pathol* 1990;10:837–41.

35. Byard RW. Mechanisms of unexpected death in infants and young children following foreign body ingestion. *J Forensic Sci* 1996;41:438–41.

36. Byard RW, Bourne AJ, Moore L, Little KET. Sudden death in infancy due to delayed cardiac tamponade complicating central venous line insertion and cardiac catheterisation. *Arch Pathol Lab Med* 1992;116:654–6.

37. Reay DT, Eisele JW, Ward R, Horton W, Bonnell HJ. Investigation of anesthetic deaths. *J Forensic Sci* 1985;30:822–7.

38. Byard RW, Bourne AJ, James RA. Childhood deaths and cargo barriers in cars. *J Paediatr Child Health* 1999;35:409–10.

39. Whitehead F, Couper RTL, Moore L, Bourne AJ, Byard RW. Dehydration deaths in infants and children. *Am J Forensic Med Pathol* 1996;17:73–8.

40. Byard RW, Donald T, Chivell W. Non-lethal and subtle inflicted injury and unexpected infant death. *J Law Med* 1999;7:47–52.

41. Willging JP, Bower CM, Cotton RT. Physical abuse of children. A retrospective review and otolaryngology perspective. *Arch Otolaryngol Head Neck Surg* 1992;118:584–90.

42. Sato Y, Yuh WTC, Smith WL *et al.* Head injury in child abuse: evaluation with MR imaging. *Radiology* 1989;173:653–7.

43. Levene S, Bonfield G. Accidents on hospital wards. *Arch Dis Child* 1991;66:1047–9.

44. Barlow B, Niemirska M, Gandhi RP, Leblanc W. Ten years of experience with falls from a height in children. *J Pediatr Surg* 1983;18:509–11.

45. Spaide RF, Swengel RM, Scharre DW, Mein CE. Shaken baby syndrome. *Am Fam Pract* 1990;41:1145–52.

46. Ludwig S, Warman M. Shaken baby syndrome: a review of 20 cases. *Ann Emerg Med* 1984;13:104–7.

47. Wilkinson WS, Han DP, Rappley MD, Owings CL. Retinal hemorrhage predicts neurologic injury in shaken baby syndrome. *Arch Opthalmol* 1989;107:1472–4.
48. Duhaime A-C, Alario AJ, Lewander WJ *et al.* Head injury in very young children: mechanisms, injury types, and ophthalmological findings in 100 hospitalised patients younger than 2 years of age. *Pediatrics* 1992;90:179–85.
49. Caffey J. The whiplash shaken infant syndrome: manual shaking by the extremities with whiplash-induced intracranial and intraocular bleedings, linked with residual permanent brain damage and mental retardation. *Pediatrics* 1974;54:396–403.
50. Duhaime A-C, Gennarelli TA, Thibault LE, Bruce DA, Margulies SS, Wiser R. The shaken baby syndrome. *J Neurosurg* 1987;66:409–15.
51. Bruce PA, Zimmerman RA. Shaken impact syndrome. *Pediatr Ann* 1989;18:482–94.
52. Krous HK, Byard RW. Shaken infant syndrome: selected controversies. *Pediatr Develop Pathol* 1999;2:497–8.
53. Byard RW, Krous HF. Suffocation, shaking and SIDS – can we tell the difference? *J Paediatr Child Health* 1999;35:432–3.
54. Roberton DM, Barbor P, Hull D. Unusual injury? Recent injury in normal children with supected non-accidental injury. *Br Med J* 1982;285:1399–1401.
55. Purdue GF, Hunt JL, Prescott PR. Child abuse by burning – an index for suspicion. *J Trauma* 1988;28:221–4.
56. Rossignol AM, Locke JA, Burke JF. Paediatric burns in New England, USA. *Burns* 1990;16:41–8.
57. Ryan CA, Shankowsky HA, Tredget EE. Profile of the paediatric burn patient in a Canadian burn centre. *Burns* 1992;18:267–72.
58. Byard RW, Beal SM. Munchausen syndrome by proxy: repetitive infantile apnoea and homicide. *J Paediatr Child Health* 1993;29:77–9.
59. Byard RW, Burnell RH. Covert video surveillance in Munchausen syndrome by proxy – ethical compromise or essential technique? *Med J Aust* 1994;160:352–6.
60. Rosenberg DA. Web of deceit: a literature review of Munchausen syndrome by proxy. *Child Abuse Negl* 1987;11:547–63.
61. Beal SM, Byard RW. Accidental death and sudden infant death syndrome. *J Paediatr Child Health* 1995;31:269–71.
62. Southall DP, Plunkett MCB, Banks MW, Falkov AF, Samuels MP. Covert video recordings of life-threatening child abuse: lessons for child protection. *Pediatrics* 1997;100:735–60.
63. Pinholster G. SIDS paper triggers a murder charge. *Science* 1994;264:197–8.
64. Steinschneider A. Prolonged apnea and the sudden infant death syndrome: clinical and laboratory observations. *Pediatrics* 1972;50:646–54.
65. Samuels MP, McClaughlin W, Jacobson RR, Poets CF, Southall DP. Fourteen cases of imposed upper airway obstruction. *Arch Dis Child* 1992;67:162–70.
66. Spevak MR, Kleinman PK, Belanger PL, Primack C, Richmond JM. Cardio-pulmonary resuscitation and rib fractures in infants. A postmortem radiologic-pathologic study. *JAMA* 1994;272:617–18.
67. Baum JD, Bulpitt CJ. Retinal and conjunctival haemorrhage in the newborn. *Arch Dis Child* 1970;45:344–9.
68. Wissow LS. Child abuse and neglect. *N Engl J Med* 1995;332:1425–31.
69. Gilliland MG, Luckenbach MW. Are retinal hemorrhages found after resuscitation attempts? A study of the eyes of 169 children. *Am J Forensic Med Pathol* 1993;14:187–92.

70. Gilliland MG, Luckenbach MW, Chenier TC. Systemic and ocular findings in 169 prospectively studied child deaths: retinal hemorrhages usually mean child abuse. *Forensic Sci Int* 1994;68:117–32.

71. Kantor R. Retinal hemorrhage after cardiopulmonary resuscitation or child abuse? *J Pediatr* 1986;108:430–2.

72. Sandramouli S, Robinson R, Tsaloumas M, Willshaw HE. Retinal haemorrhages and convulsions. *Arch Dis Child* 1997;76:449–51.

73. Weedn VW, Mansour AM, Nichols MM. Retinal hemorrhage in an infant after cardiopulmonary resuscitation. *Am J Forensic Med Pathol* 1990;11:79–82.

74. Fackler J, Berkowitz I, Green W. Retinal hemorrhages in newborn piglets following cardiopulmonary resuscitation. *Am J Dis Child* 1992;146:1294–6.

75. Krous HF. The differential diagnosis of sudden unexpected infant death. In: Rognum TO (ed.) *Sudden Infant Death Syndrome. New Trends for the Nineties.* University of Scandinavia Press, Oslo, 1995, pp. 74–80.

76. Handy TC, Buchino JJ. Sudden natural death in infants and young children. *Clin Lab Med* 1998;18:323–8.

77. Byard RW, Bourne AJ, Adams PS. Subarterial ventricular septal defect in an infant with sudden unexpected death: cause or coincidence? *Am J Cardiovasc Pathol* 1990;3:333–6.

78. Byard RW. Ventricular septal defect and sudden childhood death. *J Paediatr Child Health* 1994;30:439–40.

79. Stahl J, Couper RTL, Byard RW. Oncocytic cardiomyopathy – a rare cause of unexpected childhood death associated with fitting. *Med Sci Law* 1997;37:84–7.

80. Byard RW, Smith NM, Bourne AJ. Incidental cardiac rhabdomyomas: a significant finding necessitating additional investigation at the time of autopsy. *J Forensic Sci* 1991;36:1229–33.

81. Byard RW. Vascular causes of sudden death in infancy, childhood and adolescence. *Cardiovasc Pathol* 1996;5:243–57.

82. Byard RW. Sudden infant death due to idiopathic arterial calcinosis. *Pediatr Pathol Lab Med* 1996;16:987–96.

83. Lipset J, Byard RW, Carpenter BF, Jimenez CL, Bourne AJ. Anomalous coronary arteries arising from the aorta associated with sudden death in infancy and early childhood – an autopsy series. *Arch Pathol Lab Med* 1991;115:770–3.

84. Moore L, Byard RW. Sudden and unexpected death in infancy associated with a single coronary artery. *Pediatr Pathol* 1992;12:231–6.

85. Lipset J, Cohle SD, Russell G, Berry PJ, Byard RW. Anomalous coronary arteries – a multicentre pediatric autopsy study. *Pediatr Pathol* 1994;14:287–300.

86. Byard RW, Jimenez CL, Carpenter BF, Cutz E, Smith CR. Four unusual cases of sudden and unexpected cardiovascular death in infancy and childhood. *Med Sci Law* 1991;31:157–61.

87. Byard RW, Edmonds JF, Silverman E, Silver MM. Respiratory distress and fever in a 2-month-old infant (Clinical Conference). *J Pediatr* 1991;18:306–13.

88. Byard RW, Moore, L. Total anomalous pulmonary venous drainage and sudden unexpected death in infancy. *Forensic Sci Int* 1991;51:197–202.

89. James CL, Keeling JW, Smith NM, Byard RW. Total anomalous pulmonary venous drainage associated with fatal outcome in infancy and early childhood: an autopsy study of 52 cases. *Pediatr Pathol* 1994;14:665–78.

90. Byard RW, Cutz E. Sudden and unexpected death in infancy and childhood due to pulmonary thromboembolism – an autopsy study. *Arch Pathol Lab Med* 1990;114:142–4.
91. Champ C, Byard RW. Pulmonary embolism in infancy. *J Paediatr Child Health* 1994;30:550–1.
92. Smith NM, Bourne AJ, Clapton WC, Byard RW. The spectrum of presentation at autopsy of myocarditis in infancy and childhood. *Pathology* 1992;24:129–31.
93. Byard RW, Bourne AJ, Silver MM. The association of lingual thyroglossal duct remnants with sudden death in infancy. *Int J Pediatr Otolaryngol* 1990;20:107–12.
94. Byard RW, Moore L. Mechanisms of sudden death in patients with congenital teratoma. *Pediatr Surg Int* 1992;7:464–7.
95. Byard RW, Silver MM. Sudden infant death and posterior lingual inflammation. *Oral Surg Oral Med Oral Pathol* 1994;28:77–82.
96. Byard RW, Kennedy JD. Diagnostic difficulties in cases of sudden death in infants with mandibular hypoplasia. *Am J Forensic Med Pathol* 1996;17:255–9.
97. Champ C, Byard RW. Sudden death in asthma in childhood. *Forensic Sci Int* 1994;66:117–27.
98. Manton NM, Smith NM, Byard RW. Unexpected childhood deaths due to hemolytic uremic syndrome. *Am J Forensic Med Pathol* 2000;21:90–2.
99. Byard RW, Bourne AJ, Hanieh A. Sudden and unexpected death due to hemorrhage from occult central nervous system lesions: a pediatric autopsy study. *Pediatr Neurosurg* 1991–92;17:88–94.
100. Byard RW. Sudden infant death, large intestinal volvulus and a duplication cyst of the terminal ileum. *Am J Forensic Med Pathol* 2000;21:176–8.
101. Byard RW, Simpson A. Sudden death and intussusception in infancy and childhood – autopsy considerations. *Med Sci Law* (in press).
102. Byard RW, Bohn DJ, Wilson G, Smith CR, Ein S. Unsuspected diaphragmatic hernia – a potential cause of sudden and unexpected death in infancy and early childhood. *J Pediatr Surg* 1990;11:1166–8.
103. Byard RW, Keeley FW, Smith CR. Type IV Ehlers–Danlos syndrome presenting as sudden infant death. *Am J Clin Pathol* 1990;93:579–82.
104. Krous HF. The international standardized autopsy protocol for sudden unexpected infant death. In: Rognum TO (ed.) *Sudden Infant Death Syndrome. New Trends for the Nineties.* University of Scandinavia Press, Oslo, 1995, pp. 81–95.
105. Mitchell E, Krous HF, Donald T, Byard RW. An analysis of the usefulness of specific stages in the investigation of sudden infant death. *Am J Forensic Med Pathol* 2000;21:395–400.

CHAPTER 13

Specific pathologic problems and possible solutions

ROGER W. BYARD AND HENRY F. KROUS

Introduction   228
Autopsy examination   229
Death-scene examination   229
Significance of 'minor' pathologic findings   230
Diagnostic conflicts   231
'Guilty until proven innocent'   232
Preventative pathology   233
References   233

Introduction

As mentioned in the previous chapter, a wide range of diseases and disorders may present identically to SIDS. Given that the diagnosis of SIDS is one of exclusion,[1,2] it is imperative that pathologists approach 'SIDS' autopsies with open minds. Death can only be attributed to SIDS once a proper investigation, including review of the clinical and family histories, examination of the death scene and performance of an autopsy has been undertaken, ideally by a pathologist with pediatric/forensic experience. A number of problems still exist, however; autopsies are not always undertaken, or are performed by doctors with no training in pathology, death scenes are not examined, and the interpretation of findings by pathologists may be contradictory.

Autopsy examination

It is recognized that cases of unexpected infant death are continually being designated as 'SIDS' in many countries where autopsies are not routinely being performed. For example, autopsy rates in infants in the past have been quoted at only 25% in Belgium, and 50 to 60% in the Netherlands.[3,4] Given that both accepted definitions of SIDS[1,2] specify that an autopsy must be performed before the diagnosis can be made, these data are disturbing. The extent of the problem of designating infant deaths as SIDS without an autopsy is, however, not known. In addition, not only are there many organic diseases that will be incorrectly diagnosed in the absence of an autopsy,[5] but many subtle injuries may also not be identified.

In the absence of mandatory autopsies the significance of research performed on cohorts of infants who were deemed to have died as a result of 'SIDS', and their families, is uncertain. This is particularly so now that the rate of SIDS has fallen, with a corresponding relative increase in the rates of other disorders.[6]

When an autopsy is performed, however, there must also be an appropriate interpretation of findings. For example, sudden death has been incorrectly attributed to such diverse and minor findings as a patent foramen ovale, a small secundum atrial septal defect, the normal narrowing of the aortic arch, and miniscule ventricular septal defects in the absence of cardiac hypertrophy. Clear understanding of normal tissue and organ growth and development is critical for a proper assessment of their possible pathophysiologic significance.

In certain parts of Australia, infant autopsies may be performed by general practitioners, with review of histologic slides being subsequently undertaken by forensic pathologists in the nearest major center. Unfortunately examination of microscopic slides in isolation, with no control over sampling sites, is a far from adequate situation.[7] In addition, complex but subtle malformations, such as cardiovascular abnormalities, will never be identified by a method such as this. There is really no substitute for a properly performed complete autopsy by a pathologist trained in the subspeciality. Increasingly there has been recognition of the need for a standardized approach to the autopsy in cases of unexpected infant death, and an International Autopsy Protocol has been formulated to provide a gold standard in this area (*see* Appendix I).[8] Each step of the proposed diagnostic pathway may yield significant information.[9] Guidelines have been proposed for the investigation of infant deaths where an autopsy is not possible,[10] however, it should be emphasized that these recommendations must be regarded as a last resort, and not a reasonable alternative to a properly conducted postmortem examination.[11]

Death-scene examination

The National Institute of Child Health and Human Development (NICHD) incorporated the need for a death-scene examination into its 1991 definition of SIDS.[2] The authors consider this to have been an extremely valuable contribution, although not all pathologists would consider that death-scene review in cases of unexpected infant death is useful. Concerns that the scene has been disturbed by the parents or child care providers, that the infant's body has been moved, and that the scene has been further violated by neighbours and ambulance personnel are all valid; however, examination of the scene by trained individuals can still be extremely informative.[5] The type of training required to undertake this examination is yet to be determined.

The infant's sleeping situation can be evaluated at death-scene examination, with assessment as to the likelihood of accidental asphyxia. Given that the autopsy findings in cases of asphyxia may be indistinguishable from those typically found in SIDS,[12] examination of the infant's cot or sleeping situation, with postmortem reconstruction of the infant's position, using a doll or the infant, may be the only way to accurately determine the cause and manner of death. The other advantage of inspecting the death scene, and/or cot and contents, is in helping to evaluate the possible contribution of furniture and toys to traumatic lesions that may be subsequently discovered at autopsy.

Significance of 'minor' pathologic findings

PETECHIAL HEMORRHAGES

Intrathoracic petechiae are well recognized in cases of SIDS and occur in from 68 to 95% of cases.[13] While the etiology has been debated, petechiae may be caused by the mechanisms that led to the terminal episode. By way of contrast, petechial hemorrhages on the conjunctiva and face are unusual in infants, and are generally only seen in cases of hanging or crush asphyxia.[14] Although they have been described very rarely in cases where the death was attributed to SIDS,[15] this has not been a general experience; for example, it has been stated that petechiae 'are never present on the conjunctiva, eyelids or on or in other soft tissues of the head or neck in SIDS'.[16]

Infants who have died in the prone position do not have facial or conjunctival petechiae.[17] This is most likely due to to the face being at approximately the same level as the body, and not in a dependent position, with no regional venous engorgement. Petechiae of the face have been described in older age groups following successful or failed resuscitation,[18] but again do not occur in infants. If facial or conjunctival petechiae are noted, the history should be carefully checked for forceful coughing or vomiting. Pertussis may result in petechiae of the face and conjunctiva,[19] which may also occur as part of a more generalized petechial rash associated with sepsis. In dark-skinned children the only observable external manifestation of generalized petechiae associated with sepsis may be conjunctival lesions.

External petechiae in cases of sudden and unexpected infant death are of greater importance than similar lesions in adults and must be regarded as a significant finding that requires explanation.[20] If no other plausible explanation can be elucidated, mechanical asphyxia, whether induced or accidental, must be seriously considered. Facial, neck, upper chest and conjunctival petechiae should not, therefore, be included among the range of pathologic lesions usually seen in SIDS infants. Cases where such lesions are found require extremely careful investigation, with close collaboration among the various agencies involved in the assessment of unexpected infant deaths.

MINOR INFLAMMATORY INFILTRATES

Although minor aggregates of chronic inflammatory cells are often found on microscopic examination of tissues from infants who have died unexpectedly, their significance remains uncertain. It has been proposed, however, that such inflammation has contributed to the majority of SIDS deaths, with a significant percentage of deaths being caused by occult myocarditis and meningitis.[21,22]

Unfortunately similar infiltrates are routinely found in infants who have died from trauma, and a plausible mechanism by which these relatively inconspicuous infiltrates could cause death has not been proven. Although it is possible that cytokines produced by these cells, in association with other factors, may increase the risk of an infant succumbing to those mechanisms that cause SIDS,[23] this remains conjectural. Until evidence can be produced demonstrating a significantly increased risk of death in association with these infiltrates, or a definite pathophysiologic link can be shown between minor cellular infiltrates and death, minor inflammatory aggregates should not be used to explain deaths that would be otherwise designated as SIDS.

Diagnostic conflicts

Marked differences in the interpretation of microscopic lesions identified at autopsy by pathologists from different countries have been noted at recent SIDS International meetings.[24] This has been particularly so in the evaluation of inflammatory infiltrates, as detailed above. The importance of consensus in this area cannot be overemphasized, as international comparisons of death rates, epidemiologic characteristics, other data and research results will be meaningless if significant diagnostic differences exist.

As in all areas of science, a new theory cannot be accepted until convincing data with appropriate controls have been produced. Corroboration from other centers is then required before the theory can be regarded as proven. Unfortunately exposing researchers in other fields and lay groups to unverified hypotheses only serves to confuse issues. Parents are also very vulnerable to new hypotheses that may offer a possible explanation for their infant's death, and so researchers should do their utmost to protect them from such material until confirmation has been achieved. The onus is, therefore, on the originators of new ideas and hypotheses to organize appropriate collaborative studies. If the results are shown to be correct by peer review and corroboration, the findings should certainly be accepted as significant, and used to help further understand the pathophysiology and etiology of SIDS.

'Guilty until proven innocent'

The occurrence of several separate incidences over the past two decades of mothers suffocating their infants, with the deaths being attributed to SIDS, has drawn attention to the fallibility of doctors in cases of Munchausen syndrome, or factitious illness, by proxy.[25,26] As detailed in Chapter 12, distinguishing between an infant who has been deliberately asphyxiated, and one who has died of SIDS may be impossible on purely pathologic grounds. Pathologists are only too aware of this significant weakness in the 'gold standard' of their diagnostic evaluation of unexpected infant death.[27]

The problem of potential misdiagnosis of inflicted suffocation has resulted in the statement that one death in a family may be accepted as SIDS, but not so with subsequent cases. If further deaths occur in the same family it is proposed that the cause should be designated as 'undetermined' for the second, and 'homicide' (until proven otherwise) for the third.[28]

Approaching a case of unexpected infant death with preconceived ideas about the cause of death may, however, result in significant errors. Deciding that a case is a likely SIDS death, or a homicide, before the autopsy, may result in important 'non-routine' investigations not being undertaken at the time. For example, more meticulous soft tissue dissection and bone sampling is required in a case with suspicious features. A metabolic assessment to diagnose or exclude inherited biochemical deficiencies requires different special tissue and fluid sampling, handling and storage, that can only be done if hospital samples are seized before they are routinely discarded, or at the time of the autopsy.

It must be remembered that more than one SIDS death may occur in the same family, and that inherited metabolic diseases may also result in serial deaths. Thus, although inflicted injury must be seriously considered in cases of unexpected infant death, this should not be to the detriment of proper pathologic investigation.

If a history of previous apparent life-threatening events (ALTEs) is obtained, a similar approach should be maintained, with serious consideration given to the possibility of each of the following: organic illness, SIDS or intentional suffocation.[29] Although it has been suggested recently (anecdotally) that previous ALTEs preclude a diagnosis of SIDS, this is an extreme position, as a minority of infants who die of SIDS may have had previous significant apneic episodes.[30] It is important that neither SIDS nor homicide are automatically assumed to be the cause of death because of the ALTEs, before proper investigation of other possibilities is undertaken.

Since the NICHD definition proposed that the term 'SIDS' could not be used for deaths of children over one year of age,[2] there has also been a trend to assume that deaths after the first year of age must also be regarded as suspicious. Again, while unexpected deaths at this age are much less common than deaths in the first 6 months, they do rarely occur. The most appropriate approach is to consider these cases as atypical, and to carefully look for other causes of death, whether organic, accidental or inflicted. It must be recognized, however, that all biological processes are continuums, often with no sharp demarcations, and that cutoff points tend to be arbitrary. For example, it is difficult to support the contention that a 'SIDS' death of an infant at 11½ months is due to entirely different pathophysiologic processes to an 'unexpected early childhood death' at 12½ months.

Preventative pathology

With the fall in SIDS numbers and the more careful evaluation of the circumstances of cases, the pathologist may find his role changing, with more involvement in infant safety issues.[31,32] This is particularly the case when death-scene examination and postmortem reconstructions have identified unsafe cots and sleeping environments as causes of, or significant contributing factors to, infant deaths.[33]

If the pathologist does not attend the death scene in South Australia cots are brought routinely to the Forensic Science Centre mortuary for evaluation prior to the autopsy. In addition, police officers and a worker from the local SIDS Association carefully assess the circumstances of the death and interview the parents before the autopsy.

Using this approach, several unsafe cot designs have been identified over the past few years which have either been subsequently modified or withdrawn from sale by manufacturers.[33] The setting up of a special interest group which produced safety pamphlets for parents and cot sellers, with lobbying of local and federal politicians, has led to improved safety standards for cots, and the introduction of new state and federal legislation.[31] Thus a pathologist's role can go well beyond purely forensic diagnostic matters in cases of unexpected infant deaths with the potential existing for major contributions being made to community health and infant safety issues.

References

1. Beckwith JB. The sudden infant death syndrome. *Curr Probl Pediatr* 1973;3:1–37.
2. Willinger M, James LS, Catz C. Defining the sudden infant death syndrome (SIDS): deliberations of an expert panel convened by the National Institute of Child Health and Human Development. *Pediatr Pathol* 1991;11:677–84.
3. Engleberts AC, de Jonge GA, Kostense PJ. An analysis of trends in the incidence of sudden infant death in The Netherlands 1969–89. *J Paediatr Child Health* 1991;27:329–33.
4. Kahn A, Wachholder A, Winkler M, Rebuffat E. Prospective study on the prevalence of sudden infant death and possible risk factors in Brussels: preliminary results (1987–1988). *Eur J Pediatr* 1990;149:284–6.
5. Byard RW, Cohle SD. *Sudden Death in Infancy, Childhood and Adolescence.* Cambridge University Press, Cambridge, 1994.
6. Mitchell E, Krous HF, Donald T, Byard RW. Changing trends in the diagnosis of sudden infant death. *Am J Forensic Med Pathol* 2000;21:311–14.

7. Byard RW, Krous HF. Suffocation, shaking and SIDS – can we tell the difference? *J Paediatr Child Health* 1999;35:432–3.
8. Krous HF. An international standardized autopsy protocol for sudden unexpected infant death. In: Rognum T (ed.) *Sudden Infant Death Syndrome. New Trends in the Nineties*. Oslo: Scandinavian University Press, Oslo, 1995, pp. 81–95.
9. Mitchell E, Krous HF, Donald T, Byard RW. An analyis of the usefulness of specific stages in the pathological investigation of sudden infant death. *Am J Forensic Med Pathol* 2000;21:395–400.
10. Bang AT, Bang RA. SEARCH team. Diagnosis of causes of childhood deaths in developing countries by verbal autopsy: suggested criteria. *Bull WHO Org* 1992;70:499–507.
11. Anker M. The effect of misclassification error on reported cause-specific mortality fractions from verbal autopsy. *Int J Epidemiol* 1997;26:1090–6.
12. Mitchell E, Krous HF, Byard RW. Pathological findings in overlaying. *J Clin Forensic Med* (in press).
13. Beckwith JB. The mechanism of death in sudden infant death syndrome. In: Culbertson JL, Krous HF, Bendell RD (eds). *Sudden Infant Death Syndrome: Medical Aspects and Psychological Management*. Edward Arnold, London, 1989, pp. 48–61.
14. Moore L, Byard RW. Pathological findings in hanging and wedging deaths in infants and young children. *Am J Forensic Med Pathol* 1993;14:296–302.
15. Kleeman WJ, Wiechern V, Schuck M, Troger HD. Intrathoracic and subconjunctival petechiae in sudden infant death syndrome (SIDS). *Forensic Sci Int* 1995;72:49–52.
16. Hilton JMN. The pathology of the sudden infant death syndrome. In: Mason JK (ed.) *Paediatric Forensic Medicine and Pathology*. Chapman & Hall Medical, London, 1989, pp. 156–64.
17. Byard RW, Stewart WA, Beal SM. Pathological findings in SIDS infants who have died in the supine position compared to the prone. *J SIDS Infant Mort* 1996;1:43–8.
18. Hood I, Ryan D, Spitz WU. Resuscitation and petechiae. *Am J Forensic Med Pathol* 1988;9:35–7.
19. Feigin RD. Pertussis. In: Vaughan VC, McKay RJ, Behrman RE (eds). *Nelson Textbook of Pediatrics*. WB Saunders, Philadelphia, 1979, pp. 766–9.
20. Byard RW, Krous HF. Petechial hemorrhages and unexpected infant deaths. *Legal Med* (in press).
21. Byard RW, Krous HF. Minor inflammatory lesions and sudden infant death – cause, coincidence or epiphenomena? *Pediatr Pathol* 1995;15:649–54.
22. Rambaud C, Cieuta C, Canioni D *et al*. Cot death and myocarditis. *Cardiol Young* 1992;2:266–71.
23. Blackwell CC, Weir DM, Busuttil A. Infectious agents and SIDS: analysis of risk factors and preventative measures. *J SIDS Infant Mort* 1997;2:61–76.
24. Krous HF, Byard R. Report from the Pathology Working Group. *J SIDS Infant Mort* 1997;2:205–9.
25. Byard RW, Beal SM. Munchausen syndrome by proxy: repetitive infantile apnoea and homicide. *J Paediatr Child Health* 1993;29:77–9.
26. Byard RW, Burnell RH, Covert video surveillance in Munchausen syndrome by proxy – ethical compromise or essential technique? *Med J Aust* 1994;160:352–6.
27. Byard RW, Donald T, Chivell W. Non-lethal and subtle inflicted injury and unexpected infant death. *J Law Med* 1999;7:47–52.

28. DiMaio DJ, DiMaio VJM. *Forensic Pathology*. Elsevier, New York, 1989, 291 pp.

29. Southall DP, Plunkett MCB, Banks MW, Falkov AF, Samuels MP. Covert video recordings of life-threatening child abuse: lessons for child protection. *Pediatrics* 1997;100:735–60.

30. Little GA, Ballard RA, Brooks JG *et al.* Concensus statement. National Institutes of Health concensus development conference on infantile apnea and home monitoring. Sept 29 to Oct 1, 1986. *Pediatrics* 1987;79:292–9

31. Byard RW. Preventative pathology. *Inj Prev* 1999;5:292–3.

32. Byard RW. Accidental death and the role of the pathologist. *Perspect Pediatr Pathol* 2000;3:405–18.

33. Byard RW. Hazardous infant and early childhood sleeping environments and death scene examination. *J Clin Forensic Med* 1996;3:115–22.

CHAPTER 14

The rise and fall of several theories

SUSAN M. BEAL

Introduction   236
Mechanical suffocation   236
The thymus   238
Thiamine   239
Vitamin C   239
Immunization   239
Bacterial toxins   240
Toxic gas from mattresses   240
Conclusion   241
References   242

Introduction

Over the centuries many theories and explanations have been put forward for the cause of sudden unexpected deaths in infancy. These have often led to huge costs for the community – emotional (e.g. overlying); health (e.g. thymic radiation, avoidance of immunization); and financial (e.g. toxic gas from mattresses). From the time an hypothesis is stated to the time it proves invalid may take many years.

It would be impossible to cover all theories in a chapter, but a few of the most costly are discussed.

Mechanical suffocation

About 600 BC, in retelling a story from the 10th century BC, Jeremiah[1] records 'and this woman's child died in the night because she overlaid it'.

The penitential of Cummean (AD 600) says 'if any layman or woman over-lays his or her child (such offenders) shall do penance for an entire year on bread and water, and for 2 years more abstain from wine and flesh'.

In 1834 Fearn[2] wrote to *The Lancet* describing autopsy findings in two infants. The first had been discovered dead in bed with its mother, but the mother stated positively that the child had not lain near her and that it was impossible for it to have been suffocated. Fearn found petechiae on the thymus, lungs and heart. He states he was 'strongly disposed to think, in spite of the evidence of the mother, that the child must have been destroyed by overlying it'. However, he subsequently performed an autopsy on a 5-month-old child, who had been 'pretty well', had been 'suckled by its mother, and laid in bed upon its side, and in about an hour and a half afterwards was discovered to be dead'. There was some frothy matter in and about the mouth, and its hands were firmly clenched. The appearances exhibited in the autopsy were strikingly the same as in the first case.

'Because the second child was lying in bed by itself, and was not obstructed in its breathing by the bed-clothes, it seemed impossible that the child could have been suffocated', Fearn says 'I became almost entirely at a loss how to account for death in either'. He further states about his findings that 'so trifling a lesion could hardly, in either instance, be supposed to be of itself sufficient to produce death'.

Despite this challenge, overlaying still seems to have been considered a common cause of infant mortality, and Templeman in 1891[3] concluded that overlaying was the commonest cause of death in a review of 258 cases of suffocation in infants.

In the same year Dr Danford Thomas gave evidence at a coroner's enquiry into an infant death which he attributed to overlaying. *The Lancet*, 1892,[4] in commenting on this enquiry made this statement:

Dr Thomas in the course of his observation offered a simple and rational explanation of the manner in which the fatal result is commonly brought about. It is due, in his opinion, either to the child slipping under the bedclothes when the mother's arm on which it lies becomes relaxed in sleep or to its being drawn too near and pressed against the breast. Either explanation is quite feasible, the former as accounting for mere accidental self-suffocation such as also occurs when an infant is put to bed closely wrapped in a shawl; the latter as explaining the purely reflex act by which a sleeping parent may turn upon and smother the infant. Clearly no person can or ought to trust herself in the circumstances with so frail a life. Cots are not so expensive but that the poorest mother, if thrifty, can usually provide one. If otherwise, even an improvised chair-couch is better for the infant than her own bed. It has been suggested that any case of fatal neglect in this particular should be held as a punishable misdemeanor.

'Accidental mechanical suffocation in the bed or cradle' was offered as an explanation for these deaths. Abramson[5] gave details of 139 infants who had died between 1939 and 1943 from accidental mechanical suffocation. Werne[6] questioned the validity of the diagnosis in most of the infant deaths attributed to mechanical suffocation; and Bowden[7] in 1950 stated that 'death in the form of natural disease sometimes strikes with great rapidity in young babies, leaving little to find at autopsy, and the death may be miscalled 'accidental suffocation,' and he concluded that 'so-called accidental suffocation by the bedclothes may be in reality swift death from undiscovered natural causes'.

By the middle of the twentieth century, at least in Australia and USA, most infants were no longer sharing a bed, but were sleeping in a 'crib or cot', and infants dying unexpectedly were described as 'crib deaths' or 'cot deaths'.

It was then felt that most infants who died had not suffocated, and this led to the erroneous corollary that infants could not suffocate. It is now recognized that occasionally infants can be overlaid, especially by a drug-affected or exhausted parent, or by a young sibling, that infants can suffocate under pillows or bed-clothes, and that although rare, intentional suffocation of infants also occurs.

The thymus

In 1614 Platerus[8] performed an autopsy on a 5-month old infant at the request of the infant's father who had previously had two sons die in a similar manner. The child was of healthy appearance having had no previous illness. He found in the region of the throat a large protruding gland 1oz in weight (now recognized as normal size for the thymus at 5 months of age in a healthy infant), and concluded the gland had compressed the blood vessels in the vicinity causing suffocation – he called the condition mors thymica.

In 1889 Paltauf[9] reported that an enlarged thymus gland was usually found in infants who had died suddenly. He felt that this caused death not by compression of the blood vessels but that the prominent thymus and lymphoid tissue was anatomical evidence of a constitutional weakness, the child had been 'so constituted that he is killed by insignificant causes' – status thymus lymphaticus.

In 1906 and 1926 Hammar[10,11] found that thymic weights were similar in those dying from 'status thymus lymphaticus' and those dying within 24 hours of an accident, and concluded that the large thymus found in infants who died suddenly was normal for the age.

A special committee of the Medical Research Council and the Pathological Society of Great Britain and Ireland was set up to study the evidence and published in 1931[12] the conclusion that 'the facts elicited afford no evidence that so-called status thymico lymphaticus has any existence as a pathological entity'.

Boyd[13] in 1932 stated that 'in spite of repeated demonstration that the thymuses of healthy well nourished children are prominent and that wide thymic shadows on roentgenograms of infants' chests are common, the belief persists that these findings represent a constitutional susceptibility to death from trivial causes'. She states that 'the situation has come to such a pass that the surgeon who does not have the child with a wide shadow treated by irradiation before the administration of an anesthetic may be held liable for malpractice if the child dies while under anesthesia'. Because of the 'tenacity of this misconception' she published details of the thymic weights in several hundred children including 137 infants dying between 24 hours and one year of life who had been ill for less than 48 hours. This confirmed that the size of the thymus varies at different ages, being relatively large in infancy and that the width of the thymus decreases with the length of illness prior to death.

Despite this, medical textbooks[14] were still describing the condition up to the 1950s, although others[15] were stating that the existence of the condition was in dispute.

Thiamine

In 1978 David Read[16] noted that infants with Leigh disease, felt to be due to a deficiency in thiamine metabolism, often presented with prolonged apnea, and that infantile thiamine deficiency in both humans and animals could cause sudden death. He suggested further studies were needed to elucidate the role of thiamine in SIDS.

In Australia this theory received wide newspaper publicity and some pregnant women began to take large doses of thiamine. By the time gestation was complete, several months later it had been shown that SIDS infants had higher levels of thiamine than infants who had died from other causes. This resulted in some panicky parents and the hypothesis that SIDS infants were unable to use thiamine, so having high levels. It was not until at least 6 months later that it was shown that SIDS infants in fact had thiamine levels which were similar to those found in living infants and infants who had died rapid accidental deaths, and that sick children, who had low thiamine levels had brought down the original control levels by their inclusion in the control series.

Vitamin C

Vitamin C deficiency in infants causes scurvy, which if left untreated can lead to death after a few months from malnutrition, exhaustion, intercurrent disease or other complications.

It was postulated that some infants with subliminal or unrecognized scurvy may die suddenly and unexpectedly from a challenge such as an intercurrent upper respiratory tract infection.[17]

Blood levels and urine levels of vitamin C vary not only from day to day, but from hour to hour, and are extremely unreliable. However, the dietary history, clinical history, autopsy findings and in some cases blood and urine levels of vitamin C have not supported low vitamin C as playing any part in SIDS.

Immunization

The age range for SIDS and infant immunization with diphtheria–pertussis–tetanus (DPT) overlap, so there was some concern that immunization may precipitate SIDS. In America several families took the manufacturers of DPT to court because their infant had died within days or weeks of immunization. Although no family won a case, the cost to the drug firm of setting up a defence was a problem, so out-of-court settlements were made. This led some people to feel there must be a relationship.

Over the last 20 years many studies have negated this relationship including:

1   Many infants who die of SIDS have had no immunization, e.g. in the NICHD study in the USA in 1978–1979,[18] comparing 840 SIDS to 1680 controls, 62% of SIDS infants had had no immunization with DPT.

2   SIDS infants are under-immunized when compared with controls, e.g. in the same NICHD study, in controls matched for age, race and birth weight only 33% had received no immunization.

3   There is no temporal relationship between SIDS and immunization, i.e. in large series SIDS occurs almost equally 1, 2, 3 and 4 weeks after immunization.

4   When the age at first immunization was lowered by 4 weeks there was no lowering of the median and mean age of SIDS.[19]

Bacterial toxins

'STRUCK'

There is a disease called 'struck' in sheep, in which suckling lambs who are apparently healthy, die suddenly and unexpectedly, especially if challenged by cold weather. Such deaths are related to *Clostridium welchii* C. If samples of upper small intestinal fluid from the lamb are injected into rats previously immunized against *Cl. welchii* C, the rats survive, while unimmunized rats die. Immunizing newborn lambs of the flock against *Cl. welchii* C prevents future lamb deaths.

Several infections and toxins have been proposed as causes of SIDS – clostridia, *E. coli*, *Hemophilus influenzae* type B, *Botulinum*, Coxsackie and herpes viruses, respiratory syncytial virus (RSV) and pertussis. While all these organisms have been responsible for occasional sudden unexpected infant deaths (in which case the deaths are not attributed to SIDS) they have not been demonstrated in over 90% of sudden deaths.

Toxic gas from mattresses

In June 1989 Barry A. Richardson, through the media, put forward a 'toxic gas hypothesis' as the cause of cot deaths. His theory suggested that toxic gases, specifically arsine, stibine or phosphine, were generated by biodeterioration caused by the mould *Scopularcopsis brevicaulis* acting on chemicals used as fire retardants, such as antimony and phosphate compounds in cot mattresses and/or their PVC coverings.

Richardson later[20,21] stated his hypothesis was not new, but that Gosio's disease, which killed many infants in the 19th century through arsine poisoning from wallpaper, involved the same biodeterioration process.

In 1994, again through the media, this time television, the 'Cook Report' broadcast that cot death infants had higher antimony levels in their blood and liver than babies who died of other causes. This report certainly convinced many people that the cause of SIDS was toxin released from cot mattresses.

In 1996 Andrew Taylor[22] had a letter published in *The Lancet* which stated that antimony was present in the liver of 37 SIDS victims (mean 7.11 ng/g) but only in the liver of one of 14 infants dying of other causes (mean <0.5 ng/g).

This contrasted with a previous report from Howatson[23] who found the mean antimony levels in the SIDS (25 infants) group to be 6 ng/g, and in the 25 infants dying of other causes to be 7 ng/g.

An expert group under the Chairmanship of Lady Sylvia Limerick was set up, following the Cook Report to investigate the suggested link between cot deaths and the emission of toxic gases from cot mattresses. The conclusion of the Group (May 1998) was that 'there is no evidence to suggest that antimony or phosphorus containing compounds used as fire retardants in PVC and other cot mattress materials are a cause of sudden infant death syndrome'. This conclusion was based on the following:

1   Cot mattress contamination with *S. brevicaulis* is rare, and no more common in mattresses used at the time of a cot death than in other used mattresses.
2   There is no evidence for the generation of gases from phosphorus, arsenic and antimony from cot mattresses, by *S. brevicaulis*, when tested using conditions relevant to an infant's cot. (The Group did, however, identify laboratory conditions, wholly unlike those that could occur in an infant's cot, in which added antimony is biovolatilized, but to the much less toxic tremethyl-antimony and not to stibine.)
3   There is no evidence of poisoning by phosphine, arsine or stibine (or their methylated derivations) in infants who have died of SIDS.
4   Low amounts of antimony can be detected in samples from the majority of live infants and even newborn infants: the concentrations in the tissues of SIDS infants were not different from those in infants dying from known causes. There are a number of sources of antimony in the domestic environment other than the fire retardants in cot mattress materials.
5   There is no evidence that the changing rates of sudden infant deaths correspond to the introduction and removal of antimony and phosphorus containing fire retardants in cot mattresses.

Conclusion

Many causes of sudden unexpected deaths in infancy have been little more than guesses; sometimes with the good intention of protecting the parents from murder or neglect charges. Such causes include teething, convulsions, silent pneumonia and overwhelming infection, the last two being so 'silent' or 'overwhelming' that they left no signs of illness.

Some disorders which account for a few relatively unexpected deaths have led to conclusions that they are responsible for most deaths, e.g. botulism, metabolic disorders, mechanical suffocation and murder.

There remain questions that still need answers, e.g. what role does long QT syndrome play in SIDS and why is there a higher incidence of SIDS in infants of tobacco smoking parents? Confirmation is needed of brain differences in SIDS infants (are they the cause or result of hypoxia, are controls accurately age-matched by days and well infants?) Why can some, but not all, infants not cope with the prone position? How do we identify such infants?

References

1. Jeremiah. A story from the 10th century BC and recorded about 7th century BC. *The Bible*, 1 Kings, Ch. 3, v. 19.
2. Fearn SW. Sudden and unexplained death in children. *Lancet* 1834;1:246.
3. Templeman C. 258 cases of suffocation in infants. *Edin Med J* 1891;38:322.
4. Thomas D. Comment. *Lancet* 1892;1:45.
5. Abramson HJ. Accidental mechanical suffocation in infants. *J Pediatr* 1944;25:404.
6. Werne J, Garrow I. Sudden deaths of infants allegedly due to mechanical suffocation. *Am J Pub Health Nat Health* 1947;37:675.
7. Bowden K. Sudden death or alleged suffocation in babies. *Med J Aust* 1950;37:65.
8. Platerus F. Observationum in hominis affectibus plerisque-libri tres. *Basillae* 1614; 172, cited in Major RH, *Classical Descriptions of Disease*. Thomas CC (ed.) The Collegiate Press of Minnesota, Springfield, USA, 1932.
9. Paltauff A. Uber die Beziehung der Thymus Zur Plotzlichen Tod. *Wien Klin Wschr* 1889;2:876 (27).
10. Hammar JA. Uber gewicht, involution and persistenz der thymus in postfotalleben des menschen. *Arch F Anbatu Phys Anat Abt (Leipzig)* 1906;91.
11. Hammar JA. Die menschenthymus in gesundheit und krankheit. 1. Das normale organ. *Ztschr Mikr-Anat Forsch* 1926;6 Suppl.:1.
12. Young M, Turnbull HM. Report of special committee of the Medical Research Council and The Pathological Society of Great Britain and Ireland. *J Pathol Bacteriol* 1931;34:213.
13. Boyd E. The weight of the thymus gland in health and disease. *Am J Dis Child* 1932;43:1162.
14. Sheldon W (ed.) *Diseases of Infancy and Childhood*. Churchill J and A, London 1955.
15. Wright S (ed.) *Applied Physiology*. Oxford University Press, London, 1952;1017 pp.
16. Read DJC. The aetiology of sudden infant death syndrome: Current ideas on breathing, sleep, possible links to deranged thiamine neurochemistry. *Aust NZ J Med* 1978;8:322–36.
17. Kalokerinos A, Dettman G. Sudden death in infancy syndrome in Western Australia (letter). *Med J Aust* 1976;2:31–2.
18. Hoffman HJ, Hunter JC, Damus K *et al.* Diphtheria – teranus pertussis immunization and sudden infant death. *Pediatrics* 1987;4:598–611.
19. Beal SM. SIDS and immunization. *Med J Aust* 1990;153:117.
20. Richardson BA. Cot mattresses, sudden infant death syndrome. *Br Med J* 1995;310:1071.
21. Richardson BA. Cot death and cot mattresses. *NZ Med J* 1995;108:370.
22. Taylor A. Antimony, cot mattresses, and SIDS. *Lancet* 1996;347:6161.
23. Howatson AG, Patrick WJA, Fell GS, Lyon TDB, Gibson AAM. Cot mattresses and sudden infant death syndrome. *Lancet* 1995;345:1044–5.

CHAPTER 15

The role of monitoring

CHRISTIAN F. POETS

Introduction   243
Who should be monitored?   243
What should be monitored?   250
For how long should infants be monitored?   253
References   253

Introduction

The application of home monitoring to specific risk groups, i.e. secondary prevention, has long been the only method widely applied to prevent SIDS. Its effectiveness in reducing the incidence of SIDS, however, has never been proven. This is largely for methodological reasons: with the current incidence of SIDS, 110,000 infants would have to be randomized in a controlled population-based trial to gain sufficient power to demonstrate (or exclude) a reduction in SIDS rate from 1 to 0.5/1000 as a result of home monitoring. Currently, this seems impractical. Efforts to reduce the incidence of SIDS on a nationwide level should, therefore, concentrate on primary prevention, namely on public information campaigns on child care practices associated with a reduced risk of SIDS. This approach was shown to have reduced the incidence of SIDS in several countries by 50 to 70%.[1–3]

Despite its unproven effect, however, there are still specific patient groups in which home monitoring appears indicated. These groups should be clearly defined, as should be the duration and the physiologic signals that are to be monitored. This chapter will deal with these issues by addressing three questions: who (or why), what, and for how long should patients be monitored?

Who should be monitored?

Indications for home monitoring depend on the goal that is to be achieved. Currently, monitors are prescribed either to prevent SIDS or to provide an early warning for situations which endanger a patient's well-being, e.g. hypoxemia in infants receiving home oxygen. With regard to SIDS prevention, one should first consider how much the risk of SIDS must be increased before home monitoring becomes indicated, given that the latter is costly, has side effects (see below) and is of unproven value. For example, it is generally accepted that monitors are not prescribed to infants whose mothers have smoked one pack of cigarettes per day during pregnancy, despite a 7- to 8-fold increase in SIDS risk in this group.[4] Why then prescribe monitors to very low birth weight (VLBW) infants, whose risk is 'only' 4- to 5-fold increased (see below)?

Because of the problems inevitably associated with defining cut-off points for risk assessment, a different approach seems plausible, namely to prescribe monitoring as a diagnostic tool or as an early warning of potentially dangerous pathophysiology (Table 15.1). Some specific aspects of this approach to defining monitor indications will be outlined.

HOME MONITORING AS A DIAGNOSTIC TOOL

Following an apparent life-threatening event (ALTE)

In approximately 30–50% of infants who survived an ALTE, defined as an episode that is frightening to the observer and that is characterized by some combination of apnea (central or obstructive), color change (usually cyanotic or pallid but occasionally erythematous or plethoric), marked change in muscle tone (usually marked limpness), choking, or gagging,[5] and that resolved only after vigorous stimulation or resuscitation, no specific cause for the event can be found.[6] Data on the risk of SIDS in these infants are conflicting, ranging from 0 to 13%.[7] It often remains unclear whether the event indeed involved potentially dangerous pathophysiology, e.g. an epileptic seizure with apnea and/or cyanosis as the only clinical signs,[8] or whether it merely reflected increased parental anxiety. For this uncertainty, documented monitoring ('event recording') seems the logical consequence in those infants in whom no treatable

Table 15.1 Indications for home monitoring

To reach a diagnosis
- In infants with unexplained ALTE
- In infants with >1 previous SIDS in the family

To warn of potentially dangerous pathophysiology
- In the technology-dependent child
- In infants with persistent AOP
- In respiratory control disorders

cause for the ALTE can be found during the initial workup (see below). If then further events occur, analysis of the data recorded may help to identify the underlying pathophysiology[9] or to reassure parents.[10] Documented monitoring should start as early as possible after the event. In an epidemiologic study from Sweden, 29% of infants had a further ALTE during the first 3 days after the first event, but only 12% had such spells later on.[11]

Patients with ALTE represent perhaps the group in which the indication for monitoring is least ambiguous, not as much with regard to SIDS prevention, but to prevent further events by identifying a specific cause for events. With regard to SIDS, it should be remembered that in the large study from the National Institute of Child Health and Development (NICHD) only 1.5% of SIDS cases (and 0.2% of controls) had an episode of apnea or cyanosis noted in their medical records.[12] Monitoring these infants will thus only have a very small impact on SIDS rates in a community.

Infants with more than one previous SIDS in the family

Documented monitoring also appears of particular value in infants from families in whom two or more SIDS have occurred. This is not only because these infants are at extremely high risk of SIDS, but also because diagnoses other than SIDS, e.g. non-accidental injury, are relatively more prevalent amongst this group. Documented monitoring may help to uncover some of these underlying diagnoses.[9,13,14]

HOME MONITORING TO PREVENT POTENTIALLY DANGEROUS PATHOPHYSIOLOGY

In these patients, home monitoring is indicated to prevent morbidity rather than mortality. Three groups can be distinguished. The first is technology-dependent infants, e.g. preterm infants discharged on home oxygen, infants who breathe through a tracheostomy, or ventilator-dependent patients. In these patients, monitoring will help to notify caregivers if tubes become disconnected or blocked or if oxygen or ventilator demands increase. The second group is preterm infants who are ready for discharge but continue to have symptoms related to apnea of prematurity (AOP). This condition is not associated with an increased risk of SIDS,[15] but monitoring may be indicated to prevent potential sequelae, e.g. cerebral palsy.[16,17] Whether monitoring at home (or in hospital) can prevent such sequelae, however, has never been proven, and this indication thus remains controversial. The third group is infants with a defined condition that is associated with a respiratory control disorder, e.g. infants with the Pierre Robin sequence,[18] cyanotic breath-holding spells involving loss of consciousness,[19] or the Arnold–Chiari malformation.[20] By definition, none of these groups is at increased risk of SIDS, but they may die from their underlying disorder.

PATIENTS FOR WHOM MONITORING IS NOT ROUTINELY INDICATED (TABLE 15.2)

Infants with one previous SIDS in family

If one infant has died of SIDS, the risk for subsequent siblings is up to five times higher.[21,22] This risk is considerably lower than that of infants born to heavy smokers; however, the situation is usually confounded by a high level of parental anxiety. It is our practice to discuss the risk factors specific to the family, ideally during the subsequent pregnancy, and to point out that the risk is extremely low if potentially amenable risk factors such as the prone sleep position, smoking during pregnancy and overheating are avoided. Helpful in this regard are recent data from The Netherlands, where monitor use is extremely uncommon, but where the annual number of SIDS cases fell from approximately 200 to 30 per year as a result of a very efficient nationwide information campaign on preventable risk factors (M. l'Hoir, personal communication). We also point out that in an Australian study on 677 SIDS families, the risk of losing a subsequent infant was only 1.6 times higher than expected in those 92% of families who had lost their previous child at between 0.5 and 12 months of age, were not severely socially deprived, and had no family history of sudden unexpected unexplained death in children or young adults.[23] We then discuss the pros and cons of monitoring, particularly that it is of unproven value and that there will always be false alarms which may give rise to new concerns. We finally explain to them that as there is no medical indication, one cannot prescribe a home monitor, just as one would not order any surgical procedure that is not medically indicated.

Increased parental concern without a family history of SIDS

Parental anxiety without a family history of SIDS is a difficult issue. Careful history taking to identify and address the underlying cause(s) of this anxiety may be helpful. Again, advice on amenable risk factors should be given, including the information that the risk of SIDS is extremely low if none of these risk factors is present. Parents must also be clearly informed about the unproven value of home monitoring. Finally, the same line of argument as outlined for SIDS siblings applies.

Table 15.2   Infants who do *not* routinely need a monitor

- Infants with one previous SIDS in family
- Twins
- Infants of drug-dependent mothers
- Asymptomatic preterm infants
- Infants with CLD without home O_2

Twins

One study reported a 4.4% risk of SIDS for the smaller twin if there was a more than 15% difference in birth weight in a pair of twins. The study involved 135 pairs of twins who fulfilled this criteria, six of whom died of SIDS.[24] It has not been confirmed, is based on relatively small numbers and is thus not sufficient evidence to justify a general recommendation for home monitoring in this particular group.

Infants of drug-dependent mothers

Earlier studies on the risk of SIDS for infants of substance-abusing mothers yielded conflicting results, with some studies showing a significantly increased risk,[25,26] whereas others did not.[27] In a recent study from New York, the risk of SIDS initially also appeared to be associated with a five- to tenfold increased risk of SIDS, but after controlling for potential confounders, relative risks were reduced to 3.6 for methadone, 2.3 for heroin, 1.6 for cocaine and 1.1 for cocaine and heroin or methadone.[28]

Probably the most complete data on this subject stem from the British Confidential Enquiry into Stillbirths and Deaths in Infancy (CESDI study). In that study, the use of illicit drugs (heroin, crack, cocaine, speed, LSD, amphetamines, barbiturates, cannabis, and glue) during pregnancy was associated with an OR of 4.3 (95% CI 1.5–12.4) after controlling for potential confounders.[29] Nevertheless, a fourfold increased risk of SIDS remains comparatively moderate and does not, on its own, justify prescription of a home monitor, particularly as there are concerns about parental compliance in this group.

Asymptomatic preterm infants

Data on the risk of death in preterm infants are conflicting, which is partly due to different ways of data acquisition. Aziz *et al.* performed a province-based follow-up study on 960 Canadian live births who weighed between 500 and 1249 g; nine of these (0.94%) died of SIDS.[30] In another study based on an analysis of linked birth/death records in California, 2962 cases of SIDS were identified. The incidence per 1000 live births was 7.5 for birth weights <1500 g, compared with 3.8 and 1.0 for those weighing 2001–2500 g and 3001–3500 g, respectively.[31] In a similar study from North Carolina, SIDS rates were 1.5, 6.9 and 3.7/1000 for birthweights of >2500 g, 1501 to 2500 g, and <1500 g, respectively.[32] This excess SIDS rate in the medium birth weight group, however, was not confirmed in a nationwide study on linked US birth/infant death data sets from 1985 to 1991, which found annual SIDS rates of 1.03 to 1.07, 3.3 to 3.5 and 3.7 for the three birth weight groups mentioned above.[33] Taken together, these data suggest that the risk of SIDS is only moderately increased in very premature or VLBW infants; however, how much the comparatively low incidence in some studies is related to diagnostic misclassification or the widespread use of home monitors in this group remains unclear. Interestingly, a Norwegian study that aimed to correct misclassification errors by carefully reviewing death certificates and autopsy reports found that the initial SIDS figure for VLBW infants increased from 4.1 to 7.6/1000 as a result of this review.[34] Nevertheless, home monitoring cannot be generally recommended for this group.

Infants with chronic lung disease (CLD) who do not require home oxygen

CLD infants, as a group, were initially considered to be at extremely high risk of SIDS. This was based on a study of 53 infants, six of whom died suddenly and unexpectedly.[35] In a similar study from 1994, however, involving 78 infants with CLD, there was no sudden death.[36] The only noticeable difference in patient management was that in the more recent study, pulse oximeter saturation (Spo_2) was strictly maintained at >93%, with 25% of infants receiving home oxygen, whereas this therapy was not used in the earlier study. A low rate of sudden death in infants with CLD, if those who require home oxygen are identified and treated, was recently confirmed in two other studies involving 700 and 141 infants, respectively; only one infant in each study died suddenly and unexpectedly.[37,38] It was not stated, however, how many of these infants received home monitoring. Nevertheless, the general assumption that infants with CLD are at particularly high risk of SIDS cannot be maintained in the light of these recent data.

THE ROLE OF SLEEP STUDIES IN DECIDING ON HOME MONITORING

Recordings of physiologic signals during sleep have long been used to help in deciding which infants require home monitoring and which do not. The data published so far, however, have not yielded any parameter that has sufficient sensitivity to be useful as a predictive marker for SIDS. The first large population-based study that prospectively collected physiologic data in future SIDS victims was carried out by Southall *et al.*, who performed 24-hour tape recordings of the electrocardiogram (ECG) and breathing movements on 9856 infants, 29 of whom subsequently died of SIDS.[39] None of the recordings in the SIDS infants showed a prolonged apneic pause (>20 s), cardiac arrhythmia, pre-excitation, or a prolonged QT-interval. Compared with surviving matched controls, the SIDS cases did not show significantly increased numbers of short apneic pauses or quantities of periodic breathing.[40] In fact, those SIDS victims that were studied after 1 month of age showed significantly *fewer* apneic pauses (>4 s) than did the control infants.[41]

Another prospective, though not population-based, study was performed by Kelly *et al.*,[42] who analysed 12-hour recordings of ECG and impedance pneumography in 17 infants who subsequently died of SIDS, drawn from a group of 11,100 infants referred for nocturnal pneumograms. They found higher mean heart rates, more periodic breathing during quiet time, and more episodes of bradycardia in the SIDS victims. However, the information from this study is limited because some of their infants were siblings of SIDS victims and some had suffered ALTE.

The same critique applies to a large prospective study reported by Kahn *et al.* They analysed polygraphic sleep studies in 30 future SIDS victims, taken from a data set of 20,750 infants who had been studied polygraphically in 10 Belgian sleep laboratories between 1977 and 1990.[43] The only two polygraphic differences between the SIDS cases and the controls were an increase in the number of obstructive apneas (defined as a pause in airflow for >2 s, and observed in 23 of 30 future SIDS victims, but in only nine of 60 controls) and a decreased number of body movements during sleep (but their data were not controlled for sleep position). All other polygraphic parameters (duration of different sleep states, number and duration of apneic pauses, heart and respiratory rates) were not significantly different in the two groups, but significantly more future SIDS victims were reported to have episodes of regurgitation after feeding (9 vs 2) or profuse sweating during sleep (7 vs 0). However, five of the 30 future SIDS victims were siblings of SIDS victims, and nine had experienced an ALTE. Therefore, caution has to be applied with inferring from these data to the pathogenesis of SIDS in infants without such a history.

The most recent attempt to predict SIDS from recordings of physiologic signals is a study on standard ECGs performed in 33,034 infants, 24 of whom subsequently died of SIDS. Twelve of these infants had a corrected QT interval (QTc) above the normal range (mean +2 SD).[44] This study is the last (and largest) in a series of similar studies, which yielded conflicting results. In an earlier study from the same group[45] a 'markedly prolonged' QT-interval was found in six of nine SIDS victims, identified in a population of 8000 infants. In contrast, Southall *et al.*, in the prospective study mentioned above[40] and in a second prospective study involving standard ECGs on 7254 infants, 15 of whom suffered SIDS, found no abnormal prolongation of the QT-interval.[46] Weinstein and Steinschneider[47] were also unable to identify a prolonged QT-interval in any of their eight prospectively studied SIDS victims. Thus, the Italian group is the only one that has yet found a prolonged QT-interval in a significant proportion of subsequent SIDS victims. Their methods and result, however, have been widely criticized.[48] Thus, it was not stated in their study how blinding was achieved, how the QRS complexes on which measurements were performed had been chosen, or what the precise criteria for diagnosing SIDS were. Also, if the death mechanism supposedly induced by a prolongation of the QT-interval is fatal ventricular arrhythmias,[49] and such a prolonged interval can be found in 50% of subsequent SIDS victims, it is surprising that these arrhythmias have never been found in cardiorespiratory recordings obtained during SIDS.[50] Recordings of ECG and/or breathing movements plus ECG can thus not be recommended for SIDS prediction in otherwise asymptomatic infants.

Sleep studies, however, play an important role in symptomatic infants, e.g. following an ALTE, but only to identify the underlying pathophysiology, not to assess the risk of SIDS. Recordings that include measurements of oxygenation are also helpful in identifying preterm infants that require oxygen at home or in the nursery. The issues related to these studies, however, are beyond the scope of this chapter.[51]

What should be monitored?

Three types of monitors are used at home: devices that monitor breathing efforts ('apnea monitors'), ECG plus breathing efforts ('cardiorespiratory monitors'), or oxygenation monitors (mostly pulse oximeters).

APNEA MONITORS

Apnea monitors register breathing efforts via impedance plethysmography, piezo belts, pressure capsules, or motion-sensitive pads placed underneath the infant. The devices are comparatively cheap and easy to use. Their concept, i.e. the sole monitoring of respiration, is based on the so-called apnea hypothesis which assumes that apnea is an early component of the sequence of events leading to SIDS.[52] This hypothesis, however, was based on two infants who were later found to have been murdered by their mother; not on SIDS.[53] More recent studies have shown that in the majority of cases, prolonged apnea occurs in fact rather late during SIDS, namely when the infants are already gasping.[50] It may thus not be surprising that a large number of deaths on apnea monitors have been reported. In a questionnaire study which was sent to all members of the British Paediatric Association, a total of 80 deaths was reported in infants on apnea monitors; in 48 of these deaths the infants were reported to have died at home despite the monitor being connected and functioning at the time of death; 16 additional deaths occurred in infants monitored in hospital (mostly in the low-dependency area of the neonatal unit).[54] Moreover, in the recent Confidential Enquiry into Sudden Deaths in Infants (CESDI) study, covering one-third of births in England, the usual use of an apnea monitor was associated with an OR of 7.7 (95% CI 2.3–25.9); it was used in 10% of cases and 2.1% of controls. During the last/reference sleep, 5% of SIDS infants (vs 2% of controls) had been on an apnea monitor.[55] These data clearly suggest that the use of apnea monitors cannot be recommended.

CARDIORESPIRATORY MONITORS

Cardiorespiratory monitors register both heart rate and respiratory efforts, the latter mostly via impedance. They were introduced to overcome the inability of apnea monitors to detect obstructive apnea; however, it has never been conclusively shown that bradycardia occurs regularly and/or early during obstructive apnea. In contrast, there is evidence that bradycardia may occur extremely late during episodic upper airway obstruction and/or hypoxemia. For example, in older infants and children with obstructive sleep apnea, only two out of 209 episodes of hypoxemia, defined as a fall in SpO_2 to <85% lasting for >30 s, were associated with a fall in heart rate to below 50/min.[56] Similarly, during recordings of unexplained ALTE in infants on transcutaneous PO_2 memory monitors, only 18% of events with a fall in transcutaneous partial pressure of oxygen

($P_{Tc}O_2$) to <20 mmHg for >40 s were associated with a bradycardia (defined as a fall in heart rate to <60–80/min depending on age), and 22% with prolonged apneic pauses (>20 s).[9] These data on spontaneously occurring events are confirmed by experimental data. During 46 episodes of induced airway occlusion lasting 4–19 s (mean 13 s) in healthy term and preterm infants, no bradycardia was observed during any occlusion.[57] Also, in six patients with congenital central hypoventilation syndrome who had diaphragmatic pacers, bradycardia was not elicited in any patient in response to airway occlusion, despite desaturation with a mean $Sp o_2$ of 61% (SD 12%).[58]

In a recent analysis of cardiorespiratory recordings obtained during sudden infant deaths, seven of nine infants were already gasping at or around the time the monitor sounded a bradycardia alarm.[50] Since gasping only occurs if a subject is severely hypoxemic ($Pa o_2$ <10 mmHg), it must be assumed that bradycardia occurred very late during the sequence of events leading to these deaths, whatever their precise pathophysiology. Moreover, cardiorespiratory monitors may have an extremely high false alarm rate. Using an event recording system in conjunction with a standard cardiorespiratory monitor, a total of 12,980 false alarms were reported during a total of approximately 2100 days of monitoring in 83 infants, giving an average of six false alarms per day per infant.[59] Besides being a nuisance to parents, this feature bears the risk of non-compliance, i.e. of not using the monitor. In summary, the data summarized above raise doubts as to whether cardiorespiratory monitors will alarm early enough during potentially life-threatening situations. These doubts are substantiated by recent epidemiologic data obtained from the National Maternal and Infant Health Survey.[60] In this case–control study, national prevalences for home cardiorespiratory monitor use in infants with birthweights of 500 to 1499 g, 1500 to 2499 g and 2500 g or more were 19.9, 2.6 and 1.1% for black and 44.0, 8.8 and 1.2% for non-black infants. In this study, black VLBW infants who had a monitor prescribed were four times more likely to die of SIDS than non-monitored control infants (OR 3.93, 95% CI 1.09–14.17). In all other birthweight groups, monitor use was not associated with a significant increase or reduction in SIDS rates. Hence, use of a cardiorespiratory monitor did again not result in a reduced SIDS rate.

OXYGENATION MONITORS

The concept of monitoring oxygenation is based on the consideration that whatever causes SIDS, will lead to hypoxemia and/or circulatory failure, both of which will be sensed by an oxygenation monitor. This has already been shown for the transcutaneous $P o_2$ monitor, which detected hypoxemia reliably[61] and, since it depends on adequate skin perfusion, is also very sensitive to reductions in cardiac output.[62] However, the instruments are difficult to use, require heating of the skin and therefore frequent re-siting of the sensor and have to be calibrated in regular intervals. Perhaps for these reasons there has never been a device designed for home use, and $P_{Tc}O_2$ monitoring has never gained wide acceptance. Its applicability is now declining even further since production of the 'home' monitor used in published studies[61] has ceased.

An alternative device for monitoring oxygenation is the pulse oximeter. Conventional instruments, however, do not appear suitable for home use because of an unacceptably high rate of false alarms. New developments, however, promise considerably fewer such alarms. One such development (Masimo Signal Extraction Technology (SET), Masimo Corp., Irvine, CA) reduces false alarms by mathematically manipulating the pulse oximeter's red and infrared light absorbance to identify and subtract the noise components associated with these signals.[63] Compared with a conventional pulse oximeter, it had 93% fewer alarms in one study.[64] Another instrument (Nellcor OXISMART, Mallinckrodt, Pleasanton, CA) relies predominantly on an improved identification of periods where the pulse waveform signal deviates from a pre-defined template and suppresses any audible alarm for up to one minute during such periods.[65]

We recently investigated the reliability of these new devices, compared with a conventional pulse oximeter and a $P_{Tc}O_2$ monitor, in detecting hypoxemia and bradycardia.[66] The former was defined as a fall in $P_{Tc}O_2$ to <40 mmHg, confirmed by manual determination of arterial oxygen saturation from analysis of the raw red and infrared light absorption signal, the latter as a fall in heart rate to <80/min. We found that the conventional oximeter had alarmed during all 185 hypoxemic episodes thus identified; however, in 15 episodes it only alarmed because it had zeroed out due to signal loss. One of the new instruments (Masimo SET) only missed one hypoxemic episode where it had stayed 1% above the alarm threshold. In contrast, the other new generation instrument (Nellcor OXISMART) failed to alarm in 5.4% of episodes where there was definite hypoxemia, despite the latter lasting for up to 32 s. The pulse oximeters' ability to identify bradycardia differed even more widely, with more than two thirds of episodes missed by the new Nellcor and one third missed by the conventional oximeter. The Masimo SET again performed significantly better, but still missed four of 54 bradycardias. Thus, the reduced false alarm rate of one of the two new generation instruments investigated in that study appeared to have been achieved at the expense of a reduced ability to identify true alarms, i.e. hypoxemia and particularly bradycardia. Nevertheless, if detection of hypoxemia rather than bradycardia is the primary aim, some new generation oximeters appear to offer a sufficiently good trade-off between a low number of false alarms and a high sensitivity to true alarms to appear suitable for use as home monitors. Also, their reliability in detecting circulatory failure has yet to be tested.

DOCUMENTED MONITORING

Documented monitoring means the storage of physiologic data before, during and following a monitor alarm. It can help (1) to assess parental compliance with home monitoring[67]; (2) to put parental perceptions of alarms into perspective[68,69]; and (3) to identify the pathophysiology leading to true alarms.[9] The first two aims can usually be achieved with the devices currently available, and published data show that between 71 and 89% of alarms regarded by parents as true are in fact false alarms.[68,69] However, the 30–90 s pre-alarm window of these monitors is usually not sufficient to identify the pathophysiology leading to true alarms. For example, in a recent analysis of recordings obtained during sudden infant deaths, 30% of infants were already gasping at the time the recording started.[50] It thus remained entirely unclear what had led to this gasping. In contrast, we were able to identify causes for alarms in 19 of 34 infants (56%) with documented events about who had been monitored for recurrent ALTE using monitors that had a 10 minute pre-alarm window.[9] Often, the changes that led to the diagnosis occurred 2 to 5 minutes before the monitor alarm. At current prices for storage media, a longer pre-alarm recording interval should not be denied for financial reasons, and documented monitors should thus generally have a 5 to 10 minute pre-alarm window. Also, there are now investigative devices that can record not only physiologic data but also video images, so that any changes in physiologic waveforms can be validated against what the infant actually did during these changes.[70] Such devices are obviously particularly valuable for diagnostic monitoring, e.g. in infants with ALTE or two previous SIDS in the family.

For how long should infants be monitored?

Recommendations for monitoring duration should be based on epidemiologic data. In infants who have suffered an ALTE, the risk for further events ceases to be increased if no true alarms have occurred for one month. Monitoring can thus be discontinued after that period. The same applies to infants with persistent apnea of prematurity. In technology-dependent patients, monitoring should continue until 1–2 months after the measures for which surveillance has been ordered, e.g. home oxygen, have been discontinued. This recommendation, however, is based on personal experience rather than on systematic studies.

Finally, it must be stressed that prescription of a home monitor must always be accompanied by careful training of parents and/or other caretakers, which must include training in cardiopulmonary resuscitation. During monitoring, technical and medical support for problems with either the patient or the monitor must be available on a 24-hour basis. Only then can home monitoring be expected to contribute to an improved outcome in selected patient groups.

References

1. Willinger M, Hoffman HJ, Wu KT *et al*. Factors associated with the transition to nonprone sleep positions of infants in the United States. *J Am Med Ass* 1998;280:329–35.
2. Wennergren G, Alm B, Oyen N *et al*. The decline in the incidence of SIDS in Scandinavia and its relation to risk-intervention campaigns. *Acta Paediatr* 1997;86:963–8.
3. Court C. Cot deaths. *Br Med J* 1995;310:7–10.

4. Poets CF, Rudolph A, Schlaud M, Kleemann WJ, Diekmann U, Sens B. Maternal cigarette smoking and sudden infant death syndrome: Results from the Lower Saxony Perinatal Working Group. *Eur J Pediatr* 1995;154:326–9.

5. National Institutes of Health consensus development conference on infantile apnea and home monitoring, Sept 29 to Oct 1, 1986. *Pediatrics* 1987;79:292–9.

6. Kahn A, Montauk L, Blum D. Diagnostic categories in infants referred for an acute event suggesting near-miss SIDS. *Eur J Pediatr* 1987;146:458–60.

7. Brooks JG. Apparent life-threatening events and apnea of infancy. *Clin Perinat* 1992;19:809–38.

8. Hewertson J, Poets CF, Samuels MP, Boyd SG, Neville BGR, Southall DP. Epileptic seizure-induced hypoxemia in infants with apparent life-threatening events. *Pediatrics* 1994;94:148–56.

9. Poets CF, Samuels MP, Noyes JP *et al*. Home event recordings of oxygenation, breathing movements and electrocardiogram in infants and young children with recurrent apparent life-threatening events. *J Pediatr* 1993;123:693–701.

10. Steinschneider A, Santos V. Parental reports of apnea and bradycardia: temporal characteristics and accuracy. *Pediatrics* 1991;88:1100–5.

11. Wennergren G, Milerad J, Lagercrantz H *et al*. The epidemiology of sudden infant death syndrome and attacks of lifelessness in Sweden. *Acta Paediatr Scand* 1987;76:898–906.

12. Damus K, Pakter J, Krongrad E, Standfast SJ, Hoffman HJ. Postnatal medical and epidemiological risk factors for the sudden infant death syndrome. In: Harper RM, Hoffman HJ (eds). *Sudden Infant Death Syndrome*. PMA Publishing, New York, 1988, pp. 187–201.

13. Samuels MP, Poets CF, Noyes JP, Hartmann H, Hewertson J, Southall DP. Diagnosis and management after life threatening events in infants and young children who received cardiopulmonary resuscitation. *Br Med J* 1993;306:489–92.

14. Southall DP, Plunkett MCB, Banks MW, Falkov AF, Samuels MP. Covert video recordings of life-threatening child abuse: Lessons for child protection. *Pediatrics* 1997;100:735–60.

15. Hoffman HJ, Damus K, Krongrad E, Hillman L. Apnea, birth weight, and SIDS: Results of the NICHD cooperative epidemiological study of sudden infant death syndrome (SIDS) risk factors. In: US Department of Health and Human Services (eds). *Infantile Apnea and Home Monitoring*. NIH Publication No. 87–2905, Bethesda, 1987, pp. B53–B69.

16. Jones RAK, Lukeman D. Apnoea of immaturity. 2. Mortality and handicap. *Arch Dis Child* 1982;57:766–8.

17. Marlow N, Hunt LP, Chiswick ML. Clinical factors associated with adverse outcome for babies weighing 2000 g or less at birth. *Arch Dis Child* 1988;63:1131–6.

18. Williams AJ, Williams MA, Walker CA, Bush PG. The Robin anomalad (Pierre Robin syndrome) – a follow up study. *Arch Dis Child* 1981;56:663–8.

19. Southall DP, Samuels MP, Talbert DG. Recurrent cyanotic episodes with severe arterial hypoxaemia and intrapulmonary shunting: a mechanism for sudden death. *Arch Dis Child* 1990;65:953–61.

20. Cochrane DD, Adderley R, White CP, Norman M, Steinbok P. Apnea in patients with myelomeningocele. *Pediatr Neurosurg* 1990;16:232–9.

21. Guntheroth WG, Lohmann R, Spiers PS. Risk of sudden infant death syndrome in subsequent siblings. *J Pediatr* 1990;116:520–4.
22. Irgens LM, Skjaerven R, Peterson DR. Prospective assessment of recurrence risk in sudden infant death syndrome siblings. *J Pediatr* 1984;104:349–51.
23. Beal SM, Blundell HK. Recurrence incidence of sudden infant death syndrome. *Arch Dis Child* 1988;63:924–30.
24. Beal S. Sudden infant death syndrome in twins. *Pediatrics* 1989;84:1038–44.
25. Davidson-Ward SL, Bautista D, Chan L *et al*. Sudden infant death syndrome in infants of substance-abusing mothers. *J Pediatr* 1990;117:876–81.
26. Durand DJ, Espinoza AM, Nickerson BG. Association between prenatal cocaine exposure and sudden infant death syndrome. *J Pediatr* 1990;117:909–11.
27. Baucher H, Zuckerman B, McClain M, Frank D, Fried LE, Kayne H. Risk of sudden infant death syndrome among infants with *in utero* exposure to cocaine. *J Pediatr* 1988;113:831–4.
28. Kandall SR, Gaines J, Habel L, Davidson G, Jessop D. Relationship of maternal substance abuse to subsequent sudden infant death syndrome in offspring. *J Pediatr* 1993;123:120–6.
29. Blair PS, Fleming PJ, Bensley D *et al*. Confidential Inquiry into Stillbirths and Deaths Regional Coordinators and Researchers. Smoking and the sudden infant death syndrome: results from 1993–5 case–control study for confidential inquiry into stillbirths and deaths in infancy. *Br Med J* 1996;313:195–8.
30. Aziz K, Vickar DB, Sauve RS, Etches PC, Pain KS, Robertson CMT. Province-based study of neurologic disability of children weighing 500 through 1249 grams at birth in relation to neonatal cerebral ultrasound findings. *Pediatrics* 1995;95:837–44.
31. Grether JK, Schulman J. Sudden infant death syndrome and birth weight. *J Pediatr* 1989;114:561–7.
32. Dollfus C, Patetta M, Siegel E, Cross AW. Infant mortality: a practical approach to the analysis of the leading causes of death and risk factors. *Pediatrics* 1990;86:176–83.
33. Bigger HR, Silvestri JM, Shott S, Weese-Mayer DE. Influence of increased survival in very low birth weight, low birth weight, and normal birth weight infants on the incidence of sudden infant death syndrome in the United States: 1985–1991. *J Pediatr* 133;1998:73–8.
34. Oyen N, Irgens LM, Skjaerven R, Morild I, Markestad T, Rognum TO. Secular trends of sudden infant death syndrome in Norway 1967–1988: application of a method of case identification to Norwegian registry data. *Paediatr Perinat Epidemiol* 1994;8:263–81.
35. Werthammer J, Brown ER, Neff RK, Taeusch HW. Sudden infant death syndrome in infants with bronchopulmonary dysplasia. *Pediatrics* 1982;69:301–4.
36. Gray PH, Rogers Y. Are infants with bronchopulmonary dysplasia at risk for sudden infant death syndrome? *Pediatrics* 1994;93:774–7.
37. Moyer-Mileur LJ, Nielson DW, Pfeefer KD, Witte MK, Chapman DL. Eliminating sleep-associated hypoxemia improves growth in infants with bronchopulmonary dysplasia. *Pediatrics* 1996;98:779–83.
38. Gregoire LM, Levebvre F, Glorieux J. Health and neurodevelopmental outcome at 18 months in very preterm infants with bronchopulmonary dysplasia. *Pediatrics* 1998;101:856–60.

39. Southall DP, Richards JM, de Swiet M *et al*. Identification of infants destined to die unexpectedly during infancy: evaluation of predictive importance of prolonged apnoea and disorders of cardiac rhythm or conduction. *Br Med J* 1983;286:1092–6.

40. Southall DP, Richards JM, Stebbens V, Wilson AJ, Taylor V, Alexander JR. Cardio-respiratory function in 16 full-term infants with sudden infant death syndrome. *Pediatrics* 1986;78:787–96.

41. Schechtman VL, Harper RM, Wilson AJ, Southall DP. Sleep apnea in infants who succumb to the sudden infant death syndrome. *Pediatrics* 1991;87:841–6.

42. Kelly DH, Golub MD, Carley D, Shannon DC. Pneumograms in infants who sub-sequently died of sudden infant death syndrome. *J Pediatr* 1986;109:249–54.

43. Kahn A, Groswasser J, Rebuffat E *et al*. Sleep and cardiorespiratory characteristics of infant victims of sudden death: a prospective case–control study. *Sleep* 1992;15:287–92.

44. Schwartz PJ, Stramba-Badiale M, Segantini A *et al*. Prolongation of the QT interval and the sudden infant death syndrome. *N Engl J Med* 1998;338:1709–14.

45. Schwartz PJ. The quest for the mechanisms of the sudden infant death syndrome: doubts and progress. *Circulation* 1987;75:677–83.

46. Southall DP, Arrowsmith WA, Stebbens V, Alexander JR. QT interval measurements before sudden infant death syndrome. *Arch Dis Child* 1986;61:327–33.

47. Weinstein SL, Steinschneider A. QTc and R-R intervals in victims of the sudden infant death syndrome. *Am J Dis Child* 1985;139:987–90.

48. Lucey JF. Comments on a sudden infant death article in another journal. *Pediatrics* 1999;103:812–20.

49. Southall DP, Arrowsmith WA, Oakley JR, McEnery G, Anderson RH, Shinebourne EA. Prolonged QT interval and cardiac arrhythmias in two neonates; sudden infant death syndrome in one case. *Arch Dis Child* 1979;54:776–9.

50. Poets CF, Meny RG, Chobanian MR, Bonofiglo RE. Gasping and other cardio-respiratory patterns during sudden infant death. *Pediatr Res* 1999;45:350–4.

51. Poets CF. Polygraphic sleep studies in infants and children. In: Carlsen KH, Sennhauser F, Warner JO, Zach MS (eds). *New Diagnostik Techniques in Paediatric Respiratory Medicine. European Respiratory Monograph*, 1997;2:179–213.

52. Steinschneider A. Prolonged apnea and the sudden infant death syndrome: clinical and laboratory observations. *Pediatrics* 1972;50:646–54.

53. Little GA, Brooks JG. Accepting the unthinkable. *Pediatrics* 1994;94:748–9.

54. Samuels MP, Stebbens VA, Poets CF, Southall DP. Deaths on infant 'apnoea' moni-tors. *J Maternal Child Health* 1993;18:262–6.

55. Fleming PJ, Bacon C, Berry J. *Sudden Unexpected Deaths in Infancy: The CESDI Study 1993 to 1996*. The Stationary Office, London, 2000.

56. D'Andrea LA, Rosen CL, Haddad GG. Do children with airway obstruction during sleep have significant changes in heart rate during severe desaturations? *Pediatr Pulmonol* 1993;16:362–9.

57. Warburton D, Stark AR, Taeusch HW. Apnea monitor failure in infants with upper airway obstruction. *Pediatrics* 1977;60:742–4.

58. Marzocchi M, Brouillette RT, Weese-Mayer DE, Morrow AS, Conway LP. Compar-ison of transthoracic impedance/heart rate monitoring and pulse oximetry for patients using diaphragm pacemakers. *Pediatr Pulmonol* 1990;8:29–32.

59. Weese-Mayer DE, Morrow AS, Conway LP, Brouillette RT, Silvestri JM. Assessing

clinical significance of apnea exceeding fifteen seconds with event recording. *J Pediatr* 1990;117:568–74.

60. Malloy MH, Hoffman HJ. Home apnea monitoring and sudden infant death syndrome. *Prevent Med* 1996;25:645–9.

61. Poets CF, Samuels MP, Noyes JP, Jones KA, Southall DP. Home monitoring of transcutaneous oxygen tension in the early detection of hypoxaemia in infants and young children. *Arch Dis Child* 1991;66:676–82.

62. Tremper KK, Waxman K, Bowman R, Shoemaker WS. Continuous transcutaneous oxygen monitoring during respiratory failure, cardiac decompensation, cardiac arrest, and CPR. *Crit Care Med* 1980;8:377–81.

63. Dumas C, Wahr JA, Tremper KK. Clinical evaluation of a prototype motion artifact resistant pulse oximeter in the recovery room. *Anesth Analg* 1996; 83:269–72.

64. Bohnhorst B, Poets CF. Major reduction in alarm frequency with a new pulse oximeter. *Intens Care Med* 1998; 24:277–8.

65. Technology overview: SpO_2 monitors with Oxismart advanced signal processing and alarm mangement technology. Reference Note Number 9. Nellcor Puritan Bennett, Pleasanton, CA, 1997.

66. Bohnhorst B, Peter CS, Poets CF. Pulse oximeters' reliability in detecting hypoxemia and bradycardia: Comparison between a conventional and two new generation oximeters. *Crit Care Med* 2000;28:1565–8.

67. Silvestri JM, Hufford DR, Durham J *et al*. Assessment of compliance with home cardiorespiratory monitoring in infants at risk of sudden infant death syndrome. Collaborative Home Infant Monitoring Evaluation (CHIME). *J Pediatr* 1995;127: 384–8.

68. Nathanson I, O'Donnell J, Commins MF. Cardiorespiratory patterns during alarms in infants using apnea/bradycardia monitors. *Am J Dis Child* 1989;143:476–80.

69. Steinschneider A, Santos V, Freed G. Cost implications of event recordings in apnea/bradycardia home monitoring: a theoretical analysis. *Pediatrics* 1995;95:378–80.

70. Brouillette RT, Tsirigotis D, Cote A, Morielli A. Computerized audiovisual event recording documents infant behavior preceding bradycardia/apnea spells. *Pediatr Pulmonol* 1998;26:443.

CHAPTER 16

Mother–infant cosleeping: toward a new scientific beginning

JAMES J. MCKENNA AND SARAH MOSKO

Introduction   258
Clarifying definitions   259
Cosleeping in form, function and outcome   260
The origins of mother–infant cosleeping   263
Mother–infant bed-sharing and breastfeeding   264
Conclusions   269
References   272

'Breastfeeders are three times more likely to bed share and appear to differ from non-breastfeeding bed-sharers on several characteristics. These data do not link bed-sharing to risk of SUDI'.[1]

The findings suggest that it is not bed-sharing *per se* that is hazardous, but rather particular circumstances in which bed-sharing occurs.[2]

Introduction

This chapter examines several important conceptual issues related to the biological functions of mother–infant cosleeping, as well as critical aspects of the controversy surrounding the relationship between bed-sharing and SIDS. A definition of safe mother–infant cosleeping (as distinct from safe and unsafe bed-sharing) is proposed to potentially reconcile and make more precise the nature of discourse in this research area. Just as most researchers accept without question the necessity of distinguishing between safe and unsafe cribs, and safe and unsafe ways to place infants to sleep alone in cribs, we call attention to the need to distinguish between safe and unsafe beds and bed-sharing. Short-term beneficial physiological effects of cosleeping are reviewed, and results from a NICHD-funded behavioral and physiological study of Latino mother–infant bed-sharing are presented to illustrate why blanket recommendations against bed-sharing[3–5] are inappropriate and scientifically unjustified. Data collected among low risk mother–baby pairs provide the basis for speculations that, in otherwise safe physical and social circumstances, routine bed-sharing with breastfeeding might reduce the risks of SIDS among some infants, in some cultural groups.[6–9]

Clarifying definitions

TAXONOMY OF COSLEEPING, BED-SHARING AND DANGEROUS CONDITIONS

Mother–infant cosleeping represents the preferred and obligatory sleeping arrangement for most contemporary people, and under most circumstances this arrangement continues to provide maximum protection and nutrition (through night-time breastfeeding) for the highly neurologically immature and slow developing human infant. As breastfeeding rates push to all time highs in Western countries[10] mother–infant cosleeping is rapidly becoming the arrangement of choice for many urban Western parents, as it appears that breastfeeding and bed-sharing are mutually reinforcing.[1,11,12]

Despite this fact, so variable is the range of 'factors' associated with especially one type of cosleeping, i.e. bed-sharing, which significantly influences outcomes, no single recommendation to bed-share either as a way to reduce SIDS or to enhance the night-time attachment behaviors shared between parents and their children is appropriate at this time; but neither is it appropriate, we argue, to recommend in an unqualified way against bed-sharing, or to advise that infants should 'never' sleep with their parents. Such an unqualified recommendation confuses species-wide normal, healthy human behavior, i.e. forms of mother–infant cosleeping practiced safely by millions of human beings, with dangerous pieces of furniture, and/or dangerous social conditions, and confuses adaptive behavior (cosleeping) with behavioral pathology.

In the context of SIDS and pediatric sleep research we propose that the term cosleeping be used generically to describe a diverse, but proactive, generalized class of sleeping arrangements, and not be limited to any one particular 'type' of cosleeping arrangement as, for example, bed-sharing *per se* (see below). One step toward standardizing a definition of safe mother–infant cosleeping that can be extended to include situations where high levels of mother or caregiver–infant body contact occurs during sleep is to apply the description safe cosleeping to particular 'types' of sleeping arrangements, in which at least one proactive, responsible, adult cosleeper (whether mother or not) takes safety precautions unique to the particular 'type' of cosleeping practiced; and, regardless of whether sleeping occurs on the same or a different surface with another adult present, the cosleeping dyads potentially are able to communicate through multiple, but minimally two mutually reinforcing sensory modalities as, for example, through a combination of at least tactile and visual, or auditory and olfactory, or visual and auditory, and/or auditory and vestibular sensory channels.

Safe mother–infant cosleeping can be applied to bed-sharing situations where the overall bed-sharing context (physical setting and social circumstances including triadic situations) are made as safe as current knowledge permits, and where at least one adult cosleeper/caregiver not only is present, but in addition to being physically capable of potentially detecting and responding to changes in the baby's status, the cosleeper is motivated and willing to do so. Sleep location *per se* such as infants sleeping alone on an adult bed without a parent present *sensu* Drago and Dannenberg[3] and Nakamura et al.[4] is not considered bed-sharing, using this operational definition.

As proposed, a safe cosleeping environment must always provide the infant with the opportunity to 'sense' and respond in turn behaviorally and/or physiologically to the caregiver's signals and cues as, for example, to the mother's smells, breathing sounds, infant directed speech, sleep or breathing movements, invitations to breastfeed, touches or to any as yet unidentified 'hidden' sensory stimuli, whether intended or not. In this way, bed-sharing is not necessarily excluded from being considered one type of safe 'cosleeping' but nonetheless, like other specific 'types' of cosleeping, bed-sharing needs further to be taxonomically differentiated into one of two sub-types: safe or unsafe. Although the same can be said for almost any sleeping arrangement such as solitary crib sleeping, bed-sharing is probably practiced slightly differently in each household. Yet, now we can identify specific, modifiable 'bed-sharing risk factors' as well as 'crib risk factors'[2–4,13] that should help to eliminate unnecessary risk regardless of location or arrangement.

Cosleeping in form, function and outcome

We maintain that sleep location is but the beginning, not the end point, for analysis in studying sleeping arrangements, and that all 'types' of cosleeping must be distinguished by the condition and composition of sleeping structures or pieces of furniture or materials which are used, including characteristics of the sleep surface (hard, soft, fibrous, textured or smooth), and by the bedding materials including infant sleep wrappings, nightclothes and/or blankets, as well as by who, and/or how many people, are sleeping close to, with or by, the infant or child.

Compared with solitary infant sleep, analytically important features of the cosleeping environment are more numerous and more complex. For example, in the bed-sharing environment it appears that the quality of care the infant receives from the caregiver once in bed is partially determined by the nature of their social relationship outside of the bed, which often helps to explain the parent's reasons for cosleeping. For example, mandatory, non-elective bed-sharing by smoking mothers that occurs in socially chaotic households where bed-sharing is the only option leads to outcomes quite different from those situations in which bed-sharing is chosen by a non-smoking mother specifically to protect, nurture and breastfeed her infant, under more routine and stable social circumstances.[1,2,14–16]

Only recently have we started to address the impact of particular adverse circumstances on the bed-sharing environment. Amongst parents of infants who have died unexpectedly in Great Britain the prevalence of alcohol consumption, cigarette smoking and the use of illegal drugs was also higher, whilst the infants exhibited adverse clinical features at birth (prematurity, low birth weight). Moreover, during their short lives these doomed infants experienced more infections and lower daily weight gains, suggesting increased vulnerability from the beginning.[2,17] Treating bed-sharing as a starting point in which risks occur, rather than as a crude end-point, Blair *et al.*[2] found no evidence to suggest that bed-sharing was a risk amongst parents who did not smoke, or among infants 4 months or older (*see* Ref. 1 for corroborating USA data).

In another study in St Petersberg, Russia, compromised maternal attachment was associated with many babies who died while bed-sharing. Physicians of the dead infants indicated that the mothers of deceased infants had been less eager 'to quiet or comfort' their infants in general, and while their infants were being examined (by the physician) before their deaths these mothers 'paid less attention to the baby's responses' and were less willing or likely to touch or look at them, compared with matched control mothers whose babies lived.[18]

PARTICULAR 'TYPES' OF COSLEEPING

Bed-sharing, room-sharing, sofa and recliner use

Bed-sharing is just one of many forms of cosleeping, and while all bed-sharing represents a more intimate type of cosleeping, not all cosleeping takes the form of bed-sharing. Moreover, safe bed-sharing can now be distinguished from unsafe bed-sharing. For these reasons 'cosleeping' and 'bed-sharing' are not synonymous and should not be used interchangeably, a distinction not acknowledged by Drago and Dannenberg[3] and Nakamura *et al.*[4] in their recent condemnation of 'cosleeping' and 'bed-sharing'.

Bed-sharing is complicated because it involves different furniture components sometimes articulated but sometimes not. Adult beds mostly include mattresses, usually but not always surrounded by other pieces of furniture, such as wooden or metal frames. Sleeping in or on a bed represents one of the major contexts within which cosleeping among Westerners is likely to take place. Bed-sharers sleep on at least one, and sometimes two types of mattress, (a box spring under a cloth mattress in many Western societies) although cloth mattresses can sit on the floor without a frame, which for infants may prove dangerous if positioned next to a hard wall or surface. The space between a wall and a mattress can lead to the infant's head becoming wedged causing asphyxiation, a major category of mechanical death reported by Drago and Dannenberg.[3]

In Western societies cosleeping can also occur on sofas, recliners, on child beds, or daybeds, or even while the adult sits or sleeps on chairs which recline, or rock. In some areas in the United States (e.g. Michigan), these types of infant death are lumped into the category of bed-sharing/cosleeping deaths which makes less precise the understanding of the dangers posed by any one sleep environment, and significantly misrepresents and exaggerates the numbers of deaths associated with true bed-sharing. However, cosleeping on a sofa, couch, waterbed or recliner, may be highly risky.[2,4]

ROOM-SHARING AS A FORM OF COSLEEPING

Room-sharing between infants and parents increasingly is the norm in many Western countries and is associated with increased protection against SIDS, although studies showing the protective effects of room-sharing did not include data on the actual proximity of infants to their caregivers, or if mothers were breastfeeding. Nevertheless, depending on whether or not the infant and parent can see, and/or hear, and/or smell, each other, and if the caregiver intends to monitor and respond to an infant, room-sharing can be considered another form of safe cosleeping, although there is, of course, a spatial distance outside of which caregiver–infant sensory exchanges which define cosleeping (as proposed here) are impossible.

Epidemiologic data show that in the presence of an adult caregiver room-sharing infants are four times less likely to die from SIDS than are infants sleeping either alone, or in the same room with siblings[19]; similar results are reported from the CESDI study conducted in the UK, and reported by Blair *et al.*[2,20] Indeed, the CESDI study suggests that infants who sleep in a separate room alone are more likely to die from SIDS than are those infants who bed-share for part of the night, and who remain in the room close to the mother.[2] For example, in a univariate analysis of the CESDI data set, in which separate room sleeping in a cot/crib was the reference group (OR 1.00) with 95% CI, the odds ratio for babies room-sharing was 0.51 (0.35,0.74). Partial bed-sharing was 0.33 (0.19,0.57), while for those infants found bed-sharing the OR was 1.49 (0.99,2.24). The highest odds ratio was calculated for sofa sleeping, 15.79 (4.43,56.24).[16]

SIDS BED-SHARING EPIDEMIOLOGY

SIDS bed-sharing epidemiology and catastrophic 'overlays' occur mostly, (often exclusively) in the context of extreme high risk–infant-friendly adult beds and the elimination of dangerous 'factors' are called for.

Blair *et al.*[2,20] argue against a simplistic analysis of expected 'outcomes' associated with bed-sharing. Using data collected during the CESDI study in Great Britain that includes 325 SIDS and over 1300 controls, Blair[20] proposes an *a priori* epidemiologic model which examines bed-sharing behavior *not as a risk factor itself, but as a particular kind of environment within which specific risks may or may not appear*. An analogy is that, merely because some parents lay their baby in a crib prone with a covered head, loose coverings and a poorly fitted soft mattress, it is not appropriate to conclude that crib sleeping is a risk factor for SIDS, only that there are safe and unsafe ways to use cribs.

No data support the idea that bed-sharing among non-smoking parents increases the risks of SIDS.[21] In fact, similar to other epidemiologic studies, a high percentage (84%) of SIDS mothers in the CESDI study smoked after the infant was born. A high percentage (66%) smoked during pregnancy, (68% afterwards), while 28% of SIDS mothers breastfed their babies for at least 4 weeks, compared with 40% of the controls.[2] This means that it could not be determined if bed-sharing in combination with breastfeeding among non-smoking mothers might prove protective,[2] as our research team has hypothesized. Non-smoking, breastfeeding and bed-sharing mother–baby pairs are consistently under-represented in SIDS populations especially in urban settings, making it difficult to assess the potential protective effects of multiple positive factors which promise, we argue, improved outcomes associated with bed-sharing.

The origins of mother–infant cosleeping

How do we know that 'cosleeping' remains 'biologically appropriate'? The cultural near-universality of the supine infant sleep position, the single most important factor known to reduce the chances of an infant dying from SIDS, can best be explained by understanding that it functions to facilitate breastfeeding, when expressed within the micro-environment within which it evolved: the mother–infant cosleeping/breastfeeding context. That is, the supine infant sleep position evolved in tandem with breastfeeding, and indeed studies show that without instruction the supine infant sleep position by the infant is chosen by the breastfeeding mother nearly 100% of the time, compared with instances in which the infant is placed in a crib to sleep alone.[22] Hence, supine infant sleep likely emerged to facilitate breastfeeding during night-time mother–infant cosleeping.

Human infants appear pre-sensitized, as if biologically 'expecting' to receive sensory signals linking them to a cosleeping partner, to signals such as breathing sounds,[23] chest movements,[24–26] smell of mother's breast milk[22] and touches.[27] All of these factors have been shown to change human infant physiology, including heart rate and breathing patterns in clinically advantageous ways, and to reduce excessive night-time human infant crying.[28]

Indeed, in the absence of an explanation, the best chance of determining how and why supine infant sleep might be protective should begin by first acknowledging that sleep position is but one factor in a constellation of other factors (arousals, sleep stage progression and duration, body orientations, feeding, touching and movement patterns, time asleep, time awake, body temperature, vocalizations) which mutually regulate each other when the breastfeeding mother–infant dyad sleeps in close enough proximity, changes argued by researchers other than ourselves to be protective against SIDS[29](Tables 16.1 and 16.2).

Table 16.1   Effects of bed-sharing on infant sleep**

	BNvs SN	*P* value
Total wakefulness during sleep	↓ 14%	0.008
Sleep stage percentages (of TST)		
% Stage 3–4	↓ 4%	<0.001
% Stage 1–2	↑ 3%	0.036
% Stage REM	—	—
Mean stage durations		
Stage 3–4	↓ 16%	0.027
Stage 1–2	↑ 16%	0.005
Stage REM	↑ 26%	0.001
Waking	—	—
Arousal frequency (per hour)		
Stage 3–4		
EWs	↑ 38%	0.014
TAs	—*	—
Stage 1–2		
EWs	—	—
TAs	—	—
Stage REM		
EWs	↓ 35%	<0.001
TAs	—	—

Table reflects results of 2 × 2 repeated measures ANOVA (laboratory sleeping condition × routine sleeping condition). Entries show significant (*P* < 0.05) effects of laboratory condition (BN vs SN).
*For frequency of TAs in Stage 3–4, there was a significant effect of routine sleeping condition, reflecting 76% more frequent TAs in RB infants, irrespective of laboratory condition. The only other significant effects of routine sleeping condition or significant interaction effects were for percentage Stage 3–4 sleep and total wakefulness during sleep, and these reflected greater effects in routine bed-sharers.
**See Refs 8, 9 and 34.
BN: bed-sharing night; SN: solitary night.

Mother–infant bed-sharing and breastfeeding

From the perspective of the breastfeeding mother–infant dyad, what does it mean to 'bed-share'? Over a 15-year period our research team conducted three separate studies of mother–infant bed-sharing.[6–9,30–35] These empirical studies challenge the validity of many widely-held models concerning what constitutes 'normal and healthy' infant sleep and under what conditions 'normal infant sleep' can be quantified and defined. In our most recent laboratory study our research team quantified differences in the sleep behavior and physiology of 70 mothers and infants. This study involved over 105 separate nights in the laboratory, 155 eight-hour infrared video recordings, and 210 separate mother and

Table 16.2   Effects of bed-sharing on maternal sleep*

	BN vs SN	*P* value
Total sleep time (TST)	—	—
Total wakefulness during sleep	—	—
Sleep Stage percentages (of TST)		
% Stage 3–4	↓ 4%	0.001
% Stage 1–2	↑ 4%	0.014
% Stage REM	—	—
Mean stage durations		
Stage 3–4	↓ 25%	0.002
Stage 1–2	↓ 30%	<0.001
Stage REM	—	—
Waking	↓ 62%	<0.001
Arousal frequency (per hour)		
Stage 3–4		
EWs	↑ 67%	<0.001
TAs	—	—
Stage 1–2		
EWs	↑ 37%	<0.001
TAs	↑ 28%	<0.001
Stage REM		
EWs	—	—
TAs	—	—

Table reflects results of 2 × 2 repeated ANOVA (laboratory sleeping condition × routine sleeping condition). Entries show significant (*P* < 0.05) effects of laboratory condition (BN vs SN). The only other significant effects of routine sleeping condition or significant interaction effect was for the various Frequency of TAs in Stage 1–2, and these showed enhanced TAs in routine bed-sharers.
*See Ref 34.
BN: bed-sharing night; SN: solitary night.

infant (8-hour) polysomnographic recordings as nearly exclusively breastfeeding mothers and their infants shared a bed or slept apart (in adjacent rooms), over three successive nights per pair (*see* Ref. 5 for methods and details).

BREAST-FEEDING IN SOLITARY AND BED-SHARING ENVIRONMENTS

The 'choice' to cosleep specifically in the form of mother–infant bed-sharing was found to double not only the number of breastfeeding episodes, but increase by threefold the total nightly durations of breastfeeding and to shorten significantly the average intervals between the breastfeeding sessions[36] (Figs 16.1 and 16.2).

We have also found that without instruction, the routinely bed-sharing breastfeeding mothers almost always placed their infants in the safe supine infant sleep position, probably because it is difficult if not impossible for the mother to breastfeed a prone sleeping infant. For these reasons, we argued that bed-sharing promotes increased breastfeeding with potentially significant health gains for the baby and the mother, and possibly reduces the chance of the infant dying from SIDS, since breastfeeding while bed-sharing practically mandates the use of the safe supine infant sleep position, at least among Latino breast-feeding/bed-sharing mothers.

Increased protection from SIDS through breastfeeding is not universally established[36] but at least half the studies show it as being protective, and since no two studies use the same definition of breastfeeding, research in this area remains difficult to compare.[37] In the United States a major multicenter epidemiologic study found that 'not breast feeding' was a risk factor for SIDS for both black and white American populations.[38] Only one epidemiologic study,

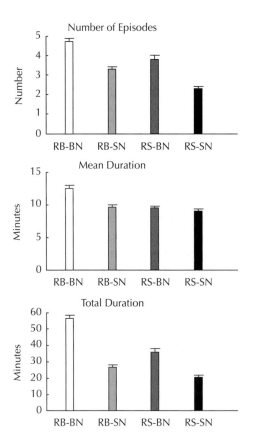

Fig. 16.1 Number of episodes of breastfeeding, mean duration per episode, and total average nightly duration of breastfeeding among routinely bed-sharing and routinely solitary sleeping mother–infant pairs, on their bed-sharing and solitary sleeping nights in the sleep laboratory. Abbreviations: RB-BN (**R**outine **B**ed-sharers on their **B**ed-sharing **N**ight); RB-SN **R**outine **B**ed-sharers on their **S**olitary **N**ight); RS-BN (**R**outine **S**olitary sleeping pairs on their **B**ed-sharing **N**ight); RS-SN (**R**outine **S**olitary sleeping pair on their **S**olitary **N**ight).

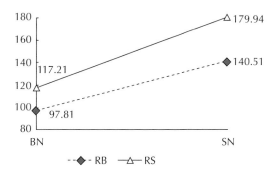

Fig. 16.2 Mean interval between breastfeeding episodes on the bed-sharing night (BN) and the solitary sleeping night (SN) for routinely bed-sharing (RB) and routinely solitary sleeping (RS) mother–infant pairs.

however, has looked at whether dose-specific response effects exist and whether this is stable across races and socioeconomic groups in relationship to SIDS. The data support the possibility that increased breastfeeding leads to increased protection from SIDS. Fredrickson *et al.*[39] found that for both black and white Americans the risk of SIDS decreased for every month of breastfeeding. Conversely, for white mothers the risk of SIDS increased by 1.19 for every month of not breastfeeding, and 2.0 for every month of non-exclusive breastfeeding. For black mothers, the risk of SIDS also increased by 1.19 for every month of not breastfeeding, but 2.3 for every month of not exclusively breastfeeding.

Sleep architecture, mother and infant arousal patterns in the bed-sharing and solitary sleep environments

The differences in feeding patterns between infants in the solitary and bed-sharing environment cannot properly be understood outside of the overall context within which they find expression. Increased breastfeeding is but one factor in a cascade of inter-dependent changes involving arousals, sleep stage duration and progression, mother–baby body orientation and sleep position in bed, breathing and infant crying. These are all mutually regulating factors as mothers and infants sleep alongside each other in bed (Figs 16.3 and 16.4). For example, we found that in general, small EEG-defined transient infant arousals are facilitated in the bed-sharing environment, albeit selectively, and that even when routinely bed-sharing infants slept alone they continued to exhibit more transient arousals than did routinely solitary sleeping infants, sleeping alone[9] (Tables 16.1 and 16.2). Furthermore, bed-sharing significantly shortened the amount of time per bout infants remained in deeper stages of sleep (Stage 3–4) compared with when they slept alone, with increases in the amount of time spent in stages 1 and 2, and more total time asleep.[8] Together, these findings justify our speculation that the increased number of arousals in the bed-sharing environment, coupled with the reduced amount of time (per bout) spent in deep stage 3–4 sleep where

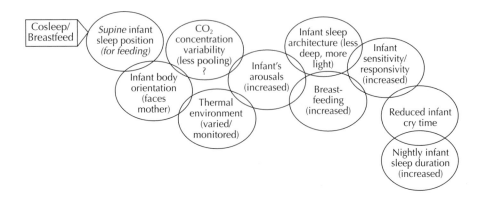

Fig. 16.3   For the breastfed infant, 'choice' by the mother to cosleep sets in motion a cascade of potentially beneficial, inter-related, bio-behavioral effects which double the amount of breastfeeding, and regulates almost every major physiologic and behavioral system. (From the infant's perspective.)

arousal thresholds for infants are highest, may reduce an infant's chances of dying from SIDS, especially among infants born with arousal deficiencies.

We also documented an acute sensitivity on the part of the routine bed-sharing mothers to their infant's presence in the bed. That is, compared to the number of temporally overlapping arousals (in which the infant aroused first), routinely bed-sharing mothers exhibited significantly more arousals than did routinely solitary sleeping mothers while bed-sharing with their infants. This finding argues against the possibility that bed-sharing mothers habituate to the presence of their babies and, thus, may pose a danger to them while asleep.[9,34]

While routinely bed-sharing mothers aroused and fed their infants more frequently while sleeping next to them, on average they received as much sleep as solitary breastfeeding mothers, and infants slept significantly longer than they did when they slept alone.[8,9,34] Moreover, 84% of the routinely bed-sharing mothers evaluated their sleep following their bed-sharing night in the laboratory as being either 'good' or 'enough', while only 64% of routinely solitary sleeping mothers evaluated their sleep as being either good or enough following their routine, solitary sleep night in the laboratory[34] (Table 16.2).

In two earlier studies we found that bed-sharing mother–infant pairs exhibited a trend toward greater simultaneous overlap in all sleep stages (i.e. stages 1–2, 3–4, and REM). This synchronization of sleep states was not explained by chance and is not found when the sleep/wake activity of infants is compared with randomly selected mothers with whom they did not cosleep.[30,40]

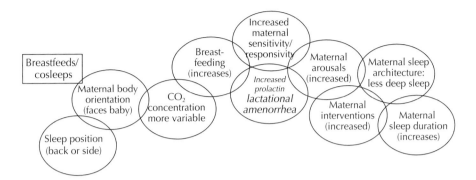

Fig. 16.4   For the breastfeeding mother, the choice to cosleep sets in motion a cascade of short-term potentially beneficial, inter-related bio-behavioral effects, that can in addition to suppressing mother's ovulation through increased breastfeeding, provide long-term increased protection from breast and ovarian cancers. (From the mother's perspective.)

Conclusions

FROM DEBATE TO DISCOURSE

The argument over bed-sharing, i.e. to bed-share or not to bed-share, should be transformed from debate to discourse. Discussions about infant and childhood sleeping arrangements by pediatricians, pediatric sleep researchers, SIDS researchers, health and government authorities should move away from the assumption that a singular recommendation is appropriate, and away from the mistaken belief that bed-sharing (as one type of cosleeping) is a uniform practice with any predictable, singular outcome. To be specific, this new discourse on bed-sharing needs to reject the traditional epidemiologic categorization of 'bed-sharing' as a discrete unitary variable, which carries a fixed, relative risk across all circumstances, leading invariably either to good or bad outcomes.

THE CONTINUUM OF PARENT–INFANT SLEEP PROXIMITY

This new discourse needs also to reject the assumption that any particular sleeping arrangement is necessarily practiced in an all-or-nothing manner, all night and every night, in the same way, throughout each stage of infancy or childhood development across the first 5 or so years of life. Ample evidence exists to now suggest that even where parents consider themselves either cosleepers or solitary sleepers there are often a variety of sleeping arrangements which can vary from night to night, and/or from one part of a night to another.[41–44] *Infants do not sleep in the same place, all night, every night.* In conjunction with the infant/child's changing social, emotional, and cognitive needs and sleep behavior, and changing parental attitude, experiences, and understandings of their own and their child's needs, sleeping arrangements more or less fluctuate (in many families) around what is perhaps best conceptualized as a continuum of parent–infant sleep proximity. This continuum can be conceptualized as ranging from the most intimate, high contact forms of sleeping arrangement i.e. parent–infant cosleeping occurring on the same surface, side-by-side, often with baby-controlled breastfeeding, to infants sleeping physically distant from the caregivers, routinely in a crib in his or her own room, all night, every night. Health educational programs and written materials aimed at teaching parents how to arrange a safe sleep environment should appreciate and accommodate the potential fluidity of sleeping arrangements in any given family. Furthermore, they should entertain the possibility that many, perhaps most, infants are likely to experience diverse sleep locations and arrangements, and, therefore encounter a rich variety of sensory and physical circumstances hypothetically imagined by this model. Sometimes, parents never make a firm decision about where their baby will sleep[41]; however they should be alert to, and made knowledgeable of, the special precautions that they need to take as different points on this continuum of parent–infant sleep proximity is encountered.

IDENTIFIABLE BED-SHARING AND COSLEEPING 'PROBLEMS'

It is important that health and governmental authorities understand that there are different ways to approach and solve the 'problems' or hazards associated with any given sleep environment, and that how, or if, certain hazards are thought worth solving, will depend on one's own values and preferences, as well as on one's own early childhood sleeping experiences, which may differ from the experiences of others. It is not so much tolerance, but respect, that is called for in reaching consensus on relevant areas of this controversy. This specifically involves respect for scientific and parental positions which differ from, and legitimately challenge, the more traditional culturally-based views which disparage and recommend against every and all kinds of cosleeping or bed-sharing. This means that the preparation of written materials on safe infant sleep environments needs to include the participation of diverse health professionals and scientists whose training and experiences reflect the needs of the diverse communities for whom recommendations are intended. Those families who elect to bed-share deserve every bit as much support, encouragement and education as those parents who choose to place their infants to sleep in cribs.

'FACTORS' – NOT PRACTICE

By distinguishing between cosleeping in a generic sense and particular forms of cosleeping such as sofa cosleeping and safe and unsafe bed-sharing, health professionals can preserve and acknowledge the importance of parents and infants sleeping within arms reach (cosleeping), perhaps on different but sometimes on the same surfaces, while simultaneously recognizing that under specific conditions, especially among the urban underclass where most of the bed-sharing deaths occur, specific types of cosleeping can be dangerous; just as placing infants in specific types of cribs under specific types of conditions, in certain kinds of ways (prone, for example) is also dangerous. Hence, there are dangerous conditions – not necessarily dangerous parental bodies.

That catastrophic accidents can and do occur in the bed-sharing or cosleeping environment is not an affirmation of the legitimacy of anti-bed-sharing rhetoric, or evidence that such catastrophes must occur, or likely will occur, for any given mother–infant pair. The existence of catastrophic accidents cannot be used as the argument against all bed-sharing, any more than catastrophic accidents associated with crib sleeping should constitute an argument against all crib sleeping. Risks are dependent on who is involved and how, and why, the practice takes place. One thing is certain, it is only when health professionals and governmental regulatory agencies agree that cosleeping can be a good choice for parents that there will ever be attention paid to designing safe child–adult beds with associated supportive bedding, structures and furniture.

The first step in reconciling social and scientific biases is to acknowledge that they exist. We have argued that scientific and social bias have dominated and severely limited the discourse in regards to the question: where should infants and children sleep? It is hoped that this chapter will facilitate a major shift away from traditional thinking about legitimate sleeping arrangements among infants and children, particularly concerning the larger issue of what constitutes healthy, safe and satisfying infant–child sleep. This shift will include the idea that cosleeping can be one of several 'healthy' choices, especially where parents are provided supportive education as to how to make and practice that choice safely. Educating parents about bed-sharing and crib risk 'factors', rather than condemning either practice, is in our opinion the best public health strategy. Surely, health professionals have a responsibility to provide the type of educational context within which a comfortable exchange of information between interested parents and health professionals can occur. Indeed, a century of psycho-biological studies documenting developmental benefits associated with maternal–infant contact among primates indicate that there is no scientific justification for beginning co-sleeping or SIDS studies with the *a priori* concept that increased sleep contact between the human mother and infant (when in a bed) is inherently dangerous, and likely leads to social, emotional, or sleep-related disadvantages, disorders or death.

While some may choose to solve the hazards associated with crib sleeping, others, including parents, will continue to choose to solve the problems associated with bed-sharing. It is time to respect with equal enthusiasm and resources the alternative values that underlie the choice to cosleep – a time-tested sleeping arrangement that refuses to go away, and for good reason.[45,46]

References

1. McCoy RC, Hunt CL, Lesko SM *et al*. Population-based study of bedsharing and breast feeding. Program and Abstract and Press Release. *Pediatr Acad Soc Annual Meetings* May 5, 2000, Boston, Massachusettes.
2. Blair PS, Fleming PJ, Bensley D *et al*. Where should babies sleep – alone or with parents? Factors influencing the risk of SIDS in the CESDI Study. *Br Med J* 1999;319:457–62.
3. Drago DA, Dannenberg AL. Infant mechanical suffocation deaths in the United States, 1980–1997. *Pediatrics* 1999;103:59.
4. Nakamura S, Wind M, Danello MD. Review of hazards associated with children placed in adult beds. *Arch Pediatr Adoles Med* 1999;153:1018–23.
5. Scheer NJ. Safe sleeping environments for infants: a CPSC perspective. *Program and Abstracts Sixth International SIDS Conference, Auckland, New Zealand.* February 8–11, 2000: Abstract.
6. McKenna JJ. An anthropological perspective on the sudden infant death syndrome (SIDS): the role of parental breathing cues and speech breathing adaptations. *Med Anthrop* 1986 10:9–53.
7. McKenna JJ. SIDS in cross-cultural perspective: is infant-parent co-sleeping protective? *Ann Rev Anthrop* 1996;25:201–16.
8. Mosko S, Richard C, McKenna JJ, Drummond S. Infant sleep architecture during bedsharing and possible implications for SIDS. *Sleep* 1996;19:677–84.
9. Mosko S, Richard C, McKenna JJ. Infant arousals during mother–infant bedsharing; implications for infant sleep and SIDS research. *Pediatrics.* 1997;100:841–9.
10. *Ross Mothers Survey, 1997.* Published and available through Ross Laboratories, Ross Products Division of Abbot Laboratories.
11. Mitchell EA, Scragg L, Clements M. Factors related to infant bedsharing. *NZ Med J* 1994;107:466–7.
12. McKenna J, Mosko S, Richard C. Breast feeding and mother–infant cosleeping in relation to SIDS prevention. In: Trevathan W, Smith N, McKenna J (eds). *Evolutionary Medicine.* Oxford University Press, New York, NY, 1999; pp. 53–74.
13. Mitchell EA, Taylor BJ, Ford RPK *et al*. Four modifiable and other major risk factors for cot death: the New Zealand study. *J Paediatr Child Health* 1992; (Suppl. 1):53–8.
14. Fleming PJ, Blair P, Bacon C *et al*. Environments of infants during sleep and the risk of the sudden infant death syndrome: results of 1993–1995 case control study for confidential inquiry into stillbirths and deaths in infancy. *Br Med J* 1996;313:191–5.
15. Fleming PJ. Infant sleep physiology: does mum make a difference? *Amb Child Health* 1998;4 (Suppl. 1):153–4.
16. Young J. *Night-time behavior and interactions between mothers and their infants of low risk for SIDS: A Longitudinal Study of room sharing and bed sharing.* 1999, Doctoral Thesis, University of Bristol.

17. Sameroff AJ, Chandler M. Reproductive risk and the continuum of caretaking casuality. In: Horowitz FD, Hetherington SM, Scarr-Salapatek S, Siegel G (eds). *Review of Child Development Research*. University of Chicago Press, Chicago, 1975;4:187–244.

18. Kelmanson I. An assessment of the microsocial environment of children diagnosed as 'sudden infant death' using the process inventory. *Eur J Pediatr* 1993;152:686–90.

19. Mitchell EA, Thompson JM. Cosleeping increases the risks of the sudden infant death syndrome but sleeping in the parent's bedroom lowers it. In: Rognum TO (ed.) *Sudden Infant Death Syndrome. New Trends In The Nineties*. Scandinavian University Press, Oslo, Norway, 1995, pp. 266–9.

20. Blair P. Where should infants sleep? Alone or with their parents? *Program and Abstracts of Sixth International SIDS Conference Auckland, New Zealand*. February 8–11, 2000.

21. Young J, Fleming PJ. Reducing the risks of SIDS: The role of the pediatrician. *Paediatr Today* 1998;6:41–8.

22. Richard C, Mosko S, McKenna JJ. Sleeping position, orientation, and proximity in bedsharing infants and mothers. *Sleep* 1996;19:667–84.

23. Stewart MW, Stewart LA. Modification of sleep respiratory patterns by auditory stimulation: indications of techniques for preventing sudden infant death syndrome? *Sleep* 1991;14:241–8.

24. Thoman EB, Graham SE. Self-regulation of stimulation by premature infants. *Pediatrics* 1986;78:855–60.

25. Korner AF, Thoman, EB. The relative efficacy of contact and vestibular-proprioceptive stimulation on soothing neonates. *Child Devel* 1972;43:443–53.

26. Korner AF, Guilleminault C, Van den Hoed J, Baldwin RB. Reduction of sleep apnea and bradycardia in pre-term infants on oscillating waterbeds: a controlled polygraphic study. *Pediatrics* 1978;61:528–33.

27. Field T. *Touch In Early Development*. Lawrence Earlbaum and Associates (eds). Malwah, New Jersey, 1995.

28. Barr R, Elias M. Nursing interval and maternal responsivity: effects on early crying. *Pediatrics* 1988;81:521–6.

29. Goto K, Miririan M, Adams M *et al*. More awakenings and heart rate variability during sleep in preterm infants. *Pediatrics* 1999;103:603–9.

30. McKenna JJ, Mosko S, Dungy C, McAninch P. Sleep and arousal patterns of co-sleeping human mothers/infant pairs: A preliminary physiological study with implications for the study of sudden infant death syndrome (SIDS). *Am J Phys Anthrop* 1990;83:331–47.

31. McKenna JJ. The potential benefits of infant–parent co-sleeping in relation to SIDS prevention; overview and critique of epidemiological bed sharing studies. In: Rognum TO (ed.) *Sudden Infant Death Syndrome. New Trends in the Nineties*. Scandinavian University Press, Oslo, Norway, 1995, pp. 256–65.

32. McKenna JJ, Mosko S, Richard C *et al*. Mutual behavioral and physiological influences among solitary and co-sleeping mother-infant pairs; implications for SIDS. *Early Hum Dev* 1994;38:182–201.

33. McKenna JJ, Thoman E, Anders T, Sadeh A, Schechtman V, Glotzbach S. Infant–parent co-sleeping in evolutionary perspective: implications for understanding

infant sleep development and the sudden infant death syndrome (SIDS). *Sleep* 1993;16:263–82.

34. Mosko S, Richard C, McKenna JJ. Maternal sleep and arousals during bedsharing with infants. *Sleep* 1997; 20(2):142–150.
35. Richard C, Mosko S, McKenna JJ. Apnea and periodic breathing in the bedsharing infant. *Am J Applied Phys* 1998;84:1374–80.
36. Gilbert R, Sigfield RE, Fleming PJ *et al.* Bottle feeding and the sudden infant death syndrome. *Br Med J* 1995;310:88–90.
37. McKenna JJ, Mosko S, Richard C. Bedsharing promotes breast feeding. *Pediatrics* 1997;100:214–9.
38. Hoffman H, Damus K, Hillman L *et al.* Risk factors for SIDS: results of the Institutes of Child Health and Human Development SIDS cooperative epidemiological study. In: Schwartz P, Southall D, Valdes-Dapena M (eds). *Sudden Infant Death Syndrome: Cardiac and Respiratory Mechanisms.* Annals of the New York Academy of Sciences, 1988;13–30.
39. Fredrickson DD, Sorenson JF, Biddle AK *et al.* Relationship of sudden infant death syndrome to breast-feeding duration and intensity. *Am J Dis Child* 1993;147:460.
40. Mosko S, McKenna JJ, Dickel M *et al.* Parent–infant co-sleeping: the appropriate context for the study of infant sleep and implications for SIDS research. *J Behav Med* 1993;16:589–610.
41. Hoffman J. Sleep like a baby: what does that really mean?. *Today's Parent* 1999;16:34–40.
42. Ball H, Hooker E, Kelly P. Where will baby sleep? Attitudes and practices of new and experienced parents regarding cosleeping with their newborns. *Am Anthrop* 1999;101:141–51.
43. Rigda RS, McMillen IC, Buckley P. Bedsharing patterns in a cohort of Australian infants during the first six months after birth. *J Paediatr Child Health* (in press).
44. Baddock S. Bedsharing Practices of Different Cultural Groups. *Program and Abstracts of Sixth International SIDS Conference Auckland, New Zealand.* February 8–11, 2000.
45. McKenna J, Gartner L. Sleep location and infant suffocation; How good is the evidence? *Pediatrics* 2000;105:917–9.
46. O'Hara M, Harruff R, Smialek J, Fowler D. Sleep location and infant suffocation: How good is the evidence? *Pediatrics* 2000;105:915–20.

CHAPTER 17

Taking a strategic approach to SIDS prevention in Maori communities – an indigenous perspective

DAVID TIPENE-LEACH, CAROLINE EVERARD AND
RIRIPETI HARETUKU

Introduction   275
Background   276
SIDS risk factors in Maori communities   277
Why has the Maori SIDS rate not fallen?   277
Strategic planning in Maori SIDS prevention   278
Conclusion   280
Acknowledgements   281
References   281

Introduction

This chapter outlines certain aspects of a New Zealand public health campaign to prevent SIDS in the indigenous Maori community. It discusses the context of SIDS as a priority Maori health area, why SIDS had such a high incidence in this community and why this persisted after the national cot death prevention campaign of 1991. The article then outlines the strategic approach taken by the Maori SIDS Prevention Program and examines some of the issues that seem to have been pivotal in the public health application of research findings to real people in real communities.

Background

Maori are the indigenous peoples of Aotearoa/New Zealand, a tribal people with at least a millennium of indigenous occupation and a more recent 160-year history of a treaty-based colonization by white settlers of mainly British stock. Since the 1840 Treaty of Waitangi, a fairly standard colonial history has ensued, namely, war, appropriation of native lands and marginalization of indigenous communities. Maori presently make up around 15% of the total New Zealand population of 3.7 million. Although living geographically among other New Zealanders in a free-market based Western democracy, the bulk of the population live in the poorer urban areas with distressingly high exposure to under-education, unemployment and poor access to health services. A decade of polit-ically conservative economic adjustment in New Zealand has seen the long standing disparity in Maori and non-Maori health indices widen.[1]

SIDS mortality in New Zealand has traditionally been higher than in the United States and Britain, and significantly higher than Asian countries like Hong Kong.[2,3] Although Maori SIDS rates have been significantly higher than non-Maori,[4] this area of post-neonatal mortality received scant attention until it was postulated that SIDS was likely to be preventable.

The risk factors for SIDS in New Zealand were established by the New Zealand Cot Death Study.[5] The relative risks associated with the prone sleeping position, a lack of breastfeeding and maternal smoking were statistically signif-icant. Further analysis of the data indicated that sharing a bed with baby was also a significant risk factor,[6] although it was later shown to be only in associa-tion with maternal cigarette smoking.[7] These four risk factors account for 82% of all SIDS mortality and they were postulated to be modifiable.[6]

Other risk factors identified in the NZ Cot Death Study were: low socio-economic status, young maternal school leaving age, young motherhood, little or late use of antenatal classes, low birth weight of baby, unmarried mother-hood, young age at first pregnancy, greater number of previous pregnancies, pre-maturity, Maori ethnicity, male sex, and admission to neonatal intensive care unit.[5] These risk factors were not postulated to be modifiable.

In 1990, the Department of Health, with the Cot Death Association and the Cot Death Study team, developed a national SIDS prevention campaign that included education updates for child and maternal health workers and the development of a national media campaign. It was put into effect before and during the winter of 1991.[8] Between 1988 and 1992 the national SIDS mortality fell by 48% from 4.4/1000 live births to 2.3/1000, with the expected decrease in post-neonatal mortality.[4] Maori SIDS rates were twice as high and, during the same period, experienced a more modest fall of 24%, from 9.1/1000 live births to 6.9/1000.

Inconsistent definitions of ethnicity used in denominator (live births/census) and numerator (death notifications/ community-based collection) data made the construction of reliable Maori SIDS rates difficult. Subsequently, gross numbers of SIDS deaths were used as the primary measure by which to compare Maori outcomes with non-Maori. In 1988 there were 197 non-Maori SIDS and this fell to 85 deaths in 1992 – a reduction of 57%. During the same time, the number of Maori SIDS deaths fell (with fluctuations) from 57 in 1988 to 50 in 1992. By this measure, the decrease in Maori mortality of only 12% is considerably smaller than that officially indicated by the New Zealand Health Information Service mortality rates.

Furthermore, the New Zealand Health Information Service at that time used the 'biological' definition of Maori ethnicity, that is, 50% or more Maori blood, rather than the more contemporary 'cultural' definition, where ethnicity is nominated by the subject. It was confirmed, by following up deaths in the community, that many Maori babies who died of SIDS were being misclassified as non-Maori for this reason. This was compounded by the details of many Maori fathers not being registered on the Birth Certificate, particularly where the mother was non-Maori. Using the more appropriate cultural definition of ethnicity redefines some non-Maori SIDS babies as Maori, and reduces the Maori health gain from the national SIDS prevention programme even further.

SIDS risk factors in Maori communities

Among New Zealand Cot Death Study participants, for both cases and controls, the prone sleeping of babies and breastfeeding were similarly prevalent behaviours for both Maori and non-Maori, but smoking amongst Maori mothers was at least twice as high.[6] In response to the SIDS prevention activities a huge reduction in the prevalence of the prone sleeping position was observed for both Maori and non-Maori but no measurable changes in breastfeeding or smoking behaviors occurred.[9] Maternal cigarette smoking is therefore the single most important risk factor for SIDS in the Maori community. It doubles the risk of cot death in an individual baby and accounts for half of the total risk of the population.[10]

In addition to cigarette smoking, Maori households have a high prevalence of multiple risk factors, that is, they are more socioeconomically disadvantaged, the mothers are younger, and the infants are of a lower birth weight.[11] Maori babies are also more likely to share a bed with another person, and where this is associated with maternal smoking, it is responsible for increased risk.[7]

Why has the Maori SIDS rate not fallen?

Philosophically, the 1991 national cot death prevention activities were based around a cheap, minimal intervention, risk reduction concept that provided simple information, and subsequently relied on individual change of behavior. We know that Maori mothers heard the SIDS prevention messages as they took up the back sleeping position readily, but this impersonal and distant approach, although economic, did not allow for community participation in such a way that they ever came to feel any commitment to dealing with the 'difficult to change' risk factor – cigarette smoking. The evidence is that anti-smoking strategies that only promote individual behavior change are not, in themselves effective and need to be complemented by a supportive environment.[12]

In retrospect, it seems that the national SIDS prevention program planners had poor public health advice all round for, there was no development of a Maori health strategy and no funding to address the Maori health need. The widely accepted convention at the time was to give priority to Maori health objectives. This had previously given rise to the use of trained community health workers (CHWs) in the Auckland meningococcal meningitis campaign of 1987[13] and the development of targeted health promotion advertising in the national hepatitis B campaign that began in 1988. Incredibly, Maori community health workers were not systematically included in the SIDS prevention program training update activities. In addition to this, the vigorous promotion of a blanket warning against bed-sharing was perceived in many Maori quarters as intrusive, insensitive and inappropriate.

Maori women have multiple maternal risk factors (young maternal school leaving age, young motherhood), and live in poverty and disadvantage (low socioeconomic status, poor education, unmarried motherhood) and, with poor access to health services (late use of antenatal care, young age at first pregnancy, multiparity), bear compromised babies (low birth weight, prematurity, male sex, admission to neonatal intensive care). All this sits alongside the high prevalence of bed-sharing, valued as a normal and cherished behavior in Maori and in other communities[14] and the sheer addictiveness of cigarette smoking.

Strategic planning in Maori SIDS prevention

While declining deaths were the national experience, the ongoing cases were noted at points of data collection, to be increasingly Maori. After some advocacy, funds from the Public Health Commission came with a brief to employ and support a national coordinator for SIDS prevention in Maori communities and the conduct of a Maori SIDS prevention campaign. The Maori SIDS Prevention Program was launched in March 1994 with a three pronged strategic approach to decreasing SIDS mortality in the Maori community.

The dissemination of SIDS risk factor information in Maori communities began in 1992 with a series of regional and tribal *hui* (community meetings) where the SIDS issues were discussed with mothers, CHWs and community leaders at dozens of *marae* (traditional meeting grounds) around Aotearoa/New Zealand.

Maori language SIDS prevention messages were chosen to be played on the Maori radio stations, two television advertisements were made and there was also a small national television presence. In addition, there was either advertising or articles in all the Maori newspapers and magazines. Pamphlets, posters, training packages and videos as resources for SIDS prevention in Maori communities were also developed.

In workforce development, that is, the training of Maori CHWs in strategies that prevent SIDS and support SIDS families, specific skills training programs in breastfeeding promotion, smoking cessation, grief support and crisis counseling were developed. Maori CHWs were also trained to reorganize their schedule of activities in order that the identification and servicing of at-risk families became a priority.

It was also very obvious that the strategic approach in communities needed to be cognizant of the wider picture of Maori mothers and their children, and of the need to address a wide variety of the so-called 'non-modifiable' risk factors. It was proposed that mobilizing Maori CHWs could facilitate measures to deal with issues like access to care, and that some risk factors, like low birth weight, prematurity, admission to neonatal intensive care, might be avoided. Similarly, that the provision of simple resources like good budgeting advice could help to fill the gaps created by early school leaving and unemployment.

The third strategy was to identify the important disempowering factors in the lives of Maori mothers and babies, and to induce structural changes within primary health care services such that gaps in services were eliminated and families were strengthened and supported. This long-term strategy has involved the collection of data around Maori SIDS cases, a service audit of the subsequent process, the development of a systematic review of those deaths, and a feedback of recommendations to the bureaucracy.

Cigarette smoking was one obvious primary target for SIDS prevention efforts in the Maori community. The initial approach to smoking was to provide a goal that was attainable – *Smoke Free Zones for Babies* was used, and then to provide further resources and support for smoking cessation amongst pregnant women and mothers of babies. Toward that end an auricular mini-acupuncture smoking cessation resource for Maori community health workers was piloted. It is a cheap, easy to use, locally available, repeatable intervention without side effects that is looking, potentially, very effective.

Breastfeeding became an effective vehicle for all the risk reduction messages – 'natural, holistic and under the immediate control of women' and this led to the later development of the Whangai U (professional Maori lactation consultants) and the Ukaipo (traditional Maori childcare) training programs for Maori midwives and community health workers. In addition a 'Maori friendly' video on breastfeeding for mothers and health workers was produced.

In considering the modifiable risk factor messages there was an attempt to construct a useful position based around the support of 'traditional' Maori child-raising behaviors like breastfeeding and lying babies on their backs, and the re-evaluation of behaviors 'influenced or imposed' by the dominant non-Maori culture, like modern beds, sleeping conditions and cigarette smoking.

Later, a strict policy to recommend only change that was clearly consistent with a Maori world view was adopted. This policy caused controversy, for instance, when postmortem examination as a mandatory part of the diagnosis of SIDS was challenged. To the Maori mind the body is tapu (sacred beyond compare) and is thoroughly desecrated by necroscopy and, unless it has a direct SIDS diagnostic value, then there is no reasonable thesis to support the usefulness of the mandatory process.

The team also ran foul of their colleagues in SIDS prevention because they consistently refused to sanction an open message against bed-sharing, believing that it would alienate the Maori audience to whom they were trying to appeal. Instead they opted for 'stop smoking' to be the public media line, with the Maori program training Maori CHWs to deal with the sensitive bed-sharing issues with smoking mothers in a one-on-one fashion.

Successful policy advocacy is based on accurate information and the Maori SIDS prevention team remain well informed, collecting vital information, particularly on ethnicity, about SIDS cases in communities by talking to the families, and to pathologists and Coroners. This has led to the development of the national SIDS Register which is housed in the Department of Maori and Pacific Health at the University of Auckland School of Medicine. This is used to follow up cases in the community as they occur and the team is developing the capacity to operate a national SIDS Register database.

SIDS prevention however, needs to be based in an even wider context and a series of projects have been undertaken that have anchored the Maori team securely in the mainstream of SIDS developments in New Zealand. They have fostered projects as diverse as the development of a SIDS event scene protocol with roles for each acute response worker, the sponsoring of grief resolution training workshops, the expansion of the SIDS Register to include all SUDI (Sudden Unexpected Death of an Infant) and the development of a pilot project for a child health mortality review system.

They have also developed a program of expansion, devolving the activities of the national Maori SIDS prevention coordinator to five new regional Maori SIDS coordinators and their local delegated workers. The regional coordinators are responsible for SIDS health promotion and the training of local health workers, and also for the support of Maori SIDS families. In order to strengthen the support for SIDS families they have developed a SIDS/SUDI Professional Support Team in each of the regions. This team includes the Maori SIDS regional coordinator, the pediatrician, the pathologist, the inquest officer, the local health nurse, the social worker, the counselor and the parent support worker. The team will provide information for a SIDS family, coordinate and debrief the acute response workers, follow up the case to its diagnosis, ensure that the case is reviewed, develop an active local service audit and then ensure that data are stored safely and utilized usefully for systematic mortality review.

A multidisciplinary, multicultural and multicentered team has regrouped to carry out further research into SIDS. Maori and Pacific researchers alongside most of the original NZ Cot Death Study researchers are involved in the planning of this new research thrust. The painful lessons from the previous case–control study are being incorporated into the present research process.[15]

Finally, it is worth saying that the Maori SIDS has dropped significantly. Despite the inadequacies of the NZHIS measure, Maori SIDS have fallen from the 1988 level of 9.1/1000 live births to 6.9/1000 in 1992 and to 4.6/1000 in 1996. This is a reduction of 50% over this period.[4]

Conclusion

SIDS, by its tragically and uniquely quantifiable outcome, has provided an unprecedented opportunity to observe how Maori health outcomes are influenced by the strategic approach taken. The whole process of SIDS death management is designed to suit health professionals and statutory processes with little understanding of the impact on parents and families. The Maori SIDS prevention workers have developed insights and made changes simply by listening to people – the SIDS parents, the families, the acute response workers, the Police, the Coroners, and the grief counselors – and getting them all talking to each other. Although the Maori SIDS Prevention Team began its life as a small information dissemination project, it grew to become a significant player in the SIDS environment and in the child health scene.

The following are the pivotal issues that characterize a community development approach to this problem. Firstly, there was wide consultation in Maori communities and a commitment to a philosophical approach that keeps the program thinking and operating within a Maori world view. Secondly, the management and organizational processes are effective, that is, they are able to advocate effectively in the policy cycle, they have financial accounts and other management processes handled professionally and they are positioned well in the Medical School close to academic resources. In addition, a capacity to run a national health database is being developed and they are facilitating the development of an integrated SIDS/SUDI team of local health professionals in order to establish medical and social support for families and a service audit process. These initiatives have led to Maori SIDS becoming a major focus of public health attention that has attracted significant funding for the project and wide research interest.

SIDS is the worst outcome scenario in child health. The Maori SIDS prevention team have consistently advocated that health activity which addresses the prevention of SIDS is a step towards the development of a Maori well child health service that supports pregnant women and mothers with young babies. This paper shares our understanding of the need for a clearly structured and well-funded Maori approach to health planning in Maori communities. A project designed and promulgated by Maori will be the one that saves Maori babies.

Acknowledgements

We would like to acknowledge the families and workers who take part in SIDS prevention initiatives throughout New Zealand.

References

1. Te Puni Kokiri. *Progress towards closing social and economic gaps between Maori and non-Maori – A Report to the Minister of Maori Affairs*, 1998.
2. Gantley M, Davies DP, Murcott A. Sudden infant death syndrome: links with infant care practices. *Br Med J* 1993;306:16–20.
3. Davies DP. Cot Death in Hong Kong: a rare problem. *Lancet* 1985;ii:738–9.
4. *Fetal and Infant Deaths 1987–1992*. National Health Statistics Centre/New Zealand Health Information Service, Department/Ministry of Health, Wellington.
5. Mitchell EA, Scragg R, Stewart AW *et al*. Results from the first year of the New Zealand Cot Death Study. *NZ Med J* 1991;104:71–6.

6. Mitchell EA, Taylor BJ, Ford RPK *et al*. Four modifiable and other major risk factors for cot death: The New Zealand Cot Death Study. *J Paediatr Child Health* 1992;28 (Suppl. 1): S3–8.
7. Scragg R, Mitchell EA, Taylor BJ *et al*. Bedsharing, smoking and alcohol in the sudden infant death syndrome. *Br Med J* 1993;307:1312–18.
8. Mitchell EA, Alley P, Eastwood J. The National Cot Death Prevention Programme in New Zealand. *Aust J Pub Health* 1992;16:158–61.
9. Scragg LK, Tonkin SL, Hassal IE. Evaluation of the Cot Death Prevention Programme in South Auckland. *NZ Med J* 1993;106:8–10.
10. Mitchell EA, Stewart AW, Scragg R *et al*. Ethnic differences in mortality from sudden infant death syndrome in New Zealand. *NZ Med J* 1993;306:13–16.
11. Mitchell EA, Scragg R. Observations on ethnic differences in SIDS mortality in New Zealand. *Early Hum Dev* 1994;38:151–7.
12. Abel S, Wyllie A, Casswell S. *The primary prevention of alcohol and other drug related problems amongst women: a literature review*. Alcohol and Public Health Research Unit, School of Medicine, August 1992.
13. Lennon, D, Gellin B, Hood D *et al*. Control of epidemic group A meningococcal disease in Auckland. *NZ Med J* 1993;106:3–6.
14. Abel S *et al*. *Infant Care Practices: A qualitative study of the practices of Auckland Maori, Tongan, Samoan, Cook Island, Niuean and Pakeha caregivers of under 12 month old infants*. Department of Maori and Pacific Health, March 1999.
15. Everard C. Managing the New Zealand Cot Death Study – lessons from between a rock and a hard place. *Pacific Health Dialogue* 1997;4:146–52.

CHAPTER 18

Recurrence of sudden unexpected infant death in a family

SUSAN M. BEAL

Introduction   283
Incidence of recurrence in families   284
Causes of sudden unexpected deaths in infancy   284
Disorders with familial recurrence diagnosed as SIDS   286
Twins   287
Genetic predisposition to SIDS   287
Prevention of recurrence of SIDS   288
Conclusion   288
Summary   288
References   288

Introduction

The incidence of SIDS has changed dramatically over the past decade, with many countries more than halving their SIDS rates, as a result of avoiding the prone sleeping position. Accompanying this has been a change in the epidemiology, including changes in age incidence,[1,2] seasonal distribution,[1,2] socioeconomic status[3] and intra-country racial proportions. This means the recurrence of SIDS in families must be re-examined, using data from after 1990, or even later in some countries. Ideally infants found prone or with the head covered, both powerfully associated with infant death, should be excluded. The incidence of SIDS in supine with the head uncovered in South Australia is <0.1 per 1000 live births, so it will require at least national, but preferably international, cooperation to produce significant figures of recurrence.

The incidence of recurrence also relates to family size. With the reduction in family size in many Western countries the incidence of recurrence of SIDS is likely to fall. On the other hand, families who have had an infant die of SIDS often rethink their priorities, recognizing more clearly the importance of children and family. This may increase the size of these families.

Incidence of recurrence in families

PRIOR TO 1990

Prior to 1990, the incidence of SIDS in prior siblings of SIDS victims, most of whom would be expected to be prone, varied between 1.3% (G. Molz personal communication, 1991) and 2%[4,5] and in subsequent siblings between 0.5%[6] and 2.2%.[7] In Norway the incidence in the mother's next child[6] was four in 712 or 0.6%. A review of recurrence prior to 1990 was published in 1992.[8]

SINCE 1990

In the CONI (Care of the Next Infant)[9] study in Sheffield in the years 1988–1996, of 3431 subsequent siblings there were 26 unexpected deaths. In four of these a parent has been convicted of filicide and one case is pending. The remaining 21 'cot deaths' is a rate of 0.6%, which is six times the expected UK rate.

In a previously reported series from the same team[10] excluding explained deaths and deaths with insufficient information to draw a conclusion, 31 of 43 recurrences (72%) were thought to be due to filicide. If those deaths that were partly explained are excluded, 31 of 36 (86%) were due to filicide. This included 9 of 11 (82%) from the 22 health districts included in the original study, and 22 of 25 (89%) of those referred by pediatricians outside the designated health districts.

Between January 1990 and December 1995 in South Australia, the 123 infants who died suddenly and unexpectedly without autopsy evidence of disease sufficient to account for death had 118 prior full siblings and 40 prior half siblings. Of the full siblings three had previously died, one from filicide, one from suspected filicide and one from SIDS. Of the half siblings one had previously died from SIDS. If the filicide and suspected filicide and their siblings are removed, two in 115 (1.7%) of previous siblings and half siblings had died of SIDS. In Seattle, Washington, USA, since 1990, only one family has had two sudden unexpected infant deaths, occurring in a family with known central hypoventilation syndrome (Nora Davis, personal communication, 1998).

Causes of recurrent sudden unexpected deaths in infancy

The two most important factors in recurrence of sudden infant death in apparently healthy infants are dangerous infant care practices and filicide.

INFANT CARE PRACTICES

Parents tend to care for their infants in a similar way, unless a practice can be shown to be dangerous. For example, in South Australia between 1973 and 1997 there were 13 families who had a sudden unexpected death in which a prior sibling had died of SIDS, and where there was no suspicion of filicide or metabolic disorder. Of these 13 families, nine had both infants prone, one had both infants on the side, one family had both infants supine with the head buried under bedclothes, and for two families both infants were sharing a bed.

It is possible that there is a familial susceptibility to SIDS in prone related to an underslung lower jaw[11] or a narrow pharyngeal airway,[12] and this could account for the high South Australian incidence of nine in 328 families with a prone SIDS death (2.7%) having a SIDS death in a future prone sibling. In South Australia over the past 24 years only 50 infants died on the back or side with the face free (if suspected filicide and metabolic disorders are excluded). Two of these infants were siblings (Table 18.1). These numbers are too small for any conclusion to be drawn.

FILICIDE

Filicide is recognized as being recurrent. In one family nine siblings died, several diagnosed as SIDS, before filicide was proven.[13] In other families, although filicide is suspected it may be difficult to prove[14] and if unproven the deaths are likely to be attributed to SIDS.

One of the problems with recognizing filicide is that it is often not suspected until a second 'SIDS' occurs in a family, i.e. the index of suspicion rises with a second death. In South Australia since 1970, 20 families who have had an infant die of SIDS, have had a recurrence of sudden unexpected death. Two of these were proven, four others suspected filicides. In only one of these families was filicide suspected after the first death. The incidence of proven filicide is therefore two in 20 (10%) and proven and suspected filicide six in 20 (30%). In the Wolkind study[10] the incidence of suspected filicide was 31 of 43 recurrences (72%) and in the CONI study[9] the incidence of proven filicide was 4 in 26 (15%) or if the pending case is included five in 26 (19%).

Table 18.1   SIDS, South Australia 1974–1997

	Total SIDS	2nd Sibling	Suspected filicide	Suspected metabolic
Bed-share	61	2	–	–
Head covered	148	1	–	–
Head not covered				
Prone	338	10	1	
Back or side	54	5	3	1
Total	601	18	4	1

Clues to filicide

- Abuse in other infants and children in the family.
- Recurrent apparent life-threatening events (ALTE) in index or other children, especially if commencing in presence of same person.
- Munchausen syndrome in the mother (or perpetrator).
- Reluctance to be visited by SIDS Association counselors (or occasionally obsessive involvement with such associations).
- Suspicion expressed by other family members.
- Conflicting statements about the circumstances surrounding the death.

Disorders with familial recurrence that may be diagnosed as SIDS

CARDIAC DISORDERS

Some cardiac anomalies that may have a genetic basis can be responsible for sudden unexpected infant death.[15] When an infant with a known family history of such a disorder as long QT syndrome, Wolff–Parkinson–White syndrome, or congenital heart block dies suddenly and unexpectedly, other family members, including subsequent siblings, can be investigated for such disorders and be managed appropriately.

CENTRAL HYPOVENTILATION SYNDROME (ONDINE'S CURSE)[16]

This disorder can be familial,[17] and, although rare, it may be suspected from the parents' story after a sudden unexpected infant death. Investigation of future siblings may lead to necessary aggressive management for this disorder. Fatal apneic familial disorders responsible for neonatal deaths[18] could have less acute forms causing post-perinatal infant deaths and may be related to congenital hypoventilation syndrome. The only recurrence of sudden unexpected death in Seattle, Washington, in the past 7 years has been in a family in whom congenital hypoventilation syndrome has been demonstrated in siblings and first cousins (N. Davis, personal communication, 1999).

RESPIRATORY TRACT ANOMALIES

Upper respiratory tract narrowing[11,12] may be familial and could be a factor in some SIDS deaths, and lower respiratory tract dysplasias may be a genetic problem in others.[4,19]

INBORN ERRORS OF METABOLISM (IEM)

Inborn errors of metabolism can result in sudden collapse and death.[20,21] Such disorders are usually recessively inherited, so it is possible that two infant deaths could occur in one family. A search for IEM in 200 consecutive SIDS deaths in Avon, UK, identified two families with IEM, but in both cases these were felt to be coincidental rather than a cause of death. In South Australia, an infant of 5 days of age collapsed and died within an hour. His death was not attributed to SIDS. His sister was subsequently diagnosed as having an IEM.

INFANTILE SPINAL MUSCULAR ATROPHY (WERDNIG–HOFFMANN DISEASE)

Muscle biopsy for diagnosis of spinal muscular atrophy has now been largely superseded and is only used if SSPC gel test is negative. The most common tests now are:

- SSPC (**s**ingle **s**tranded **c**onfirmative **p**olymorphism) gel test; *or*
- mutation analysis.

Prenatal testing is now possible for sibling fetuses.

This disorder is recessively inherited and usually results in death in the first 2 years of life. In most cases, the diagnosis is made during life by muscle biopsy examination after a classical clinical presentation of diminishing physical ability and strength. Routine muscle microscopy is not usual in sudden unexpected infant death, and it is possible that a few cases of spinal muscular atrophy could be classified as SIDS.[19] At this stage of medical knowledge, future deaths from the same disorder in the family cannot be prevented, but genetic counseling may result in the parents deciding to have prenatal testing for further infants from the same union.

Other genetic disorders such as malignant hyperpyrexia[22] and anhidrotic dysplasia[23] may play a role in, or be misdiagnosed as, SIDS in a few cases.

Twins

Too little time has elapsed since the halving of SIDS rates in any individual state for the risk for a twin of an infant who has died of SIDS to be assessed. Malloy[24] reports that in the USA, 1987–1991, of 760 twin pregnancies in which a twin died of SIDS, seven had a subsequent death of a twin. This is an incidence in a co-twin of 0.9%. Over the longer term, including those deaths associated with prone sleeping, the risk for a twin of an infant who has died is probably similar to the risk for any sibling.[25]

Genetic predisposition to SIDS

Rognum[26] has shown differences in DNA sequence patterns of maternally inherited D-loop in six of 24 SIDS victims, but none of 31 controls. Familial traits such as face[10] and upper airway structure[11] may predispose to apnea and SIDS. Apart from this there seems to be little genetic predisposition to SIDS. Several genetic disorders, e.g. central hypoventilation syndrome, infantile spinal muscular atrophy and metabolic disorders may be misdiagnosed as SIDS, and these obviously have a tendency to recur.

Prevention of recurrence of SIDS

Infant care practices are similar for siblings and identification of potentially dangerous practices should result in reduction in both the incidence of and recurrence of SIDS.

Filicide is responsible for recurrent infant deaths. Careful history, including family history, death-scene investigation and autopsy may indicate which families need close follow-up of future children, even if filicide cannot be proven.

Correct diagnosis of the few genetic disorders which may cause sudden death in infancy using specific investigations as indicated by a thorough clinical history, should lead to genetic counseling and appropriate management of siblings.

Conclusion

It is important to try to make an accurate diagnosis in all cases of sudden unexpected deaths, as this will help prevent recurrence in a family. Recognized disorders which tend to recur, such as metabolic disorders, central hypoventilation syndrome and filicide need careful clinical history, death-scene investigation and autopsy using specific added investigations when history and death-scene investigation indicate this. Such investigations may be metabolic, x-rays, toxicology or muscle biopsy.

If no proof of filicide is obtained, but the suspicion remains, it may be better to categorize the cause of death as 'undetermined' rather than SIDS.

The classical SIDS of the 1970s and 1980s, and still the largest proportion of SIDS, is the death of an infant who finds prone position life-threatening.

For the few remaining SIDS, expected to be less than one in 10,000 live births, it will take many years, or international cooperation, to establish the risk of recurrence for these families. The present evidence suggests the incidence of recurrence is less than 2%, which is reassuring for most families.

Summary

Several genetic disorders and filicide can cause recurrent sudden unexpected infant death and may be misdiagnosed as SIDS. Exclusion of these from SIDS diagnosis, and prevention of death due to unobserved prone position, or having the face covered, should result in an incidence of SIDS of <0.1 per 1000 live births. The incidence of recurrence for this group has not yet been established.

References

1. Beal S, Need M, Byard RW. Which infants are no longer dying because of avoidance of prone sleeping? *Med J Aust* 1994;160:660.
2. Wigfield R, Fleming PJ. The prevalence of risk factors for SIDS : Impact of an intervention campaign. In: Rognum TO (ed.) *Sudden Infant Death Syndrome: New Trends in the Nineties*. Scandinavian University Press, Oslo, 1995, pp. 124–128.
3. Beal S. Changes in the epidemiology of SIDS in South Australia. In: *Abstracts of 5th SIDS International Conference*, Rouen, France, 1998, p. 25.
4. Beal SM, Blundell HK. Recurrence incidence of sudden infant death syndrome. *Arch Dis Child* 1988;63:924.
5. Engelberts A. *Cot Death in the Netherlands, Amsterdam*. VU University Press, 1991, 80 pp.
6. Irgens LM, Skjaerven R, Peterson DR. Prospective assessment of recurrence risk in sudden infant death syndrome in siblings. *J Pediatr* 1984;104:349.
7. Peterson DR, Sabotta EE, Daling JR. Infant mortality among subsequent siblings of infants who died of sudden infant death syndrome. *J Pediatr* 1986;108:911.
8. Beal SM. Siblings of sudden infant death syndrome victims. Hunt C (ed.) *Clin Perinatol*. 1992;19:839–48.
9. Waite AJ. Repeat cot deaths in families enrolled onto a support programme. In: *Abstracts of the 4th SIDS International Conference*. Washington, USA, 1996, p. 36.
10. Wolkind S, Taylor EM, Waite AJ *et al*. Recurrence of unexpected infant death. *Acta Paediatr Scand* 1993;82:873–6.
11. Guielleminault C, Heldt G, Powell N *et al*. Small upper airway in near-miss sudden infant death syndrome infants and their families. *Lancet* 1986;1:402.
12. Tonkin S. Sudden infant death syndrome. Hypothesis of causation. *Pediatrics* 1975;55:650.
13. Egginton J. *From Cradle to Grave*. William Morrow, USA, 1989.
14. Diamond EF. Sudden infant death syndrome in five consecutive siblings. *Illinois Med J* 1986;170:33.
15. Schwartz PJ. The quest for the mechanisms of the sudden infant death syndrome. *Circulation* 1987;75:677.
16. Mellins RB, Balfour HH, Turino GM *et al*. Failure of automatic control of ventilation (Ondine's curse). *Medicine* 1970;49:487.
17. Haddad GG, Mazza NM, Detendine R *et al*. Congenital failure of automatic ventilation, gastrointestinal motility and heart rate. *Medicine* 1978;57:517.
18. Vogel F. Sudden and unexplained death of two newborn siblings. *Humangenetik* 1974;22:89.
19. Emery JL. Families in which two or more cot deaths have occurred. *Lancet* 1986;1:313.
20. Hallock J, Morrow G, Karp LA *et al*. Post-mortem diagnosis of metabolic disorders. The finding of maple syrup urine disease in a case of sudden and unexpected death in infancy. *Am J Dis Child* 1969;188:649.

21. Allison F, Bennett MJ, Variend S *et al.* Acyl coenzyme A dehydrogenase deficiency in heart tissue from infants who died unexpectedly with fatty change in the liver. *Br Med J* 1998;296:11.

22. Denborough MA, Galloway GJ, Hopkinson, KC. Malignant hyperpyrexia and sudden infant death. *Lancet* 1982;2:1068.

23. Testard H, Soto B, Wood C. Dysplasie ectodermique anhidrotique. *Arch Fr Pediatr* 1991;48:343.

24. Malloy M. SIDS and infanticide among twins. In: *Abstracts of 5th SIDS International Conference*. Rouen, France, 1998, p. 42.

25. Beal S. Sudden infant death syndrome in twins. *Pediatrics* 1989;84:1038.

26. Rognum TO, Vege Å, Opdal SH *et al.* MTDNA D-loop sequence in SIDS differs from controls. In: *Abstracts of 4th SIDS International Conference*. Washington, USA, 1996, Abstract 2–06–07, p. 96.

CHAPTER 19

SIDS and infanticide

RICHARD FIRSTMAN AND JAMIE TALAN

Introduction   291
The SIDS movement: infanticide as taboo   292
Caution and evaluation   293
The recognition of infant abuse   294
Munchausen by proxy   295
SIDS diagnosis masking child abuse   296
Multiple deaths   296
Single deaths: causes for concern   297
Conclusions   299
Further reading   300

Introduction

The casual observer might imagine that what our modern, acronym-laden society calls SIDS is something of a twentieth-century phenomenon. In fact, in one sense, it is just that. True, babies have always died suddenly and inexplicably – consider the classic biblical story of King Solomon and his sword, an episode triggered by the sudden death of an infant in the night, leaving two mothers to fight over a surviving child. But it wasn't until 1969, when two dozen physicians and scientists gathered on a small island in North Puget Sound, that the world came to call these tragic and vexing occurrences sudden infant death syndrome, thereby giving some measure of medical legitimacy – a label, in any case – to an otherwise enigmatic death.

That same casual observer might imagine that the even more horrifying notion of an infant dying not of unknown causes but at the hands of a parent – the kind of tragedy that seems to pop up in the media with disturbing regularity – is also something of a modern discovery. True again, human history is burdened with the murder of children by their parents, with factors ranging from poverty to insanity playing a role. But not until recent years has the medical community summoned the intellectual fortitude necessary to explore infanticide, and to openly suggest that the murder of babies might be more than a legal matter, but – in its occasional confusion with SIDS – a medical one as well.

These two inscrutable entities of sudden infant death and infanticide – one an aberration of the undeveloped body, the other a riddle of the contorted mind – have lived parallel lives through the ages, shadowing each other, occasionally intersecting, but only recently forcing us to finally confront the reality that they are inevitably attached. For it has become clear that any broad discussion of SIDS must now include the infanticide factor – in spite of how vague it is, but more important, *because* of how vague it is.

The SIDS movement: infanticide as taboo

In researching a book that examines the question of SIDS and infanticide, and in numerous subsequent case reviews, we have accumulated significant evidence, matched by others who have studied these issues, that some unknown number of infant murders – perhaps hundreds a year in the United States alone – occur under the guise of sudden infant death syndrome and remain undetected or unresolved. But which ones are they? How can they be identified, taken out of the SIDS statistics, their parents brought to justice and prevented from visiting the same fate upon other children? And exactly how extensive is this problem?

In many quarters, even considering these questions is a forbidding task, for complicated and sensitive reasons. Since the 1960s, a powerful movement has grown around the industry of SIDS. It is a well-meaning but often emotional bonding of physicians, researchers, social workers, businessmen, and – most significant of all – parents. This movement has done considerable good in raising awareness of SIDS, in advocating for research funds, and in providing information and emotional support to parents who have lost babies to this stealthy killer. At the same time, such a unique merger has led the larger SIDS world to be defined, in good measure, by the politics of grief. A central dynamic of this ethic has been a single-minded desire to protect parents of SIDS victims from suffering the further tragedy of unfounded suspicion. This is a laudable goal, but one that has not come without an unfortunate side effect: it has for many years been regarded as 'politically incorrect' to consider child abuse a factor of any significance in SIDS. Such a black-and-white stance has at times discouraged investigation of deaths whose circumstances suggest something more sinister than SIDS. Its victims, of course, have been children.

Almost from the beginning of the drive to establish SIDS as a legitimate medical entity and to promote research aimed at solving this ancient puzzle – a drive spearheaded by parents of SIDS victims in the 1960s and 1970s – the subject of infanticide was taboo. So, paradoxically, it was during the same decades when physical child abuse was becoming a recognized medical and legal entity, other social forces were making it unacceptable to even consider the suggestion that parents could kill their own babies and blame SIDS. This was largely – and understandably – a response to an era when many parents were unfairly suspected. At the first SIDS research strategy conference conducted by the

National Institute of Child Health and Human Development in August, 1971, the topic was quickly dismissed. A report of the meeting declared: 'Infanticide is all but discredited.' This attitude of denial remains entrenched in many quarters today, and has had two effects. First, it has made ferreting out individual cases of infanticide all the more difficult. Police investigations, including in-depth death-scene reviews, complete autopsies, and questioning of parents, where warranted, have been conducted inconsistently. Secondly, on a larger scale, it has been difficult to objectively evaluate the role infanticide may play in SIDS.

Caution and evaluation

Nevertheless, enough anecdotal evidence is now available to highlight factors and circumstances suggestive of possible infanticide. These elements include multiple unexplained deaths within a family; older children dying without explanation; and maternal behavior consistent with Munchausen syndrome by proxy, a psychiatric entity only identified in 1977. The importance of caution, thorough evaluation and due deliberation cannot be over-stressed. Nor should anyone lose sight of the fact that the vast majority of SIDS deaths are not suspicious. But at the same time, strong circumstantial evidence of child abuse cannot be ignored simply because it is the easiest thing to do. To be sure, justice is one issue. But perhaps an even more crucial consequence is the welfare of siblings in a family in which there has been one or more undetected or unresolved infanticide. The deliberate abuse of a baby is often a repetitive act, and may signal danger for subsequent infants. Recent years have witnessed any number of probable cases of multiple infanticide, suggesting that one or more children might have been saved had those in authority intervened sooner.

The debatable role of parental responsibility in sudden infant death is a difficult and entrenched question. Through the centuries, suspicious eyes have turned toward mothers, though accusation and punishment have generally been influenced more by the prevailing social attitudes of the day, and by ignorance, than by legal or medical reason. In the first century BC, Egyptian mothers who were thought to have even inadvertently smothered their children in bed were forced to hug the dead baby for 3 days and nights. Many centuries later, sudden infant death slowly evolved into a medical question with the development of pathologic anatomy. But with no cause found – despite an unlimited supply of theories, some reasonable, some preposterous – parents continued to be suspected, however unfairly.

By the middle of the twentieth century, it was not uncommon for parents of 'crib death' victims to be recklessly accused of killing their newborns. The birth of the SIDS-advocacy movement in the early 1960s was triggered, in part, by one such incident: when the infant son of Jedd and Louise Roe of Greenwich, Connecticut, died suddenly and unexpectedly in 1958, the local police initially listed the death as a 'suspected homicide.' The suspicion had no basis in fact, and the investigation was soon abandoned. But the experience did contribute to the Roes' decision to found what later became the National Sudden Infant

Death Syndrome Foundation. Four decades later, the innocence of parents remains an ingrained tenet within the culture of SIDS. That is a worthy stance in the 90 to 95% of infant deaths that can legitimately be classified as medical mysteries – as SIDS. Unfortunately, it tends to shield the remaining five to ten per cent from scrutiny.

Typically, this stance has also marked the approach of many pediatricians, who are reluctant to consider that parents could harm their children, even in cases in which such circumstances as multiple deaths within a family or repeated but unconfirmed reports of apparent life-threatening events (ALTE) point to possible Munchausen by proxy-style child abuse. In part, this is a result of ignorance: most pediatricians never encounter such cases, and have no cause to become familiar with this area. But a more important factor is denial: however unconscious, it is the instinct of many if not most pediatricians to do what is necessary, both intellectually and emotionally, to avoid casting suspicion on the parents of their patients.

It is an attitude reminiscent of a time when physicians encountering patterns of broken bones in children drew the conclusion that what they were looking at was a genetic metabolic disorder. In a seminal paper in 1946, Dr John Caffey, a radiologist at Columbia University, wrote that such fractures were the result of trauma, though he, too, was unwilling to state what now is obvious. 'The traumatic episodes and the causal mechanisms remain obscure,' he wrote. Sixteen years later, Kempe *et al.* coined the term 'battered child syndrome.' In this 1962 paper – which marked a seminal moment in our acknowledgement of child abuse as a serious national problem – these authors addressed the question of how pediatricians typically respond to child abuse: 'Physicians have great difficulty both in believing that parents could have attacked their children and in undertaking the essential questioning of parents . . . Many physicians attempt to obliterate such suspicions from their minds, even in the face of obvious circumstantial evidence.' If this is the reaction to *obvious* physical evidence, one can imagine how physicians typically might respond to the much more subtle and largely conceptual evidence that presents itself in cases of fatal infant abuse masquerading as SIDS.

The recognition of infant abuse

Perhaps the classic example of the human impulse to look away involves the case of a Philadelphia woman, Marie Noe, who lost ten children between 1949 and 1968. Nothing conclusive had been found at autopsy, and suspicions by the police did not lead to any resolution. However, many years later, in 1998, the case was reopened and Noe was charged with murder after she gave self-incriminating statements to police. No new facts had emerged; rather, archival medical and investigative records were examined under the light of modern experience, including knowledge of the patterns of Munchausen syndrome by proxy. A similar case of that period involved a Maryland woman, Martha Woods, who was not brought to justice until the seventh death of a child in her care. Her arrest and conviction, in 1972, led to a landmark article, 'A Case of

Infanticide,' by DiMaio and Bernstein, who demonstrated for the first time how easily a parent could disguise child abuse as both SIDS and so-called 'near-miss SIDS.' It is interesting to note that this article appeared in a forensic sciences journal, and the case remained obscure to the vast majority of professionals encountering SIDS.

A new era in the recognition of infant abuse traces its beginnings to 1977, when Meadow first reported the psychiatric entity he named Munchausen syndrome by proxy, a behavior in which parents – nearly always women – fabricated or caused illnesses in their own children to gain attention and sympathy, particularly from the medical establishment. In this and subsequent reports, Meadow and others described methods and outcomes that could vary in severity. An older child might be poisoned or otherwise made repeatedly ill in a way meant to baffle physicians. In severe cases, children might be forced to undergo years of misguided medical treatment and dozens of unnecessary procedures. The ruse, meanwhile, was much simpler when the victim was an infant. Some mothers might report a fictitious life-threatening incident, describing apnea and cyanosis and insisting their babies 'almost died.' Others might actually bring their babies to the brink of death by suffocating them in a way meant to mimic what had come to be known as 'near-miss SIDS,' later dubbed ALTE. Still others might actually kill their babies, intentionally or not. These were descriptions that matched the behavior of Noe and Woods – and in more modern times, of dozens of other mothers whose cases have come to light.

Munchausen by proxy

Throughout the 1980s and 1990s, the pediatric community became increasingly familiar with Munchausen by proxy (MSBP) as documented cases appeared in the literature. In 1987, Southall reported a case in which covert video surveillance was used to document a parent attempting to suffocate her 22-month-old son in the hospital. In this case, suspicion was first triggered when an event-recording monitor documented ALTEs featuring characteristics suggestive of abuse. In two of these, sudden body movements, each lasting approximately one minute, were documented. In the second episode, an oxygen monitor lead disconnected five seconds after the beginning of the event and then reconnected just after the end of the body movements. Reviews of the child's record confirmed maternal behavior consistent with MSBP. Subsequent video surveillance recorded the mother putting a tee shirt over her son's mouth and nose and forcing his head onto the mattress. The incident was viewed in real time, and medical personnel intervened. According to Southall, 'One major cause of "near-miss SIDS" is suffocation' (personal communication). Similar reports have been published in the United States. In one of the first, Rosen *et al.* reported six cases in which video surveillance was used to document parental assaults that might otherwise have been classified as 'near-miss SIDS.' Obviously, had the parents not been apprehended, these children might well have found their way into the SIDS statistics.

SIDS diagnosis masking child abuse

In a recent report, more than 20 years after he first identified the syndrome, Meadow wrote that in some cases, 'SIDS has been used as a pathological diagnosis to evade awkward truths.' He studied the cases of 81 infants who were ultimately found to have been murdered by their parents; in some instances, the true cause of death was found years after the fact, when a second child was abused or killed. In 71 of these cases – 88% – the original diagnosis was SIDS. The term is 'a barrier to the sensible and sensitive investigation of infant deaths,' Meadow said, 'and should be either revised or abandoned'.

The problem, arguably, is not with the SIDS term, but with its sometimes liberal use. The medical community must take more seriously its obligation to sift out those cases that may in fact be accidental or purposeful suffocation, or some other form of fatal infant abuse. While the question of criminal guilt in an infant-death situation is ultimately the purview of the courts, there is an increasingly vital role for members of the medical community: medical examiners, of course, but also pediatricians, nurses, and social workers. All have a responsibility to give the system of child-death review its fundamental integrity. For instance, while it has been said that pediatricians and other clinical physicians have no interest in being detectives, it is also true that the onus is on them to identify and report circumstances, incidents and reasonable suspicions suggestive of child abuse in the case of a sudden infant death. Likewise, it is the responsibility of medical examiners to go beyond the body on the autopsy table and consider circumstances that might clarify the cause and manner of death. Thus, it is incumbent on all participants to become familiar with those circumstances that might warrant further review, and to be willing to take appropriate action. The collective experience of the past two decades provides a surprisingly firm basis for deciding what constitutes a suspicious case of sudden infant death syndrome.

Multiple deaths

First and foremost is the question of multiple deaths within families. Whether SIDS is somehow familial and can strike some unfortunate families time and again is a question that has been debated for many years. However, no evidence has ever been presented to demonstrate that families that have suffered one SIDS death are legitimately at a greater risk of a second, to say nothing of a third, fourth, or fifth. On the contrary: anecdotal evidence supports the suggestion that, as Linda Norton MD, a medical examiner specializing in child abuse, said: 'SIDS doesn't run in families – murder does' (personal communication). In another report by Meadow, 27 cases of confirmed suffocation by mothers were reviewed. Nine of these cases resulted in death, and a tenth left a child with severe brain damage. Eighty-eight per cent had had previous episodes, and 40% had more than 10. Most significantly, two-thirds of these victims had siblings who had died suddenly and unexpectedly in early life.

Some published analyses have indicated a higher statistical risk of death for subsequent siblings of SIDS victims. However, the authors of these studies have never considered serial infanticide as a possible factor, one that may have skewed their data. It should be noted that the previous sentence is not speculative. It is our experience as the authors of a book on the subject of SIDS vs infanticide – and the experience of numerous forensic physicians and investigators who have devoted significant work to consideration of these issues – that a large percentage of reported cases of multiple SIDS, particularly those in which there are more than two deaths, are accompanied by strong circumstantial evidence of child abuse. Many of these cases are eventually confirmed to the satisfaction of criminal-court juries, though others remain unresolved because prosecutors in many jurisdictions are unwilling to bring such cases without a confession, a witness, or a body laden with bruises and bone fractures. Such evidence, of course, almost never presents itself in cases of infant smothering, which have sometimes been called 'gentle homicides'.

One element of this discussion that has received greater attention in recent years is the possibility that deaths attributed to familial SIDS are actually not SIDS but the result of an undetected genetic metabolic or cardiac disorder. For this reason, it is imperative in such cases to conduct a thorough review of the death – a complete medical, familial and socioeconomic history and an autopsy that includes tests for metabolic disorders, which can confirm or rule out such genetic conditions. Excluding from SIDS statistics deaths attributable to inborn errors of metabolism would seem to further erode the theory that SIDS is a recurrent condition.

It should be noted that it is statistically possible, certainly, for a family to suffer two legitimate SIDS deaths. But the same statistics tell us that such a family would be extremely rare, and that a careful review by police and medical examiners is warranted. Obviously, this need would grow with each subsequent death. Such investigations, if conducted thoroughly and properly, would clarify many cases, by revealing either the presence or absence of evidence suggestive of child abuse.

Single deaths: causes for concern

More subtle than cases of multiple deaths are those involving only a single apparent SIDS. Clearly, a death whose circumstances suggest only SIDS – a baby under a year who dies in his sleep, with nothing unusual found after a thorough autopsy, review of the history and death-scene investigation – should not be regarded as supicious. However, certain circumstances should raise red flags. Age is one important factor. It is generally agreed that the death of a child over the age of one year should not be classified as SIDS. Indeed, the vast majority of SIDS deaths occur well before a year – most between 2 and 4 months, and 90% under 6 months. Consequently, the unexplained death of an older child may be cause for concern. Previous family history, clinical history and socioeconomic and death-scene circumstances should be carefully reviewed. Some such cases may be clarified by the history. For instance, when a child over the age of one year dies after a history of being repeatedly rushed to emergency rooms with reports of apnea and cyanosis, which are then unconfirmed by medical personnel, consideration should be given to Munchausen by proxy and child abuse. Additionally, the caretaker's description of the events surrounding the death should be carefully scrutinized.

In one case investigated by the authors, a 2-year-old child died after just such a history. From an early age, she was repeatedly rushed to the local emergency room, with her mother reporting that she had stopped breathing and turned blue. The mother told one physician that between this child and an older sibling, she had performed 80 resuscitations at home. Tellingly, she said that the episodes with the older child stopped 2 weeks after his sister was born – when hers began. The father of the children confirmed that he had never been present during these episodes. Despite the suspicions of several physicians, intervention by child welfare authorities and police was undermined by a senior physician who disagreed with the Munchausen by proxy diagnosis and instead installed a pacemaker in the child at the age of approximately one year. Following this surgery, emergency room visits continued, though physicians were unable to find a cause of the supposed life-threatening events. In the final visit, the child was brought in unconscious and died 4 days later. Under questioning by police, the mother admitted to having previously pressed her child's face against her chest, but denied causing her death. She said that on the day of the fatal episode, she left the room for a moment, and when she returned, her daughter 'was having one of her spells,' which did not respond to resuscitative efforts.

The medical examiner in this case took an essentially agnostic view in listing the manner of the child's death as 'undetermined.' However, the mother's explanation was refuted by a second forensic pathologist, employed by the police, who found her account inconsistent with the child's body temperature when she was brought to the emergency room. It indicated that the 'spell' had occurred much earlier than she said. The pacemaker was also found to be working properly. In addition, the pathologist reviewed the child's troubling clinical history and considered her age, advising investigators that the case was highly suggestive of homicide and should be pursued further. The mother was eventually charged with homicide. (Nevertheless, in an interview with the authors, the senior attending physician referred to the 2-year-old's death as a SIDS, employing the kind of denial noted earlier.)

This case points up a number of crucial elements in the consideration of infanticide and SIDS. One of these may be summed up in the words of Janice Ophoven MD, one of the nation's leading pediatric forensic pathologists:

In my years of evaluating the deaths of children, there is one underlying concern that, when it presents itself, is very worrisome, and that is when there is a dead child and the story doesn't make sense. When the answers do not make medical sense then you would be making as serious a mistake not considering the possibility of foul play as it would be to say, 'Oh, I just really don't want to call this cancer. Just think how the family's going to feel.' (Personal communication).

In light of the many similar case histories in the literature, the case at hand was an obvious instance of probable child abuse – and arguably a preventable death.

Another issue illustrated by this case is the role of the medical examiner. Within this discipline are two basic views about how infant death cases should be handled. In one camp are those who believe infant deaths are no different than adult deaths; that is, the medical examiner has only one job, and that is to objectively report what is seen at autopsy, without regard to surrounding circumstances. The second camp takes a more activist approach. These medical examiners, many of whom specialize in child abuse, take the view that infant deaths are unique and require a more complex – and sometimes daring – appraisal. Most significant to this view is the fact that suffocation and SIDS are virtually indistinguishable at autopsy, and so the postmortem examination is typically the *least* important part of an infant abuse case. With absent signs of physical abuse the autopsy will be inconclusive. More important are circumstances such as those highlighted by the case at hand: age of the child, maternal behavior, family history, death-scene reports, etc. In the case above, the medical examiner chose to omit these factors from his finding. He listed the cause of death simply as 'hypoxic ischemic encephalopathy due to an apparent life threatening event', and offered no opinion indicating fatal abuse was even considered. The forensic pathologist consulted by police, on the other hand, reached his conclusion on the basis of all the information at hand.

Conclusions

The question of suspicion has historically swung like a pendulum: an era when unexplained infant deaths are routinely considered probable homicides is followed by a period when such a thought is 'verboten'. Such an all-or-nothing attitude is obviously simplistic and unproductive. Now we have arrived at a time when ambiguity is acceptable – a place to start.

Ultimately, medical as well as legal authorities must take care to avoid the kind of cruel and reckless suspicion that marked earlier eras, while still thoroughly investigating cases suggestive of child abuse. No doubt some cases will continue to challenge, or even defy, the best efforts to distinguish SIDS from infanticide. But there is also no doubt that enough knowledge now exists to significantly reduce that number. Unfortunately, authorities in many cases fail to take advantage of that knowledge. In 1996, a multi-agency task force of the government of the United States issued guidelines intended to help pathologists, medical examiners, and coroners detect child abuse as well as other causes when dealing with deaths customarily attributed to SIDS. Other task forces and investigators have helped develop standards and protocols for establishing whether a particular infant death is more or less likely to be the result of abuse.

Further reading

1. DiMaio DJ, DiMaio VJM. *Forensic Pathology*. CRC Press, Boca Raton, 1989.
2. Hausfater G, Blaffer Hardy S. (eds). *Infanticide: Comparative and Evolutionary Perspectives*. Aldine Publishing Company, New York, 1984.
3. Reece RM. *Child Abuse: Medical Diagnosis and Management*. Lea & Febiger, Philadelphia, 1994.
4. Boros SJ, Brubaker L. *Munchausen Syndrome by Proxy: Case Accounts*. FBI Law Enforcement Bulletin, June 1992.
5. Emery JL. Families in which two or more cot deaths have occurred. *Lancet* 1986;1:313–15.
6. Foreman DM, Farsides C. Ethical use of covert videoing techniques in detecting Munchausen syndrome by proxy. *Br Med J* 1993;307:611–13.
7. Hunt CA. Sudden infant death syndrome and subsequent siblings. *Pediatrics* 1995;95:430–2.
8. Kelly DH, Shannon DC, O'Connell C. The care of infants with near-miss sudden infant death syndrome. *Pediatrics* 1978;61:511–14.
9. Krugman, Richard D *et al*. Committee on Child Abuse and Neglect. Distinguishing sudden infant death syndrome from child abuse fatalities. *Pediatrics* 1994;94.
10. Meadow R. Munchausen syndrome by proxy - the hinterland of child abuse. *Lancet* 1977;ii:343–5.
11. Meadow R. Suffocation, recurrent apnea and sudden infant death. *J Pediatr* 1990;117:351–7.
12. Norton L. Child abuse. *Clin Lab Med* 1983;3:321–42.
13. Oren J, Kelly DH, Shannon DC. Identification of a high-risk group for sudden infant death syndrome among infants who were resuscitated for sleep apnea. *Pediatrics* 1986;77:495–9.
14. J Kelly DH, Shannon DC. Familial occurrence of sudden infant death syndrome and apnea of infancy. *Pediatrics* 1987;80:355–8.
15. Rosen CT *et al*. Two siblings with recurrent cardio-respiratory arrest: Munchausen syndrome by proxy or child abuse? *Pediatrics* 1983;71.
16. Southall DP *et al*. Apnoeic episodes induced by smothering: two cases identified by covert video surveillance. *Br Med J* 1987;294:1637–41.
17. Southall DP *et al*. Covert video recordings of life-threatening child abuse: lessons for child protection. *Pediatrics* 1997;100:537–60.
18. Steinschneider A. Prolonged apnea and sudden infant death syndrome: clinical and laboratory observations. *Pediatrics* 1972;50:646–54.
19. Talan J, Firstman R. *The Death of Innocents*. Bantam, 1997.

CHAPTER 20

SIDS years later – how families survive

DEBBIE GEMMILL

Introduction   301
Marriage and relationships   302
Surviving and subsequent children   304
How lives change   306
How research affects us   308
How we remember   309
Revisiting a loss   309

Introduction

I live in a brush fire danger zone in Southern California. From midsummer through to late autumn we sniff the air when we pick up the morning newspaper, wondering where and when the next fire will be. We have reason to worry. We have seen the destruction.

Two years ago a small brush fire quickly grew and hopscotched into an established neighborhood a few miles from ours. We could see the huge black clouds from our home, and we worried about the speed and the direction of the wind. We were glued to the television, watching as the fire spread rapidly.

A good friend of mine lives in that neighborhood. She wasn't home when the fire started, and once her family learned of it, the neighborhood had been evacuated and there was nothing she could do.

It was a terrible fire, destroying 51 homes and taking the life of one man. My friend's house miraculously survived intact, while those quite close to hers were completely destroyed. She felt grateful, she said, but also stunned by the randomness of terrible things.

Six months later we walked the hillside behind her house which had been completely blackened by the fire. We climbed carefully through the ruins; trees that had been tall and majestic were just charred skeletons. Bushes and shrubs were just sticks poking out of the ashen gray ground. How quickly things change, we said; how at morning you have a view of everything beautiful, and how in the afternoon you can't see anything because of the smoke from a fire. How frightening it is to wonder what it is you will see when the smoke clears.

How does anyone survive this destruction, we wondered out loud. How do people rebuild, reconstruct? How do we manage to live after loss? *And how,* my friend whispered to me as we walked through the remains of what was once beautiful, *does anyone survive the loss of a child?*

It's a question I've been asking myself for nearly 18 years, since the death of my son Tyler from sudden infant death syndrome. The answers are as personal as our grief, but the more I thought about it the more questions I had. Clearly, we have survived, but both the tragedy of losing our son, as well as surviving his death have changed us. How? I wonder.

I began to ask my long time SIDS support group friends. *How has your life changed? How would our lives be different had our children lived?* It was a topic worth exploring, I quickly discovered. Just how does the death of a child affect us individually, as a family, as a society? There's a saying that one child's death affects 100 people. Who are those people and how have they been changed?

What kinds of things change long after it appears to the outside world that we have recovered? My questions soon expanded outside my SIDS group by way of a questionnaire circulated through newsletters and the internet, and the responses came pouring in. SIDS families whose loss ranged from 2 to 40 years ago were eager to share and grateful for the opportunity to try to explain just what their child's life and death has meant to them. As one mother said, 'This is the first time in 28 years anyone has asked me about her. It's like she never existed to anyone but me.'

I asked 15 questions, the major ones dealing with the effects on a marriage and friendships, surviving and subsequent children, decisions about education and/or vocation, personal philosophy and their reaction to current SIDS research. This is not intended to be a scientific study, but an opportunity for SIDS families to share their experiences as they have learned to live after loss. Their stories are both inspirational and heartwrenching; tragic and hopeful.

Marriage and relationships

Within 2 weeks of our son's death, my husband and I visited our pediatrician. We'd received a copy of Ty's autopsy and we had many questions about the terminology. Mostly, I guess, we wanted to know *why* he had died. If there were an answer, surely it would be on these several typewritten pages.

Ty's doctor was a good one, a kind and compassionate man, a father himself. He read over the report, assured us that there was nothing we had missed as parents, (or that he, as a doctor, had missed) and then went on to talk to us about grief and marriage. He told us to keep an eye on one another, to talk about our feelings, to call him if we needed to talk. Then he gave us our term allotment for grieving: 'You should be feeling pretty much back to normal in 3 months. If you are not, call me.'

We thanked him for his time, gathered the story of our son's death as told by a coroner, and went home. Exactly 3 months later, sitting across from one another at the kitchen table, John and I peeked over the morning newspaper. 'Are you back to normal?' he asked. 'No,' I answered. 'And you?'

Of course we weren't, because the process of grief takes much longer than 3 months. No time sentences, no progress reports can accurately measure the toll that losing a child will take on a marriage. We were able to smile that morning because we had already realized and accepted that this journey through grief was not a straight line, and that there would be no marker to tell us when it was over. We have been one of the fortunate couples, but it was not easy. And it's not easy for any of us.

I've been curious about grief and its effect on marriage ever since that first person told me, shortly after my son's death, that most marriages fail after the death of a child. The statistics varied, but they ranged from 40 to 90%! *Great,* I thought, *I've lost my son, and now I'm going to lose my husband too.*

It's certainly true that a tragedy of this kind will impact on a marriage, and sadly many of the questionnaire respondents reported that their marriages did indeed end in divorce. Most reported that there were problems in the marriage to start with, and there was simply not enough strength to endure the weight of grief. The death of their child was, in many of their own words 'simply the last straw.' Here are some of their comments:

'At the time of my son's death, I was already in a bad marriage. His death was the breaking point.'

'Our daughter's dying seemed to magnify every single difference in our personalities. You can overlook those differences in day-to-day happenings, but how can you overlook them in a tragedy like this?'

'We found ways to escape reality, and without reality we could not stay with each other.'

'We grew farther apart because he could not share his grief with the rest of the family . . . we are now divorced.'

A dad shared: 'My grief forced the divorce. I did all I could to help my wife but neglected to get help myself.'

Most agreed that SIDS was not the cause of their failed marriages, but losing a child suddenly and unexpectedly and facing the issues surrounding grief were more than the relationship could bear. One father, however, was clear in his opinion that the aftermath of SIDS was the only reason his marriage failed. 'I fought it all the way,' he said, 'but she said that looking at me was just a reminder of what we had lost.' They separated immediately, and divorce soon followed.

Those who reported that their marriages had survived were a mixed group. Many said they felt their marriages had been made stronger because they had survived together. Losing the most mutually precious person in their lives – their child – often made them realize the depth of their commitment to one another.

But that wasn't always the case. Others said things have never been the same, and not for the better.

'We're together, but only because we agreed not to talk about it.'

'We stayed together,' one mother said, 'but I am more distant. I can't get close.' Reading further, I better understood: 'My husband told me I killed her. I believed him until this year.' Their baby died 11 years ago.

Recognizing that men and women often grieve differently was the first step for many of the couples who remained together. Support groups were often cited as a valuable tool in understanding the different ways in which men and women deal with loss and resultant grief. Meetings were sought out and attended more often by women, but both men and women remarked that being in a group of SIDS parents helped them better understand what one another was experiencing. Even when attended separately, group support meetings seemed to help. 'Just knowing other people survive this helped us survive it,' one mother said. 'In my meetings I heard other women talk about how their partners didn't seem to understand their need to talk and cry. That made me feel less alone, and made me realize my husband was not "the bad guy".'

A father shared this: 'When I heard other women say that their arms ached and that they sometimes thought they heard babies crying, I understood that what my wife was going through was not crazy.'

And another father: 'Up till our support group meeting, we'd felt that we were alone on an island. Meeting with other families gave us a feeling that we belonged somewhere, at least for a while.'

With few exceptions, those who participated in the survey came to this conclusion: *Men and women grieve differently.* It wasn't however, always the woman who talked and cried, and the man who kept it all inside. Both sexes reported instances of 'hiding out from grief' at their jobs or hobbies, and many said their personal ways of grieving changed from day to day. As one mother said, 'I'd have a sad day; he'd have a good day. The problem was we never knew what kind of day the other one was having.'

Because these parents lost their children several years ago, they seem to have the perspective now to see what they did and why they did it. They are eager to offer their hard-earned knowledge to newly bereaved parents. *No two people grieve the same way,* they stress. *There is no right way or wrong way. We all do it differently.*

Learning to understand and respect those differences makes all the difference, according to one father. 'She did it her way, I did it mine. We knew, somehow, we'd be okay.'

Not all marriages were 'okay'; 30 of the approximately 200 people who responded to the questionnaire reported their marriages had ended in divorce at some point after their child's death. But for those whose marriages survived, the overwhelming response was that the relationship had been made stronger and more compassionate. They had survived what had felt like the unsurvivable, and in Nancy Maruyama's words, '. . . we survived because of one another.'

Surviving and subsequent children: how parenting changes

It is impossible to put the death of a child 'behind you', especially when there are other children to parent. How can you be a 'normal' parent when you know that an apparently healthy baby can die suddenly and unexpectedly, with no warning at all? How can you take naps and quiet cribs for granted, when one moment you are a parent, and the next you are the parent of a dead baby? How can you trust well-baby checks, when within the week your child dies during the night? How could you ever let your child ride a bike, go swimming, leave your sight when you know that no matter what you do, children die?

These were the reactions of parents who have surviving children and face the challenge of ongoing nurturing and responsibility for those children. While almost all of the parents who responded said that they worked hard to be 'normal' parents after having lost their baby, almost all of them admitted it was, at best a daunting task. Overall, they felt less confident in their parenting abilities, less able to 'see' if anything is wrong, and certainly less trusting that even if they do their best, their children will be safe. For those with surviving children, it's not necessarily SIDS that's the issue; it's *everything else* that could go wrong.

Some of their comments:

'I'm very overprotective; they don't go anywhere without me. I know they are past the age of SIDS, but I also know that *my* children can die, and I know how terrible that grief is.'

'I spoil my kids. I give them everything, and as a result they do not respect me. I feel like I have to make it up to them and to the world (because) I couldn't save the baby.'

'The uncertainty – the fact that there is no answer, no solution, no prevention. How do we know that it won't happen again?'

Not everyone felt this way. 'The worst has already happened,' said one mother. 'It can't happen again. I'm not going to let my son's death ruin my other children's lives.'

And then there is the issue of subsequent children. The decision to have a child is a serious one for most people, but for those who have lost a child to SIDS, the issues surrounding that decision are often filled with unanswerable questions. Dare we have another baby? Will this baby live? Should we do anything differently? Will I be able to be a *normal* parent?

Nancy Eckert recalls her pregnancy as a time of 'sunlight and shadows.' 'I felt a little sorry for our new baby in that with each previous pregnancy there had been so much joy and anticipation. This time every time we felt happiness about the new life coming, we were hit with the sad reminder of the life we'd lost.'

Parents state fear and a sense of disloyalty as the main emotions surrounding their decision to have another child. Fear that SIDS might strike again. Fear that their desire to have another child means they are trying to replace the baby who died. Fear they won't be able to love the new baby as much as the baby they lost; fear that they will. They worry about being worried, and how their anxiety might affect their subsequent children.

'I probably wasn't a very good mother for the first few months of my subsequent daughter's life. I was afraid to leave her alone even with my husband. I had anxiety attacks and rarely slept.'

When asked how they felt the SIDS death has affected their surviving and subsequent children, many parents made the same comment. The baby who died remains a part of their family and an integral part of their family's history. As a result, in one mother's words: 'My children know they had a brother who died.

They know that babies can die. I guess that means they've lost some innocence, but they also have the understanding that even though a child dies . . . even a very small child . . . the love we have for them remains.'

How lives change

I have never talked to a SIDS parent who said their lives have not been altered in some way by the death of their child. *My life will never be the same,* I remember crying out loud at a support group meeting. The other members replied: *You are right, it never will.*

And it hasn't been the same. At the time, I'd expected that it would change for the worse. I was already feeling cynical, less trusting, and very much against the idea that anything good could come from my son's death.

I was not alone in my feelings. Many of the parents who responded said similar things, and many of them reported changes in their lives that proved those early predictions to be wrong. Some of the changes were often silent and hard for others to notice, but for some people the loss of their child resulted in very noticeable life changes.

This was particularly evident when it involved educational and/or vocational paths. A few parents reported giving up 'nicely paying, but high stress jobs' that had previously kept them away from their families. Several went back to school to become nurses, social workers, teachers, and grief counselors. One SIDS dad wrote that he returned to school to earn both a bachelors and graduate degree in social work. A mother who had been a registered nurse went back to school to become a family nurse practitioner so she could educate new families about prenatal and postnatal care. Another mother entered the seminary and is now a minister. Each one of these people cited their experience with having lost their child as the impetus for making what they considered to be meaningful, valuable changes in how they've chosen to spend their lives.

Many reported getting involved in local or national SIDS organizations in an effort to offer support to new families and to promote education and awareness of SIDS to the general public.

Chris and Dick Elliott lost their son Michael in 1973 and spent the following two years not knowing the cause of Michael's death. Determined that other families would not have to experience the same thing, Chris became active in providing support to local SIDS families and in educating the community about SIDS. Her enthusiasm and compassion brought her to the state level, where she became the first chair of the legislatively mandated California State SIDS Advisory Council. She continues today to rally for parent support and public education.

Chuck and Deb Mihalko established the SIDS Network to ensure that SIDS information and counseling was available, and that support services were provided to those affected by SIDS, including parents, extended family, friends, daycare providers, and foster parents, as well as professionals such as medical personnel, clergy, funeral directors and the community at large. Established as a local support group in Connecticut, the SIDS Network's efforts literally went worldwide when the Mihalkos created a website in 1995. At this writing, the site has been visited nearly 3 million times, providing support and education to countless individuals and groups internationally.

Barry Brokaw, a SIDS dad in California, and at the time, aide to Senator Daniel Boatwright, used his experience to help write and pass legislation which not only benefited SIDS families through education and services, but also provided a model for other states to follow.

Ned Balzer, a father who lost his first son, Willie, to SIDS in 1993, was looking for a thesis project in computer science that would combine some computer technology with something he knew about. The result was a SIDS listserver, which Ned envisioned as an opportunity for parents and professionals to communicate with one another. Its debut was in December 1995, and it currently has over 200 subscribers. It provides information and peer support to families all over the world who may not have access to local support groups, as well as an opportunity for parents to ask medical and research questions of the professionals who participate.

Gail Greener's 5-week-old son, Scott, died in 1990. She remembers her rage at the unfairness of his death. She credits family, friends and her church in giving her the strength to go on, and to volunteer as a peer contact for other Chicago area SIDS families. She recalls a strong draw to return to school. Five years later, she graduated with a Masters in Divinity, and is now an ordained minister working as a hospital chaplain. It is a result of her son's death, she says.

'I am able to minister to those in pain, because I too have been acquainted with pain. I have been able to work through my grief and in doing so have learned how to help others through grief.'

Several parents became active in their local support groups. They were grateful for the help they'd received and wanted to give something back. They set up golf tournaments, walkathons, auctions and many other fundraising events. They made themselves available as public speakers to spread SIDS awareness.

Many said there was no support group available for them, and because of that, some of them went on to form groups.

Why do all of this? Their reasons were varied, but I think it all came down to the same thing. As Deb Mihalko quietly told me, 'When we meet our Meg again, we want to be able to tell her we did all we could so that no more babies would die.'

In Gail Greener's words: 'I learned an incredible lesson from my son. I learned about my gifts. Scott was a blessing to me not only in his life, but in his death as well. I am not saying that his death was a blessing. I'm saying that a blessing came out of this little boy that I could never have foreseen.'

Not everyone, of course, had life changes this dramatic. When asked about how their personal philosophy or faith had been affected, most of the responses seemed quietly thoughtful. Many said they examined their faith system, had many questions of God, some expressed some strong anger that God had let them down.

Did they think they were better people now? Again, another mixed reaction. Most reported that they felt more sensitive, more caring, more appreciative of the little things. But a few were notably angry, even after many years, and feel that their child's death has made them more cynical and more judgmental. Some say they are still unable to hold a baby or be around newborns, even in their families.

How research affects us

I was in my garden pulling weeds one day when my backfence neighbor popped her head over the fence and said, 'Oh, Deb, I just heard what causes SIDS. Did you see the evening news?'

In nearly 18 years I have heard a lot about 'what causes SIDS'. I have listened with a careful ear, and as it turns out so have most of the families who answered the questionnaire. Most of them experienced SIDS long before the current risk reduction factors were reported; their babies died long before the Back-to-Sleep campaign was launched. I asked how current research findings have affected them.

'When the Back to Sleep campaign came out, I went into a spiral of depression, convinced I had killed my daughter because I let her sleep on her tummy. I am not yet convinced that I didn't do something wrong.'

'We had been told it was nothing we did, nothing we could have done, that it was not our fault. I never thought I was at fault and was convinced I did not cause his death. Now I know I did.'

This is a small sampling, but I wonder how many parents now struggle over what they might have done differently and if it might have made a difference. Despite the ongoing efforts to prevent risk factors as just that – *factors, not causes* – we wonder how things might have been had we had that information then. There's no way to know, of course, which was reflected in these responses:

'I support and encourage research. I need to know what causes it and won't rest till somebody has the answer.'

'I want everyone to become informed, not just those of us who have gone through it.'

'I have fully supported the Back to Sleep research. It should be used to help the babies who are alive today and let the past be history.'

Not everyone is convinced. There were several that stated their frustration at both the speed and the nature of research. They are annoyed with misleading, inaccurate information. They bristle at media reports which claim to have discovered the cause of SIDS, and they are particularly angered when highly publicized accounts of SIDS turn out to be cases of homicide.

I regret that I did not ask the question 'Do you think we will solve the SIDS mystery in our lifetime?' A parent summed it up with this: 'I feel it would do no good to know the cause unless there is a cure.'

Nonetheless, most said they enthusiastically support research, and many say they do this through personal donations or fundraising efforts. It's a way to keep the memory alive, and they want to help find an answer.

How we remember

The fact that these families wrote to me is a testimony to the importance of their children's lives. We don't forget. We remember in so many different ways. We remember by hanging an ornament on a Christmas tree, by planting a tree, by releasing a balloon. We remember by having golf tournaments, by writing poems, by speaking in front of a congressional hearing.

Sometimes we remember by keeping a baby sock in our pocket, or putting an Easter Bunny on a gravesite. Perhaps we remember by looking into our other children's or grandchildren's faces and seeing something that reminds us that we never truly *lose* anybody.

Most of us remember quietly. But the point is . . . even after all these years, we remember. We remember because it's impossible to forget. The death of a child changes our lives, the landscape of our lives, in ways that are sometimes quiet, and sometimes too loud to ignore.

Revisiting a loss

I revisited my friend's hillside, the site of that devastating fire. Early spring rains had caused some of the grass to come back, and when I looked hard I could see that a few of the trees might be getting some buds. I was excited to see the new growth, the regrowth. My friend slowed me down to see something so small I might have missed it. It was a tiny, delicate purple flower, just a couple of inches high. It was a wildflower that lays dormant for years and only sprouts under intense heat, the heat that was caused by the horrible fire a few months ago. The fire had caused it to spring from hibernation and to bloom.

I drive by that hillside once in awhile. It's beautiful with trees and shrubs, and now with an abundance of small purple flowers. From a distance the whole hillside is a soft purple, and unless you knew it you wouldn't be able to tell that not long ago everything you could see had been destroyed.

Everything you could see, but certainly not everything that was there. Some things have been taken away that can never be replaced, and some new unexpected things have grown up among the ashes, changing the way a hillside, and a life will look.

CHAPTER 21

The 'Reduce the Risks' Campaign, SIDS International, The Global Strategy Task Force and The European Society for the Study and Prevention of Infant Death

KAARENE FITZGERALD

SIDS groups and organizations 310

The development of international networks of clinicians, researchers, health professionals, bereaved parents and others interested in reducing SIDS and infant mortality has been and is continually evolving. There is no doubt that the highly motivated people who have worked together in groups and cooperatively are responsible for major changes in infant care practices leading to one of the largest drops in mortality recorded in modern times. This drop has been achieved with little or no financial support from governments in many countries. How did this wide-ranging group of advocates from disparate communities and backgrounds achieve so much with so little?

On 18th October 1985 a group of SIDS parents from eight countries, Belgium, Denmark, France, Germany, Great Britain, Holland, Luxembourg and the USA, met at the University of Brussels following an international workshop organized by Professor Andre Kahn called 'The SIDS practical management of infants at high risk'. The group agreed to stay in touch and work towards another meeting.[1]

The next meeting was held on 27th May 1987 at Lake Como, Italy following the New York Academy of Sciences meeting. This time representatives from thirteen countries, Australia, Austria, Great Britain, Canada, Denmark, France, Germany, Italy, New Zealand, Norway, Scotland, Sweden and the USA, met with the outcome being the formation of SIDS Family International (SIDSFI).[2] The aims were to facilitate the sharing of information, improve services to families, increase awareness about SIDS, improve liaison with health professionals and encourage research activities.

Recommendations were developed covering the areas of autopsies, emergency responders, recruiting new national organizations, parents working with researchers, notification to SIDS organizations, non-SIDS bereaved parents and bereaved parent contacts. Agreement was reached to pursue the adoption of recommendations in each of the participating countries.

As each country presented, statistics were collected on populations, and information on when groups first started, the average number of SIDS cases occurring, whether autopsies were performed or not, and the incidence of SIDS per thousand live births. This first summary covered 20 countries.[3] Since then, updates have been regularly prepared and circulated with the latest version, covering 35 countries, included in this chapter.

A further meeting of SIDSFI was held on 6th April 1989 in London, UK, this time with 15 countries: Australia, Austria, Great Britain, Canada, Chile, Denmark, Greece, Ireland, Italy, New Zealand, Netherlands, Norway, Scotland, Sweden and the USA. Topics for international support included using the term 'apparent life-threatening event' (ALTE) rather than 'near-miss cot death', the use of publications from other countries, and development of a newsletter with the first editor, Felicity Price, coming from New Zealand.

The two most important topics were about the development of a more formal system for international conferences including future venues and dates and a decision to advocate with the World Health Organization (WHO) to include information on SIDS in policy documents, especially 'Targets for Health For All'.

As part of the strategy to work towards achieving SIDSFI aims and increase communication it had been agreed to organize an international conference which followed the business meeting in London on 7–8th April 1989. About 350 delegates, who were primarily bereaved parents, attended.

Meetings were subsequently held with WHO in Geneva and Copenhagen and it was agreed to work towards SIDSFI developing 'Official Relations' status as a non-government organization. Despite a great deal of effort from each of the SIDSFI Chairmen, including major submissions and articles for publication, at the time of writing this has not been achieved.

In 1990 WHO did agree to adopt a 'priority issue on the subject of SIDS' and acknowledged it was 'one of the major causes of infant mortality in the industrialized countries of the world'. (However any further major activity between WHO, SIDSI and the GSTF would not occur until the SIDSI conference was held during 1998 in Rouen, France.)

A new group called the European Society for the Study and Prevention of Infant Deaths (ESPID), under the chairmanship of Professor Andre Kahn, held their Founding Congress 5–7th June 1991 in Rouen, France. It was at this meeting that the New Zealand research contingent very bravely presented the first posters opening robust discussions on the role of sleeping position.

Hazel Brooke from Scotland, the Secretary of SIDSFI, had also obtained funding to develop SIDS Europe and was coordinating efforts to support emerging interest and activities in Eastern Europe.

By the time the next SIDSFI conference was held in Sydney, Australia in February 1992, about 28 national SIDS organizations were part of the network. At the business meeting preceding the conference it was decided to alter the name to SIDS International (SIDSI) to more clearly reflect the broadened activities. In addition, a register of SIDS researchers was commenced.[4]

The Sydney conference was targeted at researchers, clinicians, health professionals and bereaved parents with over 450 delegates from 18 countries attending. One of the major foci was the emerging research activity and health promotion programs looking at safe childcare practices and ways to reduce the risks of SIDS.[5]

During informal discussions with researchers and health professionals whilst developing the Sydney conference program, it had become apparent that efforts to advance scientific activity could possibly be enhanced by a more formalized networking process.

The concept of a Global Strategy Task Force (GSTF) was then developed by Kaarene Fitzgerald. Professors Adrian Walker and Caroline McMillen provided invaluable assistance preparing a draft scientific outline for initial discussions with Dr Marian Willinger from the National Institute of Child Health and Human Development (USA) and Dr Marsden Wagner from the Copenhagen office of WHO. Both of those organizations then agreed to support the new group.

The first Global Strategy Meeting (GSM) was held following the Sydney conference on 17–18th February 1992 with 70 representatives from 16 countries divided into four workshop groups: International SIDS Diagnosis; Epidemiology and Risk Factors; Physiology, Pathophysiology, and Predictive Tests; and Community and Organization Issues.

Each group met for a day and a half to identify issues that could be addressed through international collaboration, and to identify gaps in knowledge or resources. On the last day four international working groups with multidisciplinary participation were formed covering pathology, epidemiology, developmental physiology and education.[6]

There was an enormous amount of energy in those early days. It was exciting, confronting but also salutary working on one of the major medical mysteries – why should these babies die so suddenly and, apparently, without warning?

Theories and hypotheses abounded with, at any one time, 100 or more sensible sounding ideas. Anyone could obtain coverage no matter how far-fetched his or her idea might be. Parents were confused and frightened, the media were keen to publish articles and individual research teams were passionate about their project providing the answer.

SIDS organizations at a local level were trying to develop sensible answers and stay calm whilst perhaps looking after the families of six or more deaths in a day. And, at that time, it was known that about 30,000 infants were dying from SIDS in Western countries. Who was right? Would a drop in deaths attributed to SIDS ever occur?

In the meantime, through publication of the results of several USA research projects (subsequently found to be seriously flawed), apnea monitoring had become popular. Many saw the use of monitors as the only way to 'prevent' SIDS and thriving businesses commenced. In some countries the use of monitors was described as 'a risk reduction program' and large campaigns were mounted to have 'high-risk' infants home monitored. Infant mortality did not fall significantly in most centers where these programs operated.

However, other researchers and clinicians who were visiting bereaved families, often within hours of the baby's death, realized common stories were emerging. Questionnaires were designed and case–control studies implemented. Another project looked at signs of illness in babies in the community. Stimulating papers were given on these subjects at the 1989 London conference.

Research papers had been or were being published looking at the baby's environment including overheating and sleeping position. Drs M. Lee and D. Davies from Hong Kong had written a Letter to the Editor of the *Lancet* (1988)[7] questioning the safety of prone sleeping and raised enormous interest. Susan Beal from Australia had also received significant publicity for her paper (1988).[8] In the Netherlands, Dr Guus de Jonge and Dr Adele Engelberts were also gaining significant publicity and publishing relevant articles (1989).[9]

More sophisticated questionnaires, particularly through the Avon Study (UK) led by Professor Peter Fleming[10]; the NZ Cot Death Study with Professor Ed Mitchell[11]; and the Tasmanian Prospective Cohort (Australia) with Professor Terry Dwyer,[12] were designed and implemented.

SIDS organizations were also developing brochures and articles for parents and health professionals. It is believed the first 'reduce the risk/back to sleep' publication in English was produced in May 1987 by Stephanie Cowan from the Canterbury Cot Death Society in New Zealand, called 'Cot death: you cannot predict it, you cannot prevent it, but you can reduce risks'.

The first policy change recorded for health professionals was in July 1990 when Community Services Victoria (Australia) informed all their maternal and child health nurses to advise parents to place their babies on their sides or backs to sleep and to avoid overheating. One year later (July 1991) a 12 page color brochure in English and in 10 other languages was produced and distributed by the SIDS organization, incorporating the latest research and information from the Baby Illness Research Project (later to become known as Baby Check).

As a result of the 1992 Sydney Australia conference presentations by many researchers, discussions at the SIDSI meeting and discussants' papers at the GSM, 'Reduce the Risk/Back-to-Sleep' campaigns commenced over the next few months and years in many countries. Further discussions, papers and progress to reduce infant mortality have been the focus at subsequent SIDSI meetings, conferences and GSMs held in Stavanger, Norway 1994, Washington DC, USA 1996, Rouen, France 1998, Auckland, New Zealand 2000. Future meetings will

Table 21.1 International Statistics for SIDS (August 2000)

Country	Population in millions	First SIDS group formed	National formation	SIDS/ unexpected infant deaths per annum	How often autopsy performed	Incidence per 1000 live births	Risk reduction campaign started
1. Argentina	33	1992	?	378	Sometimes	0.56	1998
2. Australia	19	1977	1986	120	100%	0.54	July 1990
3. Austria	8	1986	1986	50	70–100%	0.6	1988
4. Belgium	10	1981	1981	90	20–80%	0.6	1993
5. Canada	30	1973	1973	154	100%	0.45	Aug 1993
6. Czechoslovakia	15	None	None	?	100%	0.8–1.0	
7. Denmark	5.3	1986	1986	20	75%	0.3	1989
8. England/Wales	57	1970	1971	284	100%	0.45	Nov 1991
9. Finland	5.5	1991	1991	15	100%	0.25	1989
10. France	54	1984	1986	360	50%	0.49	1994
11. Germany	82	1984	1984	603	55%	0.78	Late 1991
12. Greece (Athens)	10.3	None	None	14	?	0.43	
13. Hungary	10	1993	planned for 2000	30	100%	0.3	Planned for 2000
14. Hong Kong	7	None	None	7	100%	0.1	Nov 1997
15. Ireland – Republic	3.5	1976	1976	42	100%	0.9	1992
16. Israel (Tel Aviv)	5.6	1999			Sometimes (30%)	0.2	1999
17. Italy	58	1979	1991	545	Sometimes	1	1994
18. Japan	122	1993	1993	360	20%	0.30	1997
19. Netherlands	15	1981	1981	27	70%	0.14	1989
20. New Zealand	3.9	1975	1979	60	Almost 100%	1.04	1990
21. Norway	4.5	1982	1985	40	90%	0.6	1990
22. Papua New Guinea	3	None	None	None	None	Zero	
23. Portugal	9.9	None	None	?	?	0.55	1992
24. Russia–St Petersburg	5	None	None	?	?	0.43	
25. Saudi Arabia	17	None	None	?	None	?	
26. Scotland	5	1976	1985	52	100%	0.6	1992
27. Singapore	2.7	None	None	None	?	Zero	
28. Slovakia	5.3	1992	1992	?	100%	0.14	
29. Slovenia	2.2	None	None	10	?	0.47	
30. South Africa	42	1989	1991	?	Sometimes	0.29–1.1	1993
31. Sweden	9	1986	1986	45	100%	0.45	
32. Switzerland	7.2					0.44	1994 & 1997
33. Turkey	65	1998	None	?	Sometimes	?	
34. Ukraine	52	None	None	?	?	?	
35. USA	249.6	1962	1987	2991	Usually	0.77	1994
36. Zimbabwe	10	1988	1988	?	No	29	

? Indicates information is being sought but is not yet available

Table 21.1 Continued

Sources (Note: The bold date in brackets represents the year of the deaths.)

1. Dr Alejandro Jenik, GIAMSI (Group of Investigation and Attention in Sudden Infant Death) Buenos Aires, Argentina. Personal correspondence **(1996)**
2. Australian Bureau of Statistics **(1998)**
3. Reinhold Kerbl, Austria. Personal communication 2000 **(1998)**
4. Professor Andre Kahn, Belgian National Observatoire for the Study and Prevention of Infant Mortality. Personal communication, 2000.
5. Statistics Canada: Canadian Statistics – Birth and birth rate, Canada, the provinces and territories: CANSIM, Matrix 5772; Statistics Canada, Canadian Vital Statistics System, 1996; Offices of the Chief Coroner, Number of Infant Deaths Recorded as Sudden Infant Death Syndrome, Alberta, British Columbia **(1998)**
6. Ministry of Health, Czechoslovakia.
7. Danish National Birth Register, The National Register of Causes of Death, 1997, Denmark **(1997)**
8. Offices for National Statistics (ONS) **(1998)**
9. Finnish SIDS Foundation **(1996)**
10. Naitre et Vivre, INSERM, 1999 **(1997)**
11. Dr Mimi Vennemann, SIDS Study Germany, University of Muenster. Personal Communication, 2000 **(1998)**
12. C. Thedosi Esopou. Athens **(1991)**
13. Eva Barko, Pro Familia Hungarian Foundation. Personal Communication, 2000 **(1998)**
14. Tony Nelson. Personal communication, 2000 **(average 1990–1996)**
15. National SIDS Register, Dublin **(1998)**
16. Dr Anat Shatz, Israeli Society for the Study and Prevention of Sudden Infant Death. Personal Communication, 2000 **(1998)**
17. Prof Gianpaolo Donzelli, Presidente of Italian Society for Perinatal and Pediatric Unexpected Deaths. Personal Communication
18. Ministry of Health and Welfare, Japan **(1998)**
19. Dutch Central Bureau of Statistics, 1999 **(1998)**
20. Professor Barry Taylor, Otago. Personal Communication, **(Provisional figures – 1998)**
21. Medical Birth Registry of Norway **(1998)**
22. World Health Organization, Manila. Personal Communication **(1990)**.
23. J Pinheiro, Temas de Medicina Legal, Ed Centro de Estudos de Pos-graduaçao em Medicini Legal, Coimbra 1998. L Guimaraes *et al.* O Sindrome Morte Subita. Inesperada e Inexplicada do Lactente (MSIL) em Portugal-Um levantamento Retrospectivo (1979–1994): Dados preliminares. *Acta Pediatr.* Port. 28:19–26, 1997 **(1994–1996)**
24. Paediatric Medical Institute, Professor I.A. Kelmanson. Epidemiological Highlights of SIDS in St Petersburg. *SIDS International Newsletter*, February 1995 **(1992)**
25. Professor Peter Herdson, King Faisal Hospital, Saudi Arabia. Personal Communication **(1990)**
26. Dr Maurice Kibel, South Africa. Personal Communication **(1998)**
27. Scottish Cot Death Trust **(1998)**
28. Dr Chew Chin Hin, Ministry of Health, Singapore. Personal Communication **(1990)**
29. Dr Jiri Jura, Chairman Slovak SIDS Foundation. *SIDS International Newsletter* 1998 **(1997)**
30. SIDS International Newsletter, No 1 1998 **(1997)**
31. Dr Joseph Milerad, Sweden. Personal Communication **(1998)**

Table 21.1 Continued

32. Federal Bureau of Statistics, Bern, 1999 **(1996)**
33. Dr Yildiz Perk, Cocuk Sağliği ve Hastaliklari Uzmani. Personal Communication
34. N Aryqev, Odessa Medical University, Odessa **(1993)**
35. Hoyert D.L., Kochanek K.D., Murphy S.L. Deaths: Final data for 1997. National Vital Statistics Report; **47** (20), Hyattsville, Maryland: National Center for Health Statistics, 1999 **(1997)**
36. National SIDS Association, Zimbabwe. Personal Communication **(1998)**

Prepared by: Kaarene Fitzgerald AC, Chairman, SIDS Global Strategy Task Force. For comments/additions/alterations contact e-mail kaarene@sidsaustralia.org.au. Please note: In many cases details in this report are based on personal communication. The purpose of these statistics is to show, where possible, infant mortality figures.

be held in Florence, Italy March 2002, Edmonton, Canada 2004 and hopefully in Japan in 2006.

Reports from SIDSI and GSM meetings and GSTF projects including the International Autopsy and Event Scene Protocols, Core Curriculum (for health professionals), details about Project RIMI (Representation Minorities and Indigenous People), International Child Care Practice study, Standardized Mortality Reporting, position statements on smoking, and other issues, minimum standards for physiological, recording, state of the art reviews, WHO, International Statistics are available on www.sidsinternational.minerva.com.au or www.sidsglobal.org.

Due to the energy and commitment by many, at this stage a significant number of countries have seen a drop of between 50–80 per cent in infant mortality. Many parents have not had to deal with the tragedy of losing a child and the world has gained many thousands of citizens who will contribute in turn to its health and well-being.

References

1. Brown M. SIDS Family International Introduction. In: Schwartz PJ, Southall DP, Valdes-Dapena M (eds) *The Sudden Infant Death Syndrome Cardiac and Respiratory Mechanisms and Interventions. Ann NY Acad Sci* 1988;427–9.
2. Fitzgerald K. SIDS Family International Minutes of Meeting. In: Schwartz PJ, Southall DP, Valdes-Dapena M (eds) *The Sudden Infant Death Syndrome Cardiac and Respiratory Mechanisms and Interventions. Ann NY Acad Sci* 1988;430–8.
3. Fitzgerald K. In: Schwartz PJ, Southall DP, Valdes-Dapena M (eds) *The Sudden Infant Death Syndrome Cardiac and Respiratory Mechanisms and Interventions. Ann NY Acad Sci* 1988:439–40.
4. Fitzgerald K, Brooke H. SIDS International Third Business Meeting Minutes. In: Walker AM, McMillen C, Barnes D, Fitzgerald K, Willinger M (eds) *Second SIDS International Conference and First Global Strategy Meeting*. Perinatology Press, 1993, pp. 449–54.
5. Walker AM, McMillen C, Barnes D, Fitzgerald K, Willinger M (eds). *Second SIDS International Conference and First Global Strategy Meeting*. Perinatology Press, 1993.
6. Barnes D, Fitzgerald K, Willinger M. First Global Strategy Meeting. In: Walker AM, McMillen C, Barnes D, Fitzgerald K, Willinger M (eds) *Second SIDS International Conference and First Global Strategy Meeting*. Perinatology Press, 1993, pp. 427–45.
7. Lee M, Davies DP, Chan TF. Prone or supine for term babies? *Lancet* 1988;1:1332.
8. Beal SM. Sleeping position and sudden infant death syndrome. *Med J Aust* 1988;149:562.
9. de Jonge GA, Engelberts AC, Koomen-Liefting AJM, Kostense PF. Cot death and prone sleeping position in the Netherlands. *Br Med J* 1989;298:722.
10. Fleming PJ, Gilbert R, Azaz Y. Interaction between bedding and sleeping position in the sudden infant death syndrome: A population based case–control study. *Br Med J* 1990;301:85–9.

11. Mitchell EA, Scragg R, Stewart AW *et al.* Results from the first year of the New Zealand cot death study. *NZ Med J* 1991;104:71–6.
12. Dwyer T, Ponsonby AL, Gibbons LE, Newman NE. Prone sleeping positions and SIDS: Evidence from recent case–control and cohort studies in Tasmania. *J Paediatr Child Health* 1991;27:340–3.

International Standardized Autopsy Protocol for Sudden Unexpected Infant Death

HENRY F. KROUS AND ROGER W. BYARD

The members of SIDS International and the National Institute of Child Health and Human Development (NICHD) jointly organized the SIDS Global Strategy Task Force (GSTF) to develop means by which the causes of sudden infant death syndrome (SIDS) and other disorders associated with sudden, unexpected infant death masquerading as SIDS could be identified and to identify and implement ways to reduce their incidence. The GSTF created five working groups among its membership to address: Epidemiology, Pathology, Developmental Physiology, Infection/Immunity and Education/Training. Each working group had international representation.

The Pathology Working Group was charged with the development and implementation of an International Standardized Autopsy Protocol (ISAP) and accompanying Instruction Manual. The use of the ISAP was intended: (1) to facilitate standardization of postmortem examination of infants whose cause of death was not apparent at the beginning of the autopsy; (2) to supplement information gained from the scene examination and medical history review; (3) to improve diagnostic accuracy and precision using an internationally accepted definition of SIDS; (4) to enhance the ability to compare accurate SIDS rates within and across countries; (5) to facilitate means by which rates of SIDS and other causes of sudden infant death could be reduced; and (6) to facilitate research not only within but also across the various medical disciplines investigating SIDS and other causes of sudden, unexpected infant death.

Following its completion and publication,[1] the ISAP and its Instruction Manual have been endorsed by the Society for Pediatric Pathology and the National

Association of Medical Examiners (USA), and is now used in numerous countries on several continents.

Reference

1. Krous H. Instruction and Reference Manual for the International Standardized Autopsy Protocol for Sudden Unexpected Infant Death. *J SIDS Infant Mortality* 1996;1:203–46.

International Standardized Autopsy Protocol For Sudden Unexpected Infant Death

Decedent's name		Local accession number
Age/sex	Ethnicity	
Date of birth	Date/time of death	
Date/time of autopsy	Pathologist	
County/District	Country	

Final anatomic diagnoses

Microbiology results:

Toxicology results:

Chemistry results:

Pathologist . . . .

Decedent's name ....

Accession number...........................

County & country ....

Pathologist...............................

	YES	NO
MICROBIOLOGY Date/Time:		
Done before autopsy:		
VIRUSES trachea stool		
BACTERIA blood CSF fluids		
FUNGI discretionary		
MYCOBACTERIA discretionary		
Done during autopsy		
BACTERIA liver lung and myocardium		
VIRUSES liver lung and myocardium		
PHOTOGRAPHS include:		
Name, case number, county, country, date		
Measuring device, color reference		
Consider front and back		
Gross abnormalities		
RADIOGRAPHIC STUDIES consider:		
Whole body		
Thorax and specific lesions		
EXTERNAL EXAMINATION		
Date and time of autopsy		
Sex (circle), Male/Female		
Observed race (circle)		
White Black		
Asian Arab		
Pacific Islander Gypsy		
Hispanic, Other (specify)		
Rigor mortis: describe distribution		
Livor mortis: describe distribution and if fixed		
WEIGHTS AND MEASURES		
Body Weight (g)		
Crown–heel length (cm)		
Crown–rump length (cm)		
Occipitofrontal circumference (cm)		
Chest circumference at nipples (cm)		
Abdominal circumference at umbilicus (cm)		

Decedent's name . . . .
Accession number. . . . .
County & country . . . .
Pathologist. . . . .

GENERAL APPEARANCE/DEVELOPMENT	YES	NO	NO EXAM
Development normal			
Nutritional status			
Normal			
Poor			
Obese			
Hydration			
Normal			
Dehydrated			
Edematous			
Pallor			
HEAD			
Configuration normal			
Scalp and hair normal			
Bone consistency normal			
Other			
TRAUMA EVIDENCE			
Bruises			
Lacerations			
Abrasions			
Burns			
Other			
PAST SURGICAL INTERVENTION			
Scars			
Other			
RESUSCITATION EVIDENCE			
Facial mask marks			
Lip abrasions			
Chest ecchymoses			
EKG monitor pads			
Defibrillator marks			
Venipunctures			
Other			
CONGENITAL ANOMALIES			
EXTERNAL			
INTEGUMENT			

Decedent's name . . . .
Accession number. . . . .
County & country . . . .
Pathologist. . . . .

	YES	NO	NO EXAM
Jaundice			
Petechiae			
Rashes			
Birthmarks			
Other abnormalities			
EYES (remove when indicated and legal)			
Color (circle) Brown/Blue/Green/Hazel			
Cataracts			
Position abnormal			
Jaundice			
Conjunctiva abnormal			
Petechiae			
Other abnormalities			
EARS			
Low set			
Rotation abnormal			
Other abnormalities			
NOSE			
Discharge (describe if present)			
Configuration abnormal			
Septal deviation			
Right choanal atresia			
Left choanal atresia			
Other abnormalities			
MOUTH			
Discharge (describe if present)			
Labial frenulum abnormal			
Teeth present			
Number of upper			
Number of lower			
TONGUE			
Abnormally large			
Frenulum abnormal			
Other abnormalities			

Decedent's name . . . .

Accession number. . . . .

County & country . . . .

Pathologist. . . . .

	YES	NO	NO EXAM
PALATE			
Cleft			
High arched			
Other abnormalities			
MANDIBLE			
Micrognathia			
Other abnormalities			
NECK			
abnormal			
CHEST			
abnormal			
ABDOMEN			
Distended			
Umbilicus abnormal			
Hernias			
Other abnormal			
EXTERNAL GENITALIA abnormal			
ANUS abnormal			
EXTREMITIES abnormal			
INTERNAL EXAMINATION			
Subcutis thickness 1 cm below umbilicus:			
Subcutaneous emphysema			
Situs inversus			
PLEURAL CAVITIES abnormal			
Fluid describe if present			
Right (ml)			
Left (ml)			
PERICARDIAL CAVITY abnormal			
Fluid, describe if present (ml)			
Other abnormalities			
PERITONEAL CAVITY abnormal			
Fluid, describe if present (ml)			
RETROPERITONEUM abnormal			

Decedent's name . . . .
Accession number. . . . .
County & country . . . .
Pathologist. . . . .

	YES	NO	NO EXAM
PETECHIAE (indicate if dorsal and/or ventral)			
Parietal pleura			
Right			
Left			
Visceral pleura			
Right			
Left			
Pericardium			
Epicardium			
Thymus			
Parietal peritoneum			
Visceral peritoneum			
UPPER AIRWAY OBSTRUCTION			
Foreign body			
Mucus plug			
Other			
NECK SOFT TISSUE HEMORRHAGE			
HYOID BONE abnormal			
THYMUS			
Weight (g)			
Atrophy			
Other abnormalities			
EPIGLOTTIS abnormal			
LARYNX abnormal			
Narrowed lumen			
TRACHEA abnormal			
Stenosis			
Obstructive exudates			
Aspirated gastric contents			
ET tube tip location			
MAINSTEM BRONCHI abnormal			
Edema fluid			
Mucus plugs			
Gastric contents			
Inflammation			

Decedent's name . . . .

Accession number. . . . .

County & country . . . .

Pathologist. . . . .

	YES	NO	NO EXAM
LUNGS			
Weight			
Right (g)			
Left (g)			
Abnormal			
Congestion, describe location, severity			
Hemorrhage, describe location, severity			
Edema, describe location			
Severity (circle)			
Consolidation, describe location, severity			
Anomalies			
Pulmonary artery			
Thromboembolization			
PLEURA abnormal			
RIBS abnormal			
Fractures			
with hemorrhages			
Callus formation			
Configuration abnormal			
DIAPHRAGM abnormal			
CARDIOVASCULAR SYSTEM			
Heart weight (g)			
Left ventricular thickness (cm)			
Right ventricular thickness (cm)			
Septal thickness maximum (cm)			
Mitral valve circumference (cm)			
Aortic valve circumference (cm)			
Tricuspid valve circumference (cm)			
Pulmonary valve circumference (cm)			
Myocardium abnormal			
Ventricular inflow/outflow tracts narrow			
Valvular vegetations/thromboses			
Aortic coarctation			
Patent ductus arteriosus			
Chamber blood (circle) fluid/clotted			
Congenital heart disease			
Atrial septal defect			

Decedent's name ....

Accession number.............................

County & country ....

Pathologist.................................

	YES	NO	NO EXAM
Ventricular septal defect			
Abnormal pulmonary venous connection			
Other			
Location of vascular catheter tips			
Occlusive vascular thrombosis locations			
Other abnormalities			
ESOPHAGUS abnormal			
STOMACH abnormal			
Describe contents and volume			
SMALL INTESTINE abnormal			
Hemorrhage			
Volvulus			
Describe contents			
COLON abnormal			
Congestion			
Hemorrhage			
Describe contents			
APPENDIX abnormal			
MESENTERY abnormal			
LIVER abnormal			
Weight (g)			
GALLBLADDER abnormal			
PANCREAS abnormal			
SPLEEN abnormal			
Weight (g)			
KIDNEYS abnormal			
Weight	████████████████		
Right (g)			
Left (g)			
URETERS abnormal			
BLADDER abnormal			
Contents, volume			
PROSTATE abnormal			
UTERUS, F. TUBES, and OVARIES abnormal			

Decedent's name . . . .

Accession number. . . . .

County & country . . . .

Pathologist. . . . .

	YES	NO	NO EXAM
THYROID abnormal			
ADRENALS abnormal			
Right (g)			
Left (g)			
Combined (g)			
PITUITARY abnormal			
CONGENITAL ANOMALIES, INTERNAL			
CENTRAL NERVOUS SYSTEM			
Whole brain weight	■■■■■■■		
Fresh (g)			
Fixed (g)			
Combined cerebellum/brainstem weight	■■■■■■■		
Fresh (g)			
Fixed (g)			
Evidence of trauma			
Scalp abnormal			
Galea abnormal			
Fractures			
Anterior fontanelle abnormal			
Dimensions			
Calvarium abnormal			
Cranial sutures abnormal			
Closed (fused)			
Overriding			
Widened			
Base of skull abnormal			
Configuration abnormal			
Middle ears abnormal			
Foramen magnum abnormal			
Hemorrhage, estimate volumes (ml)			
Epidural			
Dural			
Subdural			
Subarachnoid			

Decedent's name ....
Accession number............................
County & country ....
Pathologist...................................

	YES	NO	NO EXAM
Intracerebral			
Cerebellum			
Brainstem			
Spinal cord			
Intraventricular			
Other			
Dural lacerations			
Dural sinus thrombosis			
BRAIN: IF EXTERNALLY ABNORMAL			
FIX BEFORE CUTTING			
Configuration abnormal			
Hydrocephalus			
Gyral pattern abnormal			
Cerebral edema			
Herniation			
Uncal			
Tonsillar			
Tonsillar necrosis			
Leptomeningeal exudates (culture)			
Cerebral contusions			
Malformations			
Cranial nerves abnormal			
Circle of Willis/basilar arteries abnormal			
Ventricular contours abnormal			
Cerebral infarction			
Contusional tears			
Other abnormalities			
SPINAL CORD			
Inflammation			
Contusion(s)			
Anomalies, other abnormalities			

Decedent's name ....

Accession number.............................

County & country ....

Pathologist..................................

	YES	NO
MANDATORY SECTIONS TAKEN		
Skin, if lesions		
Thymus		
Lymph node		
Epiglottis, vertical		
Larynx, supraglottic, transverse		
Larynx, true cords, transverse		
Trachea and thyroid, transverse		
Trachea at carina, transverse		
Lungs, all lobes		
Diaphragm		
Heart, septum and ventricles		
Esophagus, distal 3 cm		
Terminal ileum		
Rectum		
Liver		
Pancreas with duodenum		
Spleen		
Kidney with capsule		
Adrenal		
Rib with costochondral junction		
Submandibular gland		
Cervical spinal cord		
Rostral medulla junction		
Pons		
Midbrain		
Hippocampus		
Frontal lobe, cerebellum choroid plexus		

Decedent's name ....

Accession number...........................

County & country ....

Pathologist. ....

	YES	NO
OIL RED O STAINED SECTIONS, IF INDICATED		
Heart		
Liver		
Muscle		
DISCRETIONARY MICROSCOPIC SECTIONS		
Supraglottic soft tissue		
Lung hilum		
Pancreatic tail		
Mesentery		
Stomach		
Colon		
Appendix		
Testes or ovaries		
Urinary bladder		
Psoas muscle		
Palatine tonsils		
Basal ganglia		
METABOLIC DISORDERS		
RETAIN ON FILTER PAPER IN ALL CASES		
Whole blood (1 drop), urine (1 drop)		
Hair (taped down)		

Decedent's name . . . .

Accession number. . . . .

County & country . . . .

Pathologist. . . . .

	YES	NO
TOXICOLOGY AND ELECTROLYTES		
FLUID AND TISSUES SAVED FOR 1 YEAR		
Whole blood and serum, save at −70°C and + 4°C		
Liver, save 100 g at −70°C		
Frontal lobe, save at −70°C		
Urine, save at −70°C Bile		
Vitreous humor		
Serum		
Gastric contents		
Analyses performed, but not limited to:		
Cocaine and metabolites		
Morphine and metabolites		
Amphetamine and metabolites		
Volatiles (ethanol, acetone, etc.)		
Other indicated by history and exam		
FROZEN TISSUES, SAVE AT −70°C		
Lung		
Heart		
Liver		
Lymph node		

Sudden Unexplained Infant Death Investigation Report Form (SUIDIRF)*

Guidelines for death-scene investigation   334
Guidelines for completing SUIDIRF   335
Page-by-page instructions   337
References   343

Guidelines for death-scene investigation of sudden, unexplained infant deaths: recommendations of the interagency panel on sudden infant death syndrome

SUMMARY

Because no uniform procedure has been developed for collecting and evaluating information on sudden, unexplained infant deaths (SUIDs) in the United States, the US Senate and US House of Representatives recommended in 1992 that the US Department of Health and Human Services Interagency Panel on Sudden Infant Death Syndrome (SIDS) establish a standard scene-investigation protocol for SUIDs. Two members of the panel, the Division of Reproductive Health of CDC and the National Institute for Child Health and Human Development of the National Institutes of Health, convened a workshop in July 1993 to gather information and ideas to use in developing such a protocol. Workshop participants, who included consultants having expertise in SIDS and representatives of

* (Reprinted from the Centers for Disease Control and Prevention *Morbidity and Mortality Weekly Report* 1996;45:1, 7–19)

public and private organizations concerned with SIDS, suggested that the Inter-agency Panel on SIDS develop both a short-form protocol and a longer, comprehensive protocol. The participants also recommended data items to include in the short-form protocol. This report includes the short form, which was developed to standardize the investigation of SUID scenes; ensure that information pertinent to determining the cause, manner, and circumstances of an infant death is considered in each investigation; and to assist researchers in accurately determining the cause of and risk factors for SIDS. It can be used by medical examiners, coroners, death investigators, and police officers. Instructions for using the protocol are also included.

Guidelines for completing the Sudden Unexplained Infant Death Investigation Report Form (SUIDIRF)

Use

SUIDIRF may be used to assess the death of any infant for whom the cause of death is not apparent before autopsy. Applicable parts of the form may also be used to collect data about the death of any infant for whom the cause of death is known. The medical examiner or coroner (ME/C) or the death investigator acting on behalf of the former should complete the SUIDIRF. Police officers who report to the ME/C may also find the form useful.

Completion

The form may be completed by using blue or black ink or a no. 2 soft-lead pencil to facilitate electronic scanning, photocopying, and fax transmission. To ensure legibility of the forms, writing on the blank side (back) of the forms is discouraged. One blank page is provided for notes. If necessary, additional sheets of blank paper may be attached.

Design

The SUIDIRF pages are designed for use on a clipboard. The pages may be separated to allow other persons to complete, scan, photocopy, or fax the pages. Each page is printed on one side for legibility.

Compatibility with other forms

CDC's Medical Examiner and Coroner Information Sharing Program has published two generic death investigation report forms (DIRFs) – one for the investigator conducting the initial phases of the investigation (IDIRF) and another for the person who certifies the death or 'closes' the investigation (CDIRF).[1,2] The SUIDIRF is compatible with the DIRFs and has many data items in common. The CDIRF may be used in conjunction with the SUIDIRF.

Although the generic IDIRF can be used for all death investigations irrespective of the age of the decedent, the SUIDIRF was designed specifically for infant deaths. On the SUIDIRF, the one-letter abbreviations in parentheses match the codes on the other DIRFs developed by CDC.

General instructions

Use military time. Military time (midnight = 0000, noon = 1200) facilitates computer applications. Midnight (0000) corresponds to the same day as 0001 (one minute after midnight). The investigator may indicate a.m. and p.m. as long as the data entry personnel converts standard time to military time.

Month and day are sufficient for many fields. Birth date, death date, and the date the case was reported to the ME/C should each contain the month, day, and year, in that order, in numeric format (e.g., 01/05/97). For other events that occur in the same year as the report, indicating the month and day only is sufficient.

Indicate answers by an X. Multiple possible answers to an item are preceded by a line or followed by a box. Indicate the correct answer by writing an X on the appropriate line or in the appropriate box.

Use NA to indicate that a specific item is not applicable. If a given item is not applicable, write NA. If the respondent refuses to answer a question, write refused. Do not leave an item blank; the reviewer needs to know that an item has not been overlooked.

Correct errors by erasing or scratching through an incorrect response. If it is not possible to erase an answer, scratch out the incorrect response and indicate the correct one by using an X or by writing text as needed.

GLOSSARY

Abbreviations used in the SUIDIRF

CPR Cardiopulmonary resuscitation
DC Death certificate
DOA Dead on arrival
DOB Date of birth
EMS Emergency medical services
IV Intravenous
ME/C Medical examiner or coroner

NA Not applicable
NOK Next of kin
OTC Over-the-counter medication
Rx Prescription medication
SIDS Sudden infant death syndrome
SS# Social security number
Unk Unknown

Terminology

EMS caller. The person who first called for emergency medical services, including an ambulance service, the police, or the fire department rescue team.

Last caregiver. The person who was last responsible for the care of the infant when he or she was discovered dead, unresponsive, or in distress (e.g. a baby-sitter, a child care custodian, or the mother).

EMS responder. The person who first responded on behalf of the emergency medical service agency.

Father. The person serving as the father at the time of the incident. The relationship as natural (birth) father, stepfather, or other should be indicated.

Finder. The person who discovered the infant dead, unresponsive, or in distress.

First responder. The first person who attempted to render aid when the infant was found dead, unresponsive, or in distress.

Health-care provider. The physician, nurse, clinician, or other medical service provider who usually gave the infant medical care or well-baby checkups.

Last witness. The person who last observed the infant alive or presumably alive in or near the area where he or she was discovered dead, unresponsive, or in distress.

Mother. The person serving as mother of the infant at the time of the incident. The relationship as natural (birth) mother, stepmother, or other should be indicated.

Placer. The person who last placed the infant in or near the area where he or she was found dead, unresponsive, or in distress.

Police. The law enforcement officer responsible for completing the police report on the death-scene investigation.

Usual caregiver. The person responsible for providing the usual, ongoing care for the infant (e.g. changing diapers and feeding).

Page-by-page instructions

Many of the information items on SUIDIRF are self-explanatory. Instructions are provided here for items that require clarification.

Page 1

Use page 1 to document the date and time of critical events as well as to describe briefly circumstances of the infant's death. If the space on the blank page provided is not sufficient, additional pages for narrative descriptions may be attached.

Home address. The primary residence of the infant at the time of his or her death.

Age. The infant's age at death. Use MI for minutes (if less than 1 hour old), HR for hours (if less than 1 day old), DA for days (if less than 1 month old), and MO for months (until 23 months). Age at death can readily be calculated from the date of birth and date of death.

Race. The infant's race (based on the race of the birth mother). Use W for white, B for black, I for American Indian or Alaskan Native, A for Asian or Pacific Islander, and O for other.

Ethnicity. Whether the infant is of Hispanic descent. Additional information about the infant's national descent may be included here (e.g. Japan, China, Philippines, South Africa, Poland, or Germany).

Receipt by. The name of the ME/C or receptionist who first received notification of the infant's death.

NOK notified. The date and time the NOK not at the scene was notified of the infant's death, who was notified, and by whom. If the family was present at the scene and already knew of the infant's death at the time of its report, write NA in the date field.

Scene visit. The date and time the ME/C or the death investigator acting on behalf of the former visited the site where the injury or illness began or the death occurred. If ME/C staff visited the site, put an X by 'ME/C staff' and name the person who went to the scene. If another agency and not ME/C staff went to the site, put an X by 'Other agency' and name the agency or person. If no scene visit took place, place an X by 'Not done'; however, use this form to collect information from telephone or in-person interviews of witnesses and from emergency medical service logs and reports.

Scene address. The address of the place where the injury or death occurred. Indicate if the scene address is the same as the home address. If the scene was not visited, give the presumed address.

Condition of infant when found. The condition of the infant at the time of his or her discovery. A dead infant is believed to be dead even after resuscitation is attempted. An unresponsive infant is unconscious but shows signs of life (e.g. has a pulse and is breathing). An infant in distress is in obvious trouble but retains some degree of responsiveness.

Sequence of events before death. A summary of the reported sequence of events leading to the infant's death. For example, 'Infant found dead in crib at 3.00 a.m. No significant history.' Use supplementary pages to detail the reported circumstances and sequence of events.

Injury. The date, time, and address of a known or suspected injury relevant to the infant's death.

Discovery. The date, time, and address of where the infant was found dead, unresponsive, or in distress.

Arrival. The date and time the infant arrived at a hospital (if such is the case).

Transport by. The mode of transport (e.g. ambulance or private motor vehicle) and the agency or person who transported the infant to the hospital.

Actual death. The specific date, time, and place where the death is believed or known to have occurred, not necessarily when or where death was pronounced. Options include where the infant was found (on scene), en route to a hospital, in a hospital emergency room, during surgery, and after being admitted to a hospital as an inpatient.

Infant placed. The date, time, and type of place where the infant was last placed as well as who placed the infant before he or she was found dead, unresponsive, or in distress. For example, a place might be listed as crib in bedroom, adult bed, sofa in living room, mattress on floor, or infant seat in vehicle.

Known alive. The date, time, and type of place where the infant was last seen or otherwise known (or assumed) to be alive as well as who believed the infant was alive.

First response. The date, time, and type of response (e.g. mouth-to-mouth resuscitation, chest compression, slapping, or shaking) rendered by the first person who attempted to aid or revive the infant as well as who rendered such aid.

EMS called. The date and time EMS was called, who called EMS, and the site from where the EMS caller called.

EMS response. The date and time EMS personnel arrived at the scene as well as the name of the EMS agency.

Police response. The date and time police arrived at the scene as well as the name of the police department.

Place of fatal event. For each choice, only one condition can apply. Indicate the correct choice with an X on the appropriate line.

Describe type of place. A concise but thorough description of the place where the events leading to death occurred. Examples include infant's bedroom at home, privately owned day care center, child restraint in back seat of moving car, and infant seat in booth at a restaurant.

The name and relationship to the infant of all involved persons referenced on page 1 should be listed in the table at the top of page 4. On page 1 of the form, generic terms (e.g. mother, sister, uncle, or neighbor) can be used to indicate 'By whom.'

Page 2

Use page 2 to document the infant's usual health-care provider, prenatal and birth history, medical history (e.g. recent symptoms, signs, and behavioral changes), and medication history as well as resuscitation attempts (including medical techniques and procedures) used in attempts to revive the infant. The letter codes can be used to identify the fields on supplementary pages and to facilitate data coding.

Medical source. The sources used to obtain medical information about the infant and the mother.

Use the section on specific infant medical history to describe relevant medical history. If further description or clarification is needed, use the space provided on the right of the form, use the blank supplement page, or attach additional pages.

Problems during labor or delivery. Includes problems with the placenta, membranes, or cord; breech or malpresentation; cephalopelvic disproportion; prolonged labor; and fetal distress.

Maternal illness or complications during pregnancy. Includes eclampsia; incompetent cervix; maternal anemia; and pregnancy-induced hypertension, diabetes, cardiac conditions, and renal diseases.

Major birth defects. Includes central nervous system defects (e.g. spina bifida or meningocele, hydrocephalus, and microcephalus), cardiac malformations, gastrointestinal defects (e.g. rectal atresia or stenosis), Down's syndrome, and cleft lip or cleft palate.

Hospitalization of infant after initial discharge. Any overnight stay of the infant at a hospital after having been discharged from the hospital of delivery. Specify the date, reason, and outcome of each hospitalization.

Emergency room visits in past 2 weeks. The date, reason, and outcome of each visit.

Known allergies. Any allergies (e.g. to cow's milk, food, medication, or vaccine).

Growth and weight gain considered normal. If not normal, clarify.

Exposure to contagious diseases in past 2 weeks. Any contact with a person who had a communicable infectious disease (e.g. a cold, hepatitis, measles, pertussis, tuberculosis, or viral or diarrheal disease).

Illness in past 2 weeks. Any observed illness the infant experienced in the past 2 weeks. Specify the condition and its outcome.

Infant has ever stopped breathing or turned blue. Any episode of apnea before the infant died.

Infant was ever breastfed. Breastfeeding was successfully initiated irrespective of whether the infant was still breastfeeding at the time of death.

Vaccinations in past 72 hours. Vaccinations against preventable childhood diseases. Specify which vaccinations were administered.

Deceased siblings. The cause and circumstances of death of the infant's deceased siblings.

Medication history. The type of medications given to the infant in the past. Place an X where it applies. List the name of the medicines and doses taken. Indicate any home remedies given to infant, such as white clay or balms.

Emergency medical treatment. The types of medical treatment rendered to revive the infant. Explain further, if necessary, in the spaces provided below.

Page 3

When completing the questions on page 3, draw on personal observations. Use the section on household environment to indicate whether the household was visited and to document the presence or absence of selected environmental and social risk factors in the primary home of the infant (even if the events leading to death occurred somewhere else). Items for which the response is yes can be clarified in the space provided on the right. The letter codes can be used to identify the fields on supplementary pages and to facilitate data coding. Also use this section to document maternal sociodemographic information.

Type of dwelling. Concise description of the type of household (e.g. single family home, apartment, or trailer).

Water source. Source of drinking water (e.g. city water, well water, bottled water, or spring water).

Number of bedrooms. The number of rooms used as night-time sleeping rooms, excluding living and dining rooms.

Estimated annual income. The estimated yearly income from all sources except public assistance.

On public assistance. Whether the householder receives public assistance (e.g. Aid for Families with Dependent Children [AFDC]).

Number of smokers in household. Includes both regular and occasional smokers in the household.

Use the section on infant and environment to document the immediate environment in which the events leading to death occurred. The immediate environment may or may not be the infant's primary home. If the infant was found in a crib or bed, put an X in the space provided. Indicate if the infant was sleeping alone or was sharing the crib or bed with others.

Temperature of area. A measured temperature where the infant was discovered. If a thermometer is not available, use subjective terms such as cold, cool, comfortable, warm, and hot.

The next items are included to help evaluate the possibility of asphyxia and external conditions as a cause of death. The questions evaluate the possibility of interference with breathing (e.g. covering of the nose and mouth) or hazards related to aspiration, choking, electrocution, excessive heat or cold, and other external factors. When possible, the manufacturer, brand, and lot or product number of relevant consumer products should be documented.

Sleeping or supporting surface. The characteristics of the crib, bed, floor, or other object that directly supported the infant when he or she was found dead, unresponsive, or in distress. Examples include sheepskin on cement floor, mesh seat of baby swing, sheeted mattress in crib, uncovered mattress on wood floor, and plastic-covered foam cushion on sofa. If the surface is easily compressed or deformed, that fact should be noted and the item should be obtained as evidence.

Clothing. A list and description of all articles of clothing worn by the infant, including diapers.

Other items in contact with infant. Any objects, other than the sleeping surface and articles of clothing, that were in contact with the infant (e.g. pacifier, dangling puppet on mobile, or plastic-covered, foam-filled bumper guard). These items should be secured as evidence.

Items in crib or immediate environment. Any other items in the immediate area to which the infant reasonably may have had access. Examples are pill on floor 16 inches from body, pacifier at opposite end of crib, and electric cord draping through crib. These items should be secured as evidence.

Devices operating in room. All electrical and mechanical devices in use in the room where the infant was found dead, unresponsive, or in distress. These devices include vaporizers, space heaters, fans, and infant electronic monitors (e.g. apnea monitor or heart rate monitor).

Cooling source in room and heat source in room. The type of cooling and heat sources in the room where the infant was found. Examples of space devices include portable heaters, window air conditioners, and ceiling fans. Central devices include gas- or electricity-powered systems that heat or cool multiple rooms or an entire house.

Use the section on items collected to document material secured as evidence for presentation to the ME/C, crime laboratory, or other expert for further observation or analysis.

Page 4

Use page 4 to document interviews and procedures related to the investigation (e.g. review of medical records and referral of the case to a SIDS services agency), provide notes to the pathologist, indicate an overall assessment of whether findings suggest SIDS or another diagnosis or injury, indicate the family's interest in organ or tissue donation, and document disposition of the body. Use the section on interview and procedural tracking to record the names of informants, their relationship to the infant, phone number, and the date and time of interview.

Relationship to infant. Specific relationship to the infant (e.g. natural [or birth] mother, adoptive mother, foster mother, stepmother, maternal aunt, or neighbor).

Alternate contact person. If the mother cannot be located, the person who would be able to provide information about her.

Doll re-enactment performed. Whether a doll was used to assist the witnesses in describing the body and face position of the infant when he or she was found dead, unresponsive, or in distress.

Detailed protocol completed. Whether the jurisdiction's detailed death investigation protocol was completed. Enter an X by 'NA' if no such protocol exists for the jurisdiction.

Use the overall preliminary summary to provide notes to the pathologist (e.g. note and evaluate subtle mark on neck), indicate whether environmental hazards or consumer products may have contributed to the infant's death, and indicate whether the family is interested in organ or tissue donation. The last line is for the investigator to indicate whether, in his or her opinion, the investigation suggests SIDS, other causes of death, or trauma or injury.

In the section on case disposition, indicate whether the ME/C declined or accepted the reported case for investigation. A case can be declined because the cause and circumstances of death do not place the case within the ME/C's jurisdiction because of the topic (subject matter) or the location of death. A case is generally accepted so that an autopsy can be performed, an external examination can be conducted, and the cause and manner of death can be certified. Diagnosis of SIDS requires a complete autopsy, including histology, toxicology, and other tests as needed.

Transport agent. The person or transport service who brings the body to the morgue from its location at the time of the death report. Enter NA if the body is not brought to a morgue.

Funeral home. The funeral home authorized to handle the disposition of the body (regardless of whether the body has been brought to a morgue).

Page 5

Use page 5 to diagram the immediate area surrounding the infant when he or she was discovered dead, unresponsive, or in distress and to record selected observations about the area.

Page 6

Page 6 is an illustration of an infant's body that may be used to note marks, bruises, discolorations, drainage from orifices, and other observations.

References

1. Hanzlick R, Parrish RG. Death investigation report forms (DIRFs): generic forms for investigators (IDIRFs) and certifiers (CDIRFs). *J Forensic Sci* 1994;39(3): 629–36.
2. National Center for Environmental Health. *McDIDS: Medical examiner/coroner death investigation data set*. US Department of Health and Human Services, Public Health Service, Atlanta, CDC, 1995.

SUDDEN UNEXPLAINED INFANT DEATH INVESTIGATION FORM (SUIDIRF)   Case number

Infant's full name	Age	DOB
Home address	Race	Sex
City, state, zip	Ethnicity	
County	SS#	

Police complaint number   Police department

I. CIRCUMSTANCES OF DEATH

Action	Date	Time	By whom (person or agency)	Remarks
ME/C notified				Receipt by:
NOK notified				Person:
Scene visit				☐ME/C staff ☐Other agency ☐Not done
Scene address				

Condition of infant when found	☐Dead(D)	☐Unresponsive(U)	☐In distress(I)	☐NA(N)

Sequence of events before death:

Event	Date	Time	Location (street, city, state, county, zip code)
Injury			
Discovery			
Arrival			Hospital: Transported by:
Actual death			☐ On scene (S) ☐ Emergency room (E) ☐Inpatient(I)
			☐ En route or DOA (D) ☐ During surgery (O)
Pronounced			By whom:
dead			License#: Where:

Event	Date	Time	By whom (person)	Remarks
Infant placed				Place:
Known alive				Place:
Infant found				Place:
First response				Type:
EMS called				From where:
EMS response			Agency:	
Police response			Agency:	

Place of fatal event	Describe type of place
☐ Witness in room or area (W) or ☐ Unwitnessed (U)	
☐ At own home (H) or ☐ Away from home (A)	
☐ Indoors (I) or ☐ Outdoors (O)	
☐ In vehicle (V) or ☐ Not in vehicle (N)	

SUDDEN UNEXPLAINED INFANT DEATH INVESTIGATION FORM (SUIDIRF)   Case number

II. BASIC MEDICAL INFORMATION

Health care provider
for infant: Phone:

| Medical history | ☐ Not investigated (X) | ☐ Unk (U) | ☐ No past problems (N) | ☐ Medical problems (P) |

| Medical source | ☐ Physician (P) | ☐ Other health care provider (H) | ☐ Other (O) |
| | ☐ Medical records (M) | ☐ Family (F) | ☐ None (N) |

Specific infant medical history	Yes	No	Unk	Remarks

A. Problems during labor or delivery
   Birth hospital:
   Birth city state:				

B. Maternal illness or complications during pregnancy Number of prenatal visits:				
C. Major birth defects				

D. Infant was one of multiple births (e.g. a twin)
   Birth weight:
   Gestational age at birth (weeks):				

E. Hospitalization of infant after initial discharge				
F. Emergency room visits in past 2 weeks				
G. Known allergies				
H. Growth and weight gain considered normal				
I. Exposure to contagious disease in past 2 weeks				
J. Illness in past 2 weeks				
K. Lethargy, crankiness, or excessive crying in the past 48 hours				
L. Appetite changes in past 48 hours				
M. Vomiting or choking in past 48 hours				
N. Fever or excessive sweating in past 48 hours				
O. Diarrhea or stool changes in past 48 hours				
P. Infant has ever stopped breathing or turned blue				
Q. Infant was ever breast-fed				
R. Vaccinations in past 72 hours				
S. Infant injury or other condition not mentioned above				
T. Deceased siblings				

Diet in past 2 weeks included: ☐ Breast milk ☐ Formula   ☐ Cows milk   ☐ Solids
   Date and time of last meal:
   Content of last meal:

Medical history ☐ Not investigated (X) ☐ Unk (U) ☐ Rx (P) ☐ OTC (O) ☐ Home remedies (H) ☐ None (N)

Emergency medical treatment   ☐ None (N) ☐ CPR (R) ☐ Transfusion (T) ☐ IV fluids (F) ☐ Surgery (S)

Medicine names and doses; if prescription, include Rx number, Rx date, and name of pharmacy:	Describe nature and duration of resuscitation and treatments used to revive infant:	Describe any known injuries or marks on infant created or observed during resuscitation or treatment:

SUDDEN UNEXPLAINED INFANT DEATH INVESTIGATION FORM (SUIDIRF)   **Case number**

III. HOUSEHOLD AND ENVIRONMENT

Action	Yes	No	Unk	Remarks
A. House was visited				
B. Evidence of alcohol abuse				
C. Evidence of drug abuse				
D. Serious physical or mental illness in household				
E. Police have been called to home in past				
F. Prior contact with social services				
G. Documented history of child abuse				
H. Odors, fumes, or peeling paint in household				
I. Dampness, visible standing water, or mold growth				
J. Pets in household				

Type of dwelling   Water source   Number of bedrooms

Main language in home   Estimated annual income   On public assistance ☐Yes ☐No

Number of adults (>18 years of age): ☐and children (<18 years of age):☐living in household. Total=☐people

Number of smokers in household: Does usual caregiver smoke? ☐Yes ☐No ☐Unk If yes,☐cigarettes/day

Maternal information	Age: ☐	☐Married (M) ☐Single (S)	☐Divorced (D) ☐Widowed (W)	Cohabiting w/partner: ☐Yes ☐No	☐Education (years)	☐Employed (E) Not employed (N)

IV. INFANT AND ENVIRONMENT

☐In crib (C)   ☐In bed (B)   ☐Sleeping alone (A)   ☐NA (N)   Temperature of area:
☐Other (O)   ☐Sleeping with others (O)

	Unk	Back	Stomach	Side	Other		
Body position when placed	☐Unk	☐Back	☐Stomach	☐Side	☐Other		
Body position when found	☐Unk	☐Back	☐Stomach	☐Side	☐Other		
Face position when found	☐Unk	☐To left	☐To right	☐Facedown	☐Face up	☐To side	
Nose or mouth was covered or obstructed	☐Unk	☐No	☐Yes				
Postmortem changes when found	☐Unk	☐None	☐Rigor	☐Lividity	☐Other		

Number of cover or blanket layers on infant: ☐Covers on infant (C)   ☐Wrapped (W)   ☐No covers (N)

Sleeping or supporting surface: Clothing:

Other items in contact with infant: Items in crib or immediate environment:

Devices operating in room: Cooling source in room: Heat source in room:
                              ☐On (+) ☐Central (C) ☐None (N)   ☐On (+) ☐Central (C) ☐None (N)
                              ☐Off (-) ☐Space (S)   ☐Off (-) ☐Space (S)

Item collected	Yes	No	Item collected	Yes	No	Number of scene photos taken:
Baby bottle			Apnea monitor			Other items collected:
Formula			Medicines			
Diaper			Pacifier			
Clothing			Bedding			

SUDDEN UNEXPLAINED INFANT DEATH INVESTIGATION FORM (SUIDIRF)   **Case number**

V. INTERVIEW AND PROCEDURAL TRACKING

Contact	Name	Date	Time	Phone	Relationship to infant
Mother					
Father					
Usual caregiver					
Last caregiver					
Placer					
Last witness					
Finder					
First responder					
EMS caller					
EMS responder					
Police					
Alternate contact person:				Phone:	

Action	Date	Time	Action	
Medical record review for infant			Doll re-enactment performed	☐ Yes ☐ No
Medical record review for mother			Scene diagram completed	☐ Yes ☐ No
Physician or provider interview			Body diagram completed	☐ Yes ☐ No
Referral to social or SIDS services			Detailed protocol completed	☐ Yes ☐ No ☐ NA
Cause of death discussed with family			Other:	

VI. OVERALL PRELIMINARY SUMMARY

Notes to pathologist performing autopsy:

Indications that an environmental hazard, drug,   Organ or tissue donation requested by family or agency
poison, or consumer product contributed to death   ☐ Yes   ☐ No   ☐ Yes   ☐ No   ☐ Unk

Cause of death: ☐ **Presumed SIDS**   ☐ **Suspect trauma or injury**   ☐ **Other**

VII. CASE DISPOSITION

Case disposition	☐ Case declined (D) due to ☐ Case accepted (J) for ☐ Topic (T) ☐ Locale (L) ☐ Autopsy (A) ☐ Inspection (I) ☐ Certification (C)
Body disposition Who will sign DC?	☐ Brought in for exam (E) ☐ Brought in for holding or claim (C) ☐ Released from site (R)
Transport agent:	Funeral home:
Investigator and affiliation:	Date: Number of supplement pages attached:

INDEX

abdominal trauma 217–18
Abramson, Harold 141
accidental death 210–14
age at death 36
airway chemoreceptors
   dysfunction 171–4
   neuroepithelial bodies (NEB) as 166–71
airway inflammation 156–81
   histopathology 158–60
   immunopathology 158–60
   model linking with airway chemoreceptor
     dysfunction 171–4
alcohol use during and after pregnancy 38–9
alveolar edema 21–2
apnea hypothesis 70, 97
apnea monitors 250
apnea of prematurity (AOP) 245
apparent life–threatening event (ALTE) 198,
     219, 232, 249, 253, 294, 295, 311
   monitoring following 244–5
Archibald, Herbert 140
arcuate nucleus 126–8
Arnold-Chiari malformation 245
Arnold-Chiari syndrome 222
arousal 96–117
arousal patterns 267–8
arousal responses to respiratory stimuli 71–2
asphyxia 62, 111, 140, 211–13, 219, 232
autopsy 4–5, 19–24, 69, 104, 118, 182, 209,
     219, 228–9, 231, 237, 238, 299
   macroscopic 19–21
   microscopic 21–4
   protocol 319–33

bacteria, potentially pathogenic 190
bacterial colonization 187–90
bacterial flora 185, 186
bacterial toxin hypothesis 185
bacterial toxins 240
battered child syndrome 294
bed–sharing 44–5, 259–61, 264–9
bed–sharing see co–sleeping
bed–sharing
   effects on infant sleep 264
   effects on maternal sleep 265
   epidemiology 262–3

problems 270–2
bedding 140, 143–4
   arrangement 46–7
   associated with face–down deaths 145
   case–control studies 143–4
   case series 144
   surface 45–6
birth weight 37, 98, 244, 247
bite marks 217
blankets 140
body temperature 20, 101, 196
   circadian rhythm of 99
Bordetella pertussis 187, 188
brain–derived neurotrophic factor (BDNF) 71
brain findings in sites rostral to brainstem
     119–25
brain homeostatic control 96–117
brain research 118–37
brain weight 121, 123
brainstem findings 119
brainstem gliosis 118, 119
breastfeeding 40–1, 183, 189–91, 264–9
   in solitary and bed–sharing environments
     265–8
broncho–alveolar lavage (BAL) 163–6
bruising 217
burns 210–11, 218

cardiac cycle length 87
cardiac disorders 286, 297
cardiac patterning during sleep 106–8
cardiopulmonary resuscitation, injuries due to
     219
cardiorespiratory control hypothesis 98
cardiorespiratory monitors 250–1
cardiovascular disease 220–1
case conferences 26
CDC guidelines 60–1, 65
central hypoventilation syndrome 286
central nervous system conditions 221–2
child abuse 298, 299
   diagnosis masking 296
chronic lung disease (CLD), monitoring 248
cigarette smoke see smoking
circadian rhythm 98–103, 196
   of body temperature 99

Clostridium botulinum 186
Clostridium perfringens 186, 188, 189, 194, 240
Clostridium welchii 240
CO_2 140, 145–51
co–sleeping 20, 258–74
    form, function and outcome 260–1
    origins 263
    particular types 261–2
    problems 270–2
    see also bed–sharing
critical developmental period 96, 130–2
cytomegalovirus (CMV) 161

dangerous conditions 259–60, 271
death scene investigation 11, 26, 58–65, 229–30
    critical aspects 61–4
    doll re–enactment 61
    guidelines 60–1, 334–47
    historical prespective 59–60
    location 59
developmental factors 197–8
developmental stage 187–8, 196–9
developmental vulnerability 75
diagnosis masking child abuse 296
diagnostic conflicts 231
differential diagnosis 209–27
diphtheria-pertussis-tetanus (DPT) immunization 239–40
documented monitoring 252–3
drowning 62, 210
drug use/abuse
    during pregnancy 38
    monitoring 247
dummies (pacifiers) 47–8
duvets 46–7

ECG 84–6, 88, 92, 248, 249
EEG 99–100, 111, 267
Ehlers-Danlos syndrome 222
electrocution 62
endotoxin 185–6
enteric bacteria 186
enterotoxin A 194
environmental factors 62, 75–7, 197–9, 214
epidemiology 31–57, 182
    and neuropathologic findings 130–2
    and rebreathing of exhaled air 150–1
    changes following reductions in rates 48–50
Escherichia coli 183, 186, 189
ethnic groups 189–90, 275–82
European Society for the Study and Prevention of Infant Death 310
exhaled air
    rebreathing of 138–55

and epidemiology 150–1
    evidence from models 145–9
    studies in infants demonstrating 149–50
exogenous stressor(s) 130–2

face–down deaths 142–3
    bedding associated with 145
face–down position 140
falls 213
familial characteristics 33
familial clustering of infant deaths 24–5
fatal injuries 210–14
feeding 194
filicide 285–6
    clues 286
foreign bodies 213
formula feeding 189
full–term infant 101

Garrow, Irene 141
gastrointestinal conditions 222
gender effects 36, 191
genetic effects 197–8
genetic metabolic disorders 297
genetic predisposition 24–5, 287
genitalia 218–19
genitourinary conditions 222
gestation 37
gestational age 98
Global Strategy Meeting (GSM) 312
Global Strategy Task Force (GSTF) 311, 312, 317
grief and grieving 302–4

H. influenzae 189, 191
haematopoeitic conditions 221
hanging 211
head trauma 215–16
heart 6, 21, 237
heart rate 106, 107
Helicobactor pylori 187
homicide 24–5, 232, 298
hospital admissions for life threatening events 24
hospital deaths 214
hyperthermia 214
hypothermia 214
hypoxia 71–4, 77

immune responses 192–3
immunization 194–5, 239–40
inborn errors of metabolism (IEM) 287
infant abuse 294–5
infant care practices 285
infant characteristics 33–7
infant deaths, familial clustering of 24–5
infant mortality rates 18

infanticide 291–300
  as taboo 292–3
  caution and evaluation 293–4
infantile spinal muscular atrophy 287
infections 39, 183, 240
infectious disease 221
inflammation 183
inflammatory changes 157–66
inflammatory infiltrates 231
inflammatory responses 192–7
inflicted injury 214–19
interferon γ (INF–γ) 196
interleukin–1 (IL–1) 196
interleukin–1ß (IL–1ß) 193, 194
interleukin–6 (IL–6) 193, 196
interstitial hemosiderin 23–4
interstitial pneumonia 22
intoxication/poisoning 62
intra–alveolar hemorrhage 23
intraparenchymal damage 216
intraseptal lymphocytes 21–2
intrathoracic petechiae 5, 69, 104, 230–1

kainate binding 128
Kawasaki disease 220

life–threatening arrhythmias 86–7
long QT syndrome (LQTS) 83–95
  molecular evidence 91–3
lung disease 68–9
lung pathology, investigation 176
lungs 6, 21–3, 156, 237
  see also specific conditions
lymphocytic choriomeningitis virus (LCMV)
  193

M. catarrhalis 191
malnourished infants 218
malocclusion 48
Maori SIDS Prevention Program 275–82
Marfan syndrome 222
marriage 302–4
maternal sleep, bed–sharing effects on 265
mattresses 45–6, 240–2
mechanical suffocation 236–8
medical examiner 299
medium chain acyl–coenzyme A
    dehydrogenase deficiency (MCAD) 62
medullary serotonergic network 125–30
microbiological aetiology 182
molecular screening 93
monitoring 243–57
  as diagnostic tool 244–5
  chronic lung disease (CLD) 248
  documented 252–3
  drug use/abuse 247
  duration 253

indications for 243–9
  morbidity prevention 245
  not routinely indicated 246
  preterm infants 247–8
  previous SIDS in family 245, 246
  sleep studies 248–9
  twins 247
  types of monitors 250–3
mother-infant co–sleeping *see* co–sleeping
motor vehicle deaths 211
multiple deaths within families 296–7
Munchausen by proxy 219, 232, 294, 295,
    298
muscarinic binding 128

natural diseases, death due to 220–2
near–miss SIDS 295
Neisseria meningitidis 188
neuroepithelial bodies (NEB) 157, 175
  as airway chemoreceptors 166–71
  general structural and functional features
    166–7
  hyperplasia 170, 172
  O_2 sensing 167–9
  pathobiology 169–71
neuropathologic findings 120–1
  and epidemiology 130–2
NIJ guidelines 60–1
non–REM (NREM) sleep 99, 102, 103, 105–6,
    109

obstructive sleep apnea syndrome (OSAS)
    196
Ondine's curse 286
overheating 21, 47
oxygen sensing in NEB cells 167–9
oxygenation monitors 251–2

pacifiers (dummies) 47–8
parental anxiety 246
parenting after SIDS 304–6
parity effect 37
partial atelectasis 22
pathologic findings 230–1
peripheral chemoreceptors 156–81
pertussis toxin 187
petechial hemorrhages 230–1
physiologic responses 75
Pierre Robin sequence 245
pillows 45–6, 140
Pneumocystis carini 164, 165
poisoning 213, 218
postconceptual age (PCA) 101
postmortem examination 299
postnatal age (PNA) 98
pregnancy
  alcohol use during and after 38–9

drug use/abuse during 38
smoking during 37–8
pregnancy–related factors 37–9
prenatal care 37
preterm infants 99, 101
monitoring 247–8
preventative pathology 233
prone sleeping *see* sleep position
pulmonary NEB 169
pulmonary neuroendocrine cell (PNEC) system
169–71
pyrogenic toxins 183, 186

QT hypothesis 83–95
arguments against 88–90
QT prolongation 83–95
and life threatening arrhythmias 86–7
clinical implications 87–8
molecular link 90–3
potential causes 90–1
see also long QT syndrome
QT syndrome 24–5
quilts 46–7

race–ethnicity 33–6
rapid eye movement (REM) sleep 99, 100,
102, 105–6, 109
rebreathing, lethality 145
rebreathing of exhaled air 138–55
and epidemiology 150–1
evidence from models 145–9
studies in infants demonstrating 149–50
Reduce the Risks Campaign 310
relationships 302–4
respiratory conditions 221
respiratory control during sleep 104–6
respiratory disorders 68–72
respiratory failure 77
respiratory mechanisms 66–82
respiratory pathogens 157–66
diagnosis 163–6
identification 161–3
respiratory stimuli, arousal responses to 71–2
respiratory syncytial virus (RSV) 161–3
respiratory system, development 66–8
respiratory tract anomalies 286
retinal hemorrhages 219
risk factors 33, 34, 183, 187–91, 193–7, 276,
277
risk reduction
campaigns 31–3
interventions 36
room sharing 45, 262
RSV 171

scalds 210–11
Scopularcopsis brevicaulis 240

season at death 36–7
seasonal incidence 184
sex differences 36
sexual abuse 218–19
shaking–impact syndrome 216
side sleeping position 43
SIDS
age distribution 5
borderline 17–19
Category I 7–8
Category II 8
Category III 8–9
change in life following 306–8
classification 13–15
decline in rates 1
definition by exclusion 9–13
definition by inclusion 5–9
definitions 4–13
diagnosis 13–15
distribution of modes 12
distribution of original and blindly revised
diagnoses 15
etiology 39, 96
exclusion (non–SIDS) 25–6
familial recurrence 283–90
family survival following 301–9
future perspectives 25–7
grey–zone 17, 25
history 1–2, 66
incidence 283
incidence in subsequent siblings 297
incidence of recurrence 283–4
incidence rates 277–8
international statistics 314–16
pathogenesis 39
philosophy 1–3
prevention of recurrence 288
rates in different countries 12–13
rates in representative countries 32
recent research 2–3
recurrence factors 284–6
remembrances following 309
research 74–7, 198–9, 308
revisiting a loss 309
risk factors 2
single deaths as causes for concern 297–9
subsequent children 304–6
support group 302, 306
syndrome question 16–17
theories and explanations 236–42
vulnerability 96, 130–2
SIDS Family International (SIDSFI) 311
SIDS prevention program, strategic approach
275–82
skeletal trauma 216–17
skin injuries 217
skull fractures 216

sleep 196–7
  architecture 267–8
  cardiac patterning during 106–8
  characteristics 104
  environment 41–8
  perspective 96–117
  proximity 269–70
  respiratory control during 104–6
  thermoregulatory control during 108–11
sleep position 41, 103, 189
  face–down 138
  prone 41–3, 104, 110, 118, 138, 150–1,
    191–2, 199
  supine 43, 104, 118
sleep studies, monitoring 248–9
smoking 72, 183, 194, 199, 276
  during pregnancy 37–8
  passive 39–40, 188, 190–2
sociodemographic factors 33–9
socioeconomic background 189–90
soft tissue trauma 217
staphylococcal enterotoxins A and B 194
Staphylococcus aureus 183, 186, 188, 189,
  191, 192, 198
starvation 218
status thymolymphaticus 2
Streptococcus mitis 191
Streptococcus pneumoniae 191
Streptococcus pyogenes 192
struck 240
sudden infant death syndrome *see* SIDS
Sudden Unexplained Infant Death
  Investigation Report Form (SUIDIRF)
  334– 47
suffocation 20, 237, 296, 299
supine sleeping 43, 104, 118
surgical intervention 214

T–cell activation 193
temperature effects 214
thermal environment 47
thermoregulatory control during sleep 108–11
thiamine deficiency 239
thymus 6, 21, 237–9
total sleep time (TST) 102
toxic gas hypothesis 240–2
toxigenic bacteria 185, 186
triple–risk model 130–2
TSST 194
tumor necrosis factor–α (TNF–α) 193, 194,
  196
twins 287
  monitoring 247

upper airway obstruction 69–70, 104, 221
upper respiratory tract infection (URI) 39,
  156, 171, 174, 175, 186, 189
upper respiratory tract narrowing 286

Valdes–Dapena, Maria 142–3
ventilatory control disorders 70–1
ventilatory muscles 69
ventral medulla 125–6
ventricular fibrillation 92
virus infection 184–5, 188, 191, 193–4
vitamin C deficiency 239

wedging 211
Werdnig-Hoffmann disease 287
Werne, Jacob 141
Wilms' tumor 222
Wooley, Paul 142

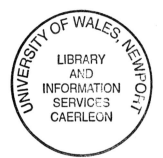